T0252956

Mind, Make-Believe and Medicine

Richard Rasker

Mind, Make-Believe and Medicine

Exploring the Divide Between Science and Wishful Thinking

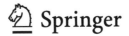 Springer

Richard Rasker
Enschede, The Netherlands

ISBN 978-3-031-29443-3   ISBN 978-3-031-29444-0   (eBook)
https://doi.org/10.1007/978-3-031-29444-0

This Springer imprint is published by the registered company Springer Nature Switzerland AG
The registered company address is: Gewerbestrasse 11, 6330 Cham, Switzerland

Acknowledgements

First and foremost, I would like to thank my wonderful partner for her patience, her critical comments and her many excellent questions when reading my work.

I also wish to thank Edzard Ernst for his encouragement to actually start writing this book, his proofreading, and for supporting me throughout the project.

Then I want to thank all those people who shared with me their experiences with both alternative and regular medicine. Even though we often disagreed, they taught me some of the most important lessons about motivations, beliefs and many other things that, right or wrong, make us human.

Introduction

This book is perhaps best described as a kind of travel guide for exploring different worlds, some of which are probably familiar, while others may be completely alien to you. Some of those worlds only exist in the minds of people, while others are very real indeed, yet often go unnoticed or have unexpected things to offer. This journey is also my personal exploration, during which I try to look through the eyes of the inhabitants of worlds that are wildly different from my own, to try and understand why those people believe certain things, and why I myself believe different things.

The main subject of this book is the human condition, from the viewpoint of some of the most precious things we have: our health and well-being, the myriad of ways that we try to maintain and/or improve this health and well-being, and how people come to have different ideas about this endlessly interesting but also very difficult subject.

Unfortunately, the recent coronavirus pandemic with its uncertain prospects and host of countermeasures limiting our freedom has shown that people quickly adopt increasingly extreme ideas. People could no longer rely on daily routine and often abandoned reason in an attempt to make sense of this loss of control over their life. Worst case, friends and even close family members became alienated from each other. What initially was a minor difference in opinion or viewpoint can quickly escalate into full-blown hostility, for instance, because one person refused to get vaccinated while their friends considered this unwise and sometimes even antisocial. Another very worrisome development was the way that political extremists quickly seized upon the opportunity to further sow distrust and confusion in attempts to have people rallying behind them and demonize any and all opposition.

However, with some exceptions, this book is not about the coronavirus pandemic, or even about the specific controversies, talking points or conspiracy beliefs that sprang up as a result. This book is mostly based on far older things that people believe affects their health and well-being, which, though already a safer subject, can still lead to heated debate. Subjects range from medicine (both the alternative and regular varieties) and health fads to conspiracies and public scares, such as the notion of 'toxins' and unhealthy 'radiation' from wireless products. Many of the subjects and principles discussed also apply to the coronavirus pandemic, but I shall leave these mostly to the reader to find out and ponder.

About Me

First off, I want to get one thing straight: I am not a scientist. I am not a doctor. I do not even have any academic credentials. I am, in other words, not a recognized authority in any field.

What I *do* have, is an insatiable curiosity for all things scientific, a very strong desire to understand how our world works, and to determine what is real and what is not. And I am strongly convinced that science is by far the best way to understand the world around us.

If this lack of credentials is already reason enough for you, as a reader, to lose interest and dismiss what I have to say out of hand, then that of course is fine with me. In all honesty, I myself also tend to value a scientist's opinion more than the opinion of the average person in the street—at least when dealing with a more or less scientific subject.

Then again, if you have an affinity with alternative medicine or similar subjects, please realize that most alternative practitioners and proponents also have no scientific or academic background. Like me, they are often laypersons who developed an interest in a particular subject, and like me, they gathered lots of information and knowledge on the subject out of curiosity and wonderment.

The main difference is that I attempt to understand phenomena with a consistently scientific mindset, without taking anything for granted. Let me put this in stronger wording: I cannot and will not take things for granted without a good explanation. An example is the homeopathic *similia* principle, which says that a substance that causes certain symptoms in a healthy person can cure a sick person with the same symptoms—and with said substance infinitely diluted, at that. How does this work, medically speaking? Does it actually work at all? Has this homeopathic principle been tested and proven correct in any scientific manner? Unfortunately, the answers to all these questions are a resounding 'NO'. There is no explanation at all how the *similia* principle is supposed to work. There is not even scientific evidence for its existence; there is not a single experiment that shows that this fundamental(!) homeopathic principle is real. The logical question then is why people still believe that it works, and yes, there are good explanations for their beliefs.

Science aficionado as I may be, I do not want to bury myself (and least of all you, the reader) in lots and lots of scientific formulas, references and jargon. I want to keep things as simple as possible, and that includes my language and my reasoning. I want to look at things and explain them from a common sense point of view (OK, *my* common sense point of view)—even though I know that 'common sense' is often wrong. Then again, I will also support my thoughts with references to proper scientific work—because sharing well-tested knowledge is the very foundation of science, making it so successful in explaining our world and everything in it.

Reasons for Writing This Book

Another reason for writing this book is to invite readers to try and think along, and use their own reasoning skills to gain new insights and viewpoints. On several occasions, I will ask you to stop reading on for a moment, and simply think about something and start asking questions for yourself.

One such example deals with conspiracies: a rather widespread conspiracy belief says that you can't trust vaccines because pharmaceutical companies stand to profit way more from sick people than from healthy people, which sounds plausible. So the reasoning goes that vaccines are actually harmful and cause all sorts of damage and misery, and that Big Pharma pays scientists, doctors and other experts to keep silent about this, in order to protect their huge profits. Could this be true? Just think about it for a moment, and perhaps do a bit of searching on the Internet to get an idea about the implications of such a conspiracy.

OK, have you made up your mind yet? And perhaps thought of some further questions to ask?

Then for starters, here is a simple, undisputed fact: there are roughly 10 million doctors worldwide. Do you think it is plausible that all these millions of smart and often quite idealistic people can be bribed into silence about harming innocent people (and in particular children!) by vaccinating them?

And is it plausible that literally none of them ever spilled the beans, in all those decades that this must have been going on? Have you made an estimate of how much money it would cost pharmaceutical companies to pay out those bribes? And have you looked up how much profits those companies actually make selling vaccines? And how they could profit from the damage that vaccines ostensibly cause? These questions and many more will return in the chapter about vaccines, together with some answers. Other answers you may have to find for yourself.

Generally, one of the most challenging things here is to question our own beliefs and assumptions. This is something that even many scientists and other smart people have serious problems with—it is very human to stick to a particular belief and seek evidence to reinforce it once it has been embraced. This problem of *confirmation bias* has been recognized by science long ago already, and one of the solutions is so-called *peer review*, where a scientist's work is judged by other scientists, who explicitly try to find errors and other shortcomings in the arguments and the work of their colleague. (And if this colleague is smart, he or she will try to prevent this from happening by asking *themselves* if they could be wrong.)

The Role and Value of Science in This Book

I just suggested that we should always be prepared to question our beliefs and assumptions. This may even go as far as to question the value of science itself in particular areas, and instead depart from human intuition and other emotions when exploring our human world. However, this area lies outside the scope of this book, except where those human traits are clearly at odds with a more science-based world view.

My primary goal is to explore the human condition with the physical reality we live in (a.k.a. 'the Real World') as the main anchor. It turns out that science is the best tool by far to describe and understand this reality— which, incidentally, also includes our physical human body and everything that may go wrong with it. This reality also dictates what we can call 'facts', as opposed to human opinions and beliefs.

About using science as a primary tool: please note that I do not simply *assume* that science is the best way to describe our world. Science has actually *proven* itself to be the best tool yet to understand our physical world. But this is explained in more detail in the second chapter, which is dedicated to science and the so-called scientific method.

How This Book is Organized

Most of the chapters in this book are organized along the same lines. Many chapters start out with an anecdote or a story on the chapter's subject. Sometimes this is written from the viewpoint of 'the other side', the side of believers in pseudoscience or alternative medicine. This gives a good taste of the subject and also demonstrates why it is quite understandable why people believe things that may sound plausible but are not supported by science. Some of the stories are based on real events, some are made up, and some others are a blend of both. I sometimes changed the names of living people to somewhat protect their privacy.

Then follows a further exploration of the core subject from the opening story, and at this point, the first questions are asked. This is also where I shall often ask you, the reader, to think along, and try to figure out what is real and what is not, and why. This part is usually easy to follow and requires little more than a bit of common sense and a willingness to set aside preconceived notions and beliefs, if only for a brief moment.

Most chapters end with more in-depth science-based information, with scientific backgrounds and explanations, perhaps a few simple formulas, and sources and references.

However, not all chapters rigidly adhere to this structure. This book is first and foremost meant as a pleasant read, intended to be understood by anyone with an interest in the various subjects, and not as a scientific reference work.

So read on, and I hope you experience the same enjoyment from reading this book that I had writing it!

Richard Rasker

Contents

1

Staying Alive

No Panic!

Monday July 29th of 2013 was balmy summer day in the Netherlands, with lots of people taking advantage of the lovely weather to visit Emmen zoo, located near the eastern border of the country.

For the zoo, it was a busy but otherwise completely uneventful day – until closing time, when zookeepers arrived at the compound where 112 hamadryas baboons spent their days. Normally, the animals would gather at the entrance to their night enclosure as soon as the zookeepers showed up, but not this time. Instead, they all huddled together on a rock and in a couple of trees in a corner of their compound, unwilling to move, refusing to budge even when the zoo's attendants tried to lure them with their favourite snacks. They were all looking intently at the neighbouring African savannah compound, where nothing out of the ordinary seemed to be going on. In the end, the animals could be persuaded to enter their night enclosure, but they did so very reluctantly, taking more than an hour to all get inside.

The next morning, things had not improved. Normally, when the doors to their daytime area opened, they would emerge and first spend some time monkeying around, engaged in play, squabbles and social grooming. After this, they typically spread out in a couple of male-led groups to go looking for morsels of food. Now, however, they did none of this. When the night enclosure opened, all the animals immediately made a frantic dash straight for the same corner they occupied the previous evening, huddling together in the trees and on the rocks below. And again, they just sat there looking scared, not eating at all, and responding to sudden sounds by drawing even closer together.

© The Author(s), under exclusive license to Springer Nature
Switzerland AG 2023
R. Rasker, *Mind, Make-Believe and Medicine*,
https://doi.org/10.1007/978-3-031-29444-0_1

Zoo personnel was mystified and could not find or think of anything that may have frightened the baboons so badly. Other animals nearby such as lemurs and kangaroos behaved perfectly normal, and to the best of anyone's knowledge, nothing strange had happened. The resident zoo biologist could not explain the animals' behaviour either, other than characterizing it as 'mass hysteria', possibly started by one of the dominant males experiencing a panic attack for reasons unknown. Still, a reassuring thought was that this was not a unique event: similar fits of mass hysteria had occurred among the zoo's baboons several times before, in 1994, 1997, and 2007. Each time, things were back to normal within a couple of days.

And just like on earlier occasions, the story of the Spooked Baboons drew a lot of public and media attention. People were e-mailing the zoo with all sorts of suggestions and theories about possible causes for the baboons' panic, ranging from the mundane to completely outlandish. One biologist pointed out that baboons were sometimes known to panic when confronted with their own reflection in water. Other people came up with causes such as a leading male mistaking a branch or a shadow for a snake, or an unusual sound that was interpreted as a threat. Some people thought that the zoo's preparations to move to another location were to blame, while others again claimed that the animals responded to an imminent earthquake or other natural disaster – which of course never materialized. One person was certain that it must have been a UFO, and even a psychic and a self-proclaimed animal interpreter turned up, offering their help – offers that were politely but firmly declined.

Instead, the zookeepers simply waited while keeping an eye on the animals, in order to intervene should anything bad happen. And as expected, things returned to normal after several more days of simply leaving the animals to themselves. To this day, no cause for the mass panic has been found.

See the Pattern

All living organisms have evolved to stay alive as best they can, at least long enough to successfully procreate as a species.

One major snag here is that most organisms need *other* organisms in order to stay alive, often as food. Every living thing not just needs to make sure that they get their dinner, but must generally also avoid *becoming* dinner, so to speak. We humans are no exception. We are, however, not really big, strong or fast, nor are we equipped with fearsome claws or fangs. We also do not have defensive body armour or spikes or venom to ward off predators. There is however one thing that more than makes up for our otherwise unremarkable defensive traits: our brain.

One of the things that our brain is exceptionally good at is pattern recognition—so good, in fact, that we tend to recognize patterns and connections even where there aren't any. This automatic pattern recognition happens especially fast when threats are involved. Now this would seem like a drawback, wasting a lot of energy on false alarms, but it makes good sense from an evolutionary point of view. When our apelike ancestors on the African savannah heard a rustling sound or thought they saw some stealthy movement in the high grass, the safest course of action was to run away or flee into a tree, even if it turned out to be false alarm for most of the time. Because those ancestors who would *not* run away every time would in fact *not end up being our ancestors*; they would most likely end up being another animal's dinner pretty quickly. To put it this way: it is still far better to needlessly run away a hundred times than to get eaten just once. This is probably also what explains the behaviour of those poor baboons in our opening story: one of the leading males saw or heard something that he thought was a serious threat, and panicked. And because baboons have a very strict social hierarchy with just a few males at the top whose will is law, the rest simply followed their leader. The most remarkable thing about this event is that the animals got stuck in panic mode for several days.

Not only is recognizing particular clues and patterns essential for our survival, we must also accomplish this *really fast*. Evolution has seen to it that we almost always err on the side of caution. Our first, automatic response to anything unexpected is an instinctive assumption that we're in danger. This is also what gives us the huge adrenaline jolt when someone suddenly jumps out at us: our brain and body immediately switch to fight-or-flight mode, even when it turns out to be just our little brother or sister giving us a scare—and even then, it takes effort not to react aggressively. Animals have similar instincts. Just look up those countless online videos of cats that are unexpectedly confronted with a cucumber surreptitiously placed near them: their instinctive fear of snakes immediately takes control, causing them to jump away. (And no, please don't do this to your own cat; you want your furry friend to feel safe and comfortable in their home environment. No matter how funny it looks to you, it is an unpleasant, scary experience for your cat.)

Our high sensitivity to patterns, regardless whether real or imagined, is even further increased when we are feeling insecure or stressed. This too is an evolved trait, and quite logical when you think about it: when first entering unfamiliar territory, there may also be unknown threats and hazards, so it pays to be extra cautious, wary for any signs of danger. Once we become familiar with our new surroundings, we can take a more relaxed approach and only respond to things that are out of the ordinary.

This influence of insecurity on pattern recognition (and also on beliefs) still applies today. We see for instance how the insecurity brought about by the

Covid-19 pandemic and its associated countermeasures have given rise to all sorts of beliefs in conspiracies and pseudoscience. One such fictitious pattern perceived by people is that official measures aimed at slowing down the spread of the disease (such as mandatory social distancing, face masks and quarantine rules) were not really meant to protect them, but were all part of one large global elite conspiracy to enslave or even eliminate ordinary citizens. Almost everything that happened over the course of the pandemic was shoehorned into this perceived pattern: Covid vaccines were not lifesaving but 'delayed genocide', face masks were 'obedience training', and of course mainstream media were not simply reporting events, but 'brainwashing' us.

These perceived patterns and beliefs all stem from a human desire to make sense of a world where major events happen that are outside of our control. Recognizing patterns and basing our beliefs on those observations provide a sense of understanding and control, even if the patterns are only imaginary. One of the problems with this is that people may find it very difficult to abandon those beliefs later on, even if they are confronted with new facts or information showing them that they are wrong after all. This new information is often ignored or even explicitly denied, in order to maintain the belief in which they have invested so much, both emotionally and in other respects. This is one of the recurring themes in this book.

Heightened sensitivity to patterns when feeling insecure is also seen in social interactions. When we find ourselves in a situation with all strangers, such as a new job or even a party with lots of people we don't know, almost all of us experience a certain level of stress. As a result, we immediately start looking for cues (read: patterns) on how to fit in with this new social environment, in order to avoid embarrassment or a bad first impression. This desire to fit in is driven by another evolutionary trait that helps us survive: our highly social nature—which we'll get to in a moment.

Invisible Threats

Protection based on pattern recognition also works in situations where a potential threat is by its nature not visible at all. Our world is full of those invisible threats, such as pathogenic microbes and toxic plants and animals.

When we eat something and start feeling sick shortly afterwards, chances are that we will not only blame this food for our illness, but also avoid it in the future. Many people will even start feeling physically unwell when they just come across that specific food again. What is more: if others around us see what happens, many of them won't touch their food either.[1] Missing a meal just leaves you hungry, whereas getting serious food poisoning may leave you dead. It does not matter if the food was the actual cause of the illness or not; it is all about taking no unnecessary risks. Because in nature, taking unnecessary risks is definitely not a good survival strategy.

This behaviour is of course not exclusive to us humans. In fact, almost all animals have some sort of instinctive response to cues that may signal danger, and many animals can learn to recognize patterns. These learned pattern recognition skills are not just used for avoiding danger, but also for other important things such as finding food and potential mates. Everyone who has ever owned a dog or a cat or another furry or feathered friend as a pet will have noticed that the animal very quickly learns to recognize patterns and cues that indicate that *Yes, Dinner is Served!* The crackle of a food bag, the sound of a tin can being opened, the rattle of a food bowl: all these things not only cause anticipation and excitement in the animal, but often even a physical response, the well-known Pavlov response. And just like humans, animals often tend to see patterns where there aren't any. One famous example is B. F. Skinner's *Superstition in the Pigeon* experiment. In this experiment, hungry pigeons were placed in a cage where a morsel of food would appear at irregular intervals. The birds quickly associated the arrival of food with whatever they were doing at that exact moment. When a pigeon happened to be turning to the left when the food appeared, it would start turning left more often in anticipation of more food. Other pigeons developed their own unique movements that they linked to getting a tasty morsel.

Later researchers contested Skinner's characterization of this behaviour as 'superstition'. However, it is of course a fact that many species of animals can be trained to perform almost any arbitrary behaviour using food as a reward. Animals that are socially adapted to humans such as dogs can even be trained by using purely social rewards: *Good Boy!*

Very Superstitious

We humans, as absolute pattern-recognition champions of the animal kingdom, are most definitely superstitious creatures. We very quickly create associations between things that often are completely unconnected, and often even develop strong emotions about these associations. Many athletes, musicians, stage performers and people in other professions where extreme performance is both essential and uncertain have their own little rituals and

---

[1] There will of course always be one reckless daredevil going 'Tastes fine to me, shame to let good food go to waste….. aaargh!'

superstitions. Some have a 'lucky shirt' or 'special bracelet' or other item that they feel they must have, while others have particular habits or rituals that make them feel more secure. What's more, the athlete or artist may even panic if it suddenly turns out that they forgot their 'lucky' item or ritual. This can certainly influence their performance—further reinforcing their superstition, even unconsciously, if their subsequent performance is indeed worse than normal. This is once again an example of how stress enhances our tendency to see patterns.

As outsiders, we usually find these things a bit silly, but mostly harmless. However, we should not forget that as children, we *all* were superstitious to some extent: almost all children at one point or other try to influence the world around them with what we could call magic, and, importantly, also believed that this can actually work. And take a critical look at yourself as an adult: do you have any little habits that serve no clear purpose, but make you feel more confident or comfortable in certain situations? Then this may also be considered superstitious, even if it is just a little bit.

Monkey See, Monkey Do, Monkey Tell

Our big, efficient brain in and of itself is already a great advantage when it comes to survival, but its full potential is unleashed in combination with two other human traits: our highly social nature and our communicative skills.

We are of course by no means the only animals to take advantage of social behaviour to increase our chances of survival, but we are definitely the ones making most extensive and effective use of our social capabilities. Not only can we attack animals that are far larger and stronger than ourselves when working together as a group, we can also plan each attack, and deliberate in detail about the best way to go about it. And, of course, we can pass on our knowledge and skills to others, and teach them about life's good and bad things. Not having to learn every important life lesson by personal experience is a *huge* survival advantage.

Things become even more interesting when we take these skills one step further: when we share knowledge, experiences and emotions, this traditionally (as in: before the invention of writing) happened in the form and stories or songs, both of which make the information a lot easier to remember, although for slightly different reasons. Stories usually follow a coherent, more or less logical progression of events, and with a good story, you can actually *see* those things happening in your mind as if you were there yourself.

Music, on the other hand, uses rhythm and repetition to get things into our head. That this sometimes works too well, is evidenced by something we all have experienced at some time or other: an 'earworm', or a piece of music that we can't get out of our head, even when it is driving us crazy. There are also combined forms, where a story is set to a particular rhythm and/or rhyme. Ancient examples are epic poems such as the Greek *Iliad*. More modern examples are opera and musicals, where large parts of the story are set to music and sung rather than spoken.

Even today, we take in most of our information in the form of stories, because we have evolved to find that an easy way to share information. Most of those stories are short and simple, with Jack telling how he just got promoted and went out with his buddies last night to celebrate (and, if Jack was a bit too enthusiastic, how he had to start the first day of his new job with a horrible hangover …). Other stories we view or read online, or if you're from the older generation, in the newspaper. And, of course, much of our entertainment is also made up of stories: books, films, and even computer games all have a kind of story line or progression that we find easy and pleasant to follow. We humans like stories so much that it prompted the late Sir Terry Pratchett and his co-authors Ian Stewart and Jack Cohen to change the name of our species from *homo sapiens* ('wise man') into *pan narrans*, or 'storytelling ape', in their wonderful series *The Science of Discworld*.

Also note that many stories are not even true, in the sense that the narrative describes real events or factual information. A lot of the stories that we enjoy are completely made up, and we have no problem with that at all. We often care a lot more about the entertainment value than actual truthfulness. In fact, most of the things we tell our children are untrue, or at best simplifications of the truth. Just think about fictional stories such as fairy tales, which are an important way to teach our children about the real world and the people in it. We come up with all sorts of evil or unpleasant characters and dangerous situations, warning children that not everyone is nice, and that the world is full of dangers and challenges. But in the end, those bad characters always end up being punished for their flaws, and challenges are always overcome. This increases trust in fellow humans and gives children the confidence to try and face their own challenges. These stories also serve as a warning, not only that we should avoid danger, but also not to become evil ourselves. So even though most stories that we tell our children aren't true, they still serve to prepare children for the very real trials and tribulations of real life later on. As adults, many of us still enjoy thrillers and horror stories, even ones that don't end well at all. Maybe we somehow need to be exposed to frightful situations every now and then? These stories can tickle our primeval senses for alertness and fear without getting us into actual trouble. Of course, real crimes, war and other horrible experiences should be avoided and prevented as much as possible, if only because these situations often traumatize people for the rest of their life.

Later in life we learn that most things don't end like fairy tales. We learn about real evil people, and also see that they do not always get the punishment they deserve—which is a valuable lesson in itself: life is not always fair, and we have to accept that sometimes, bad things happen that we can't do much about.

What the Future May Bring …

Stories are very useful to teach us about the world around us without having to learn everything by personal experience (read: trial and error). Stories are also very important for teaching us about our social and cultural roles. However, stories have yet another important function: they help us predict the future.

It should be obvious that being able to tell the future is *very* beneficial for survival and personal fortune—everyone has experienced those 'If only I had known this …' moments, and almost everyone has at one point in their life dreamed of getting rich by correctly predicting the upcoming lottery numbers. And then there is this: regardless of what will happen, good or bad, *it will all happen in the future.* This is also the reason why, throughout history, many rulers had professional fortune tellers or soothsayers in their retinue, hoping that these people could warn them and help them prevent all sorts of misfortunes. Even our modern-day leaders are sometimes caught consulting psychics and the likes. Well-known examples are former US president Ronald Reagan and his wife Nancy, who regularly consulted astrologer Joan Quigley, and the late Dutch queen Juliana, who had close ties to a psychic by the name of Greet Hofmans.

When we think of fortune tellers, we think of people who have special gifts to foresee the future. Quite often, special attributes and techniques are involved, ranging from simple items such as tea leaves, tarot cards or the obligatory crystal ball, to complex calculations involving the positions of planets and stars as in astrology. These people try to predict the future by searching for patterns and clues that most other people do not see or understand. Regardless of how they work, their most important tool is their talent for making up good stories. These stories must not only make predictions sound more plausible, but also explain the outcomes, especially if these outcomes are not exactly what was predicted. Just look at horoscopes: the predictions can look pretty detailed, but are in fact rather generic and vague, and can apply to almost anyone. This is greatly helped by people's tendency to actively try to match up those predictive stories with their own life story (the so-called *Barnum effect*).

The most successful fortune tellers are smart and careful about what they make predictions on. For instance soothsayers with a fair grasp of politics and strategy could indeed be quite successful in predicting the outcome of negotiations and battles for their master, earning them a high position in their master's court. Then again, the less successful ones often saw their career, if not their life, cut short pretty quickly, so there is definitely a sort of natural selection going on there.

But even the most successful fortune teller of course cannot really look into the future, and completely unexpected events are in fact never accurately predicted; just look at some of the major events in recent history, such as the 9/11 terrorist attacks, or natural disasters such as the 2004 Indian Ocean tsunami, killing some 230,000 people. Not a single catastrophic event like this has ever been foretold in a clear, unambiguous and well-documented prediction.

Everyday Future-Telling

When we limit ourselves to far less spectacular things, we all master the fortune tellers' trick to some degree. We all predict the future on an almost daily basis, and often quite successfully, at that. We call this 'making plans', where we think up a logical sequence of events and actions (i.e. a story) that will hopefully lead to a certain outcome—and we usually do our best to make those predictions self-fulfilling as much as possible. Just like with professional fortune tellers, our plans and predictions are often based on patterns and clues; it's just that those patterns and clues are usually more obvious. And just like in ancient times, being good at planning and successfully imagining (and steering) developments is still highly rewarded in our modern human society. (While people whose plans often fail are generally considered losers.)

A special category of self-fulfilling predictions is better known as the *laws of nature*: 'if I drop this stone here in my hand, it will fall down.' Several hundred years ago, a smart person by the name of Isaac Newton not only managed to come up with a simple formula to predict how fast it will fall, but even with the insight that this gravitational law is universal. This way of predicting the future by means of natural laws is even more successful than our planning of day-to-day activities, and is generally known as *science*. The distinguishing feature of science as a tool for predicting events is that it does not depend on humans; the laws of nature always work in the same way (which of course is why we call them *laws* in the first place), regardless of what we do. We've become so good at using science that we now live in a world dominated by the products of scientific development, aimed at taking away uncertainty and chaos as much as possible—people very much like to have control over their life. All of Chap. 2 is dedicated to science.

Equally interesting is the category of self-defeating predictions, or predictions that are supposed to prevent things from happening. This type of prediction also comes up in our daily life all the time: 'If I don't get the brakes on my car fixed, and I go out to get groceries, I will get into a bad accident at the first busy intersection.' You can literally see the events happening in your mind, even though they have not happened yet and hopefully never will. This prediction is supposed to be self-defeating: it only comes true if we do not change the future by getting our brakes fixed.

Self-defeating predictions are extremely common, and are often used to make people do things, or to stop them from doing things: 'If you fail to show up for work without a good reason, you will get fired', or 'If you keep eating too much pizza, candy and ice cream, you will become overweight and get health problems', but also the more dubious 'If you don't forward this chain letter, you will get lots of bad luck'.

Our human laws are also excellent examples of self-defeating predictions: 'If you steal someone else's money, you will be punished', in the hope that this will prevent people from committing crimes such as theft.[2]

There are lots of real-world examples where we do certain things *now* to prevent bad things from happening *later*. One major example is vaccinating people (and especially children) to prevent them from contracting serious diseases. The argument for vaccination is once again a simple story about the future: 'If we don't vaccinate our children, many of them will get very ill, and some will even die'—in other words: a self-defeating prediction.

There is, however, a snag here: as diseases we vaccinate against have become increasingly rare, people no longer feared the consequences of those diseases, but instead began to worry about the safety of the vaccines—even though those vaccines were found to be exceedingly safe after thorough testing as well as extensive use. As a result, anti-vaccine sentiments became more pronounced from the 1980s onwards, eventually leading to a noticeable decline in childhood vaccinations and an associated increase in childhood diseases (and deaths) in quite a few countries. At which point of course vaccination campaigns were again intensified in attempts to control the outbreaks.

---

[2] To which criminals often respond with a prediction of their own: 'I will steal someone's money and just make sure that I'm not caught!'

The point here is that quite often, taking action to prevent certain bad things can be too successful, exactly because people don't see those bad things happening any more, and instead start believing that those actions are no longer needed or even harmful. In other words: many self-defeating predictions tend to have an element of *negative feedback*.

When Predictive Stories Become Manipulation

Stories are often used to make people do things, but those things are not always benign. There are for instance lots of Web sites on the Internet explaining how radiation from cell phones and wireless devices supposedly causes all sorts of serious health problems, often with a lot of sciencey-sounding language. These scary stories about 'radiation' have two things in common: they're not true, and they're meant to make people buy 'anti-radiation' products which can cost anything between a couple of dollars and thousands of dollars.

More nefarious are homeopaths with scary stories about vaccination on their Web site, e.g. claiming that vaccinating children can cause brain damage—and then using this scare to sell worried parents all sorts of home-opathic products to ostensibly neutralize the damage, and even serve as a safe alternative for vaccination. In reality, vaccines don't cause brain damage, and those homeopathic products don't work at all, providing a false sense of protection.

These and other examples are discussed in more detail elsewhere in this book.

It's All About People

Virtually all the stories that we hear, tell and make up are not about things, but about people. This is to be expected: we are first and foremost social creatures, and all the things and events that shape our daily lives are dominated by people, to begin with the ones close to us: family members, colleagues, our boss, etcetera. And nowadays more than ever, we also strongly depend on lots of complete strangers, most of whom we will never even meet. Just think of all those people that we depend on to grow our food, provide services or do other things that are essential in our own life. This strong reliance on each other is one of the things that has made us hugely successful as humans.

One interesting thing is that even if we're making stories about animals and other things that aren't people, those stories are *still* about humans one way or another. Just look at stories featuring animals: those animals more often than not have strong human characteristics. Many of our fairy tales and even modern-day children's entertainment are about animals that are in fact completely human, apart from their physical appearance. And this physical appearance quickly becomes totally irrelevant. Donald Duck is a perfect example: he is a thoroughly *human* character, complete with a mix-bag of good and bad human traits. In fact, his only duck-like trait is his tendency to start quacking uncontrollably when he loses his temper. For all the rest he may still look a bit like a duck, but he does not behave like a duck at all. His anthropomorphic character takes a rather bizarre turn in one particular episode, where he goes to the park *to feed the ducks*—as in: real ducks. The really funny thing is that most people don't think anything of it when they come across this scene.

But even in serious wildlife documentaries, animals are often equipped with rather human drives and emotions through the narrative and the cut of the video. Sometimes, the animals even get names.[3]

This does not stop at animals. Everything around us that might affect our life and well-being has been explained in terms of human actors or agents at one point or other in history. We did not just passively accept natural phenomena such as night and day, or rain or sun or wind for what they were. Instead, we came up with humans as an explanation for each of these things. And because even the strongest ordinary humans turned out to be powerless against those natural forces, those human-like beings had to have superhuman properties—they were *gods*. Yet these gods, even though they had superhuman and often magical qualities, were still outright human in their behaviour: they squabbled and fought, they were jealous, they demanded that people worshipped them for no other reason than that they were the most powerful … The myths about the ancient Greek and Roman gods read just like our modern-day soap series about the rich and powerful: extremely wealthy and powerful creatures that can do almost anything they want—but for all their power, they too encounter challenges and get into trouble, just like us, mere mortals … In other words: we can still relate to them and feel better about ourselves, because in lots of ways, they too are 'only human'.

I shall leave the tricky subject of religion for others to discuss, but I think it is safe to say that any religion is not so much about gods as it is about people, just like almost everything else in life.

This human-centric view of the world will be a recurring theme throughout this book, if only because people find it difficult to accept that

---

[3] This is probably because we find people more interesting than 'just' animals doing their thing. Wildlife documentary makers can boost their success by throwing in more human elements.

things 'just happen'. This is especially the case with major events such as the recent Covid-19 pandemic. Lots of people share the belief that it was not just a virus that managed to make the jump from animals to humans, but that the virus was deliberately created (by humans) and spread (by humans) to further some obscure human agenda—an agenda by which those evil but largely anonymous humans would get absolute control over all other humans. Others even believe that there is not really a bad virus on the loose, but that we are only made to believe (by humans) that this is the case, again in order for those same humans to gain total control over us. All this bears witness to our evolution as *the storytelling ape*.

Trust and Truth

Our social nature combined with the way our stories revolve around human themes also has a profound influence on *whom* we believe, in turn dictating a lot of *what* we believe. It was already mentioned that we don't care much if a particular story is actually true or not, just as long as it's a good story. This is of course not quite correct: we *do* care about the truth if we ourselves or our loved ones are involved in any way. Being lied to can be very harmful, and betraying someone's trust is considered a grave sin in most societies.

And this is where one important aspect of information sharing emerges: we tend to trust people in our own social group more than people we don't know. Also, the less we have in common with other people, the less we tend to trust them.

The consequence of this in our modern world is that we are often more likely to listen to a friend or family member than to what an anonymous expert on a particular subject says. This can be a problem, because our modern society has become so complex that it is impossible for a single human to know everything there is to know. We really need experts to keep our society going, and lots of them, at that.

This means that we have no choice but to trust the knowledge and skills of lots of other people, most of whom we will never meet. As a result of our ancient social traits, this trust in anonymous experts is fragile. If that friendly neighbour of ours comes up with a story she read about childhood vaccines causing all sorts of horrible health problems, then chances are that some of the people who know her and trust her will believe her. These people then will *not* trust doctors and scientists who say that there is nothing wrong with those vaccines—even though the latter ones are well-educated experts who know what they are talking about, whereas your neighbour's story is more likely some piece of misinformation originating from the Internet.

Even more interesting is the social dynamic of what happens after a particular story has made its way into a social group: this shared story will often serve to increase group bonding, and contribute to the overall group identity. It also increases the likelihood of related (and often even more extreme) stories being accepted into the group, further reinforcing this process. This positive feedback mechanism causes groups of people to harbour and express increasingly extreme ideas, and has been observed quite often in our history. Chapter 12 will explore this mechanism more in-depth.

A recent example that comes to mind is QAnon, which, also due to social media algorithms, quickly developed into a grand central station where virtually all thinkable conspiracy theories, pseudoscientific ideas and political extremes came together. This looks an awful lot like how tribal societies of old reinforce their cohesion by maintaining their own mythology, complete with shared story- and music-bound rituals. The stories don't have to be true or even make sense in any objective way; their main function is to help keep the tribe together, not to provide any actual useful information.

Who Must You Trust?

Do you drive a car? Then you have to trust a *lot* of people, both experts and ordinary people, to do things right in order to get from A to B in one piece. These are just some of the parties that you need to trust to safely drive around: the designers of the car (you don't want the car to tip over in curves), the car manufacturer (you don't want any wheels to come off when cruising on the motorway), the supplier of the raw materials (you don't want unreliable nuts, bolts and other parts that can break at any moment), the petrochemical company (you don't want fuel that can make the engine explode or seize up) etcetera. And perhaps most important of all: you have to trust your fellow drivers out there to have a certain degree of expertise in actually controlling their vehicle. This is why everyone has to take driving lessons and why everyone must pass a driving test in order to show that they are capable of safely driving a car. That is a *lot* of people you have to trust, even though in all likelihood, you don't personally know any of them.

Yet oddly enough, most of us have no problem at all trusting complete strangers this way. One reason for this is that we don't so much trust these actual people themselves, but rely on *their* self-preservation instinct: if they can't be trusted and do things wrong, they are likely to suffer negative consequences. Cars that are badly designed or manufactured quickly fall out of favour and don't bring in money, and dangerous drivers usually don't last long on the road either. In fact, the ones we most distrust when it comes to cars are the only ones we meet in person: car salespeople and mechanics. This is because they can (and sometimes do) harm us financially by taking advantage of our lack of expertise, for instance by vastly overcharging us for repairs. After all, they are the experts, so when a mechanic comes up with a story(!)

explaining why that little squeaky sound ends up costing $890 to fix, we can only take their word for it ...

But generally, we just trust other people by default, simply because it is impractical or even impossible for us to check if they actually know what they're doing.

Just think about it: when was the last time when you asked an airline crew for a pilot's license and flight records before boarding an air plane?

Emotion and Information

We humans love good stories, and we saw that we accept stories more readily when they come from people we trust. Another important thing about stories is their emotional appeal. Just compare the following two (fictional) headlines:

Researchers find addictive compounds in energy drinks, urge caution with younger consumers

and

SHOCKING! Our children are made into junkies by addictive DRUGS in their soda!

Both stories provide the same basic information: energy drinks contain addictive substances, and especially younger people may be affected by this. The story from the first headline, however, will most likely be ignored by most people, whereas the second story is certain to draw the attention of lots of people.

The reason for this is of course simple: the first headline provides a more objective factual description in neutral and cautious wording, whereas the second headline evokes strong emotions. The first message looks rather dull, and even hints at some laborious reasoning, whereas the second one immediately triggers our automatic, emotional response ('Our children are in danger!'). Attention guaranteed!

This appeal to emotion is of course nothing new. Newspaper makers have known for centuries that juicy headlines attract more readers than dry, factual information. However, people are of course not just driven by on-the-spot emotions and sensation, but also by curiosity for real facts and information. Newspaper editors know that appeal to emotion should be used sparingly, at least if they want to be taken seriously as a reliable source of information. Traditionally, this led to a fairly clear distinction between serious, more respectable sources of news and information on one hand, and rather more sensationalist media outlets (tabloids, 'gutter press', certain TV channels) on the other hand.

The recent emergence of digital social media has upset this relatively simple distinction. Nowadays, almost anyone can create, spread and share almost anything they like across the world in just a few seconds. All these people generally want one thing: other people's attention—and sensational headlines are a very effective way to accomplish this. This tendency to sensationalism is further stimulated by the medium itself: as the name already implies, the main goal of social media is to stimulate social interaction, rather than spread accurate information. The companies behind those social media channels of course want people to spend as much time as possible on their particular channel, and they know that appealing to people's emotions is the most effective way to reach this goal. The algorithms used to hook visitors of a particular social media channel exploit this human tendency: once you start clicking sensational headlines, you will almost certainly receive more suggestions for sensational stories. What is worse: over time, those suggestions may get more extreme in one way or another, because the algorithm 'knows' that this is the most effective way to keep people's attention. This mechanism can be quite insidious when people are just merrily clicking around, looking for a bit of entertainment. They are usually unaware that what they 'choose' to view is not really chosen by themselves: a computer algorithm is making those choices for them, based on what they spent time on before. And because there are now literally millions of videos and tweets and other snippets of information out there even on a single subject, people can be completely overwhelmed by a deluge of one-sided information—and, even worse, misinformation and disinformation, as explained in the sidebar.

Summarized: our human social traits, our emotions and our love of stories can mess with our brain, causing even quite intelligent people to start believing things that are not true. This too is a recurring theme in this book.

Misinformation and Disinformation, and How to Spot It

Misinformation is incorrect information, usually because someone made a mistake, or misinterpreted the original information, or was just plain sloppy. *Disinformation* (a.k.a. *fake news*) is more serious, and is best defined as deliberately falsified information, aimed at changing people's opinion.

An example of accidental misinformation is found in Naomi Wolf's 1999 best-seller *The Beauty Myth*. In this book, Wolf is very critical of the pervasive social and commercial pressure leading women to be preoccupied with their physical appearance, causing lots of mental and physical health issues. She supports this with the statistic that every year in the US, some 150,000 girls and women die from anorexia. This statistic was dutifully copied by critics, other authors, journalists and even news media, often with the same outrage that Wolf expressed over this huge, senseless death toll. Except that Wolf had made a mistake: it turned out that on average, some 150,000 women per year *suffered* (not died) from anorexia. The real number of deaths was far lower, and estimated to be between 100 and 400 fatalities per year. Which is still not something to step over lightly, but by far not the horrific figure that Wolf mistakenly presented.

The moral of this story is that it pays to be critical whenever you see some rather spectacular claim or statistic, especially when it is presented with emotionally charged language. When you come across something that causes feelings of outrage, shock or horror, chances are that someone is pulling your emotional strings, and wants to *make* you feel that way, often for their own purposes, which do not necessarily align with yours. People are less critical and more susceptible to being misled when they're in an emotionally excited state.

This is how you can check news items or videos with remarkable content:

- Does it cause an emotional response, or is the language emotionally charged? If yes, be wary.
- Do other, independent sources come up with the same information? If not, be wary.
- Does a Web site sell products related to their information content? If yes, be wary.
- Does the Web site and/or author express strong political views? If yes, be wary.
- Is the Web site and/or author known for less reliable information? If yes, be wary.
- Does the content strongly match your already existing beliefs? If yes, be aware that you may be living in an 'information bubble'.

Of course you can also search online for 'Spot Fake News'.

It Stands to Reason …

Our love of stories paved the way for the next important step in cognitive development: logical reasoning, ultimately leading to the birth of science. In fact, most scientific theories and studies are still a kind of story, explaining step by step and in a logical progression how a certain phenomenon works, and how researchers have figured this out. But unlike normal human stories, those scientific stories must follow some pretty strict rules and meet special criteria before they can be considered valid scientific reasoning. But let's not get ahead of ourselves, and first take a look at reasoning as a cognitive skill.

One major difference between stories and lines of reasoning is that reasoning often takes a *lot* of conscious effort, far more than just following a story (although story plots too can sometimes also be difficult to keep track of). In his book *Thinking, Fast and Slow*, Nobel laureate Daniel Kahneman came up with the concept of two ways of thinking, which he simply named System 1 and System 2. System 1 is the fast, automatic and intuitive way of thinking that we use most of the time. It helps us to instantly recognize things in the world around us, and often makes decisions for us before we even realize that we *are* making decisions at all. It is our cognitive mode when we operate on 'auto-pilot'. System 1 thinking may be fast and easy, it is also rather inaccurate and limited as to what situations it can handle.

System 2 thinking is the far slower, more deliberate system of thinking, the one we use to figure out and learn new things, do calculations, and follow step-by-step lines of reasoning. System 2 is engaged when we are faced with a situation that System 1 cannot handle, or when we need to make a conscious effort because a situation requires all our attention. An example of the latter is cooking a gourmet meal: we really have to concentrate on getting every detail right, thinking of how much of which ingredients we have to add at which moment in time, and how to process it. And a hundred thousand years ago, getting a beef dinner could be a similar cognitive challenge involving both System 1 and System 2: planning the hunt, laying an ambush, getting a beast within reach and making sure that it couldn't escape required attentive learning and quite a few System 2 reasoning steps, especially for inexperienced hunters—although running after it and trying to catch it is typical System 1 behaviour.

We will return to Kahneman's System 1 and System 2 thinking several more times in this book, for instance when explaining why people find it much easier to just assume and believe things, instead of painstakingly figuring them out for themselves.

The discovery of agriculture, one of the most significant revolutions in human history, may also be the result of cognitive developments mentioned so far. It is quite plausible that roaming tribes of hunter-gatherers periodically ended up in the same location where they had spent some time previously, and noticed a pattern: what they abandoned a couple of years earlier as a midden with bones, inedible seeds, remains from meals and other waste had turned into a lush thicket of fruit-bearing plants. It is only a small step to deliberately bury some of the waste, and then wait a while to see what happens. Now this story about hunter-gatherers experiencing a eureka moment is of course speculation (after all, it is a story that I made up and most probably didn't actually happen this way), but we do know for a fact that some 11,500 years ago, agriculture was invented. And even more remarkable, this happened at several places around the world independently.[4]

By switching from a hunter-gatherer lifestyle to agriculture, people no longer just had to depend on chance to see if they could find or catch the next meal on a daily basis. Instead, they eventually managed to grow more food than they needed by planning ahead and putting in a good day's work (albeit very hard and tedious work). Yes, chance still played an important role, and droughts and floods and plagues could ruin a harvest,[5] but all the same, far more people could now live and survive in the same place than ever before.

And as people no longer had to constantly wander around in search of the next meal, they could turn their attention to improving agriculture and keeping animals. In these growing communities, people sometimes found time to think about other things than just the bare necessities of survival, which in turn provided increased opportunities for developments in religion and culture, and generally for System 2 thinking. This also gave rise to new developments in philosophy, architecture and technology, beginning with the ancient Babylonians and Egyptians, and culminating in the heydays of classical Greece and Rome.

Still, with all our increased reasoning skills, explanations of the world around us mostly consisted of stories—and more often than not simple stories, more compatible with System 1 than System 2 thinking.

From Reasoning to Science

The development of reasoning skills was not only a major step forward in our human success story, but also an absolute requirement for the next level of human understanding of our universe: the emergence of science. Science is an important subject in this book, for two main reasons: it is by far the most reliable and accurate way to understand the world around us and everything in it, but it is also one of the most difficult things to do properly. Because of this, science is very often misunderstood, misrepresented or even plainly abused.

---

[4] This may very well be linked to the end of the last ice age, with a gradual change to a generally milder climate making it easier to make a living in the same location for prolonged periods of time.

[5] Which was of course attributed to the gods being displeased or another anthropocentric explanation. Because humans *really* have difficulty accepting that quite often, things (and especially bad things) 'just happen'.

A major difference between science and other cognitive developments is that science doesn't come naturally to us at all. One important reason for this is that science explicitly aims to minimize the influence of lots of human traits such as beliefs, emotions and System 1 thinking in general. It almost exclusively uses Kahneman's System 2 thinking in trying to understand and explain the world around us as objectively as possible. Science is based on an important basic principle called the scientific method, plus a lot of detailed rules and guidelines on how scientific studies should and should not be conducted. All these things and more are explained in the next chapter.

Conclusion

We have come to the end of the first chapter of this book, and we have set the stage for the subjects to come. We have seen how increasing cognitive capabilities and social developments have increased our ability to survive as humans—not by being strong or aggressive, but by using our big brains in ever more sophisticated ways. We have also seen how those very same big brains can often mislead us and make us believe things that are not real. And when we look at conspiracy belief in groups such as QAnon and the likes, we see that we humans still have an awful lot in common with those poor, spooked monkeys in the opening story, huddling together in fear over an imaginary threat—all because we unthinkingly believe what people whom we trust tell us, instead of figuring things out for ourself.

In the next chapter we will see how science tries to avoid those human flaws, showing us in the most objective way possible what is true and what is not. It turns out that this is not all that easy, and that science is wrestling with quite a few flaws and problems of its own.

2

It's the Science, Stupid!

Einstein Was Wrong! Oh, Wait, Not so Fast …

Location: Laboratori Nazionali del Gran Sasso, 1400 metres below the Gran Sasso massif in central Italy

Date: September 22, 2011

A scientific experiment by the name of OPERA had been quietly humming along for several years, without anyone outside of scientific circles taking much notice. This lack of public attention was not surprising, as the experiment was not exactly spectacular: scientists in Italy were monitoring a beam of highly elusive particles called muon neutrinos, produced 730 kilometres away at the CERN institute in Geneva, Switzerland. These neutrinos then travelled right through the earth's crust in the direction of Italy. According to a hypothesis in the field of quantum physics, some of these muon neutrinos should spontaneously convert into so-called tau neutrinos along the way, and it was these tau neutrinos that scientists at Gran Sasso were looking out for. This transformation, however, happened only very rarely. Over a two-year period, only five tau neutrinos were registered. Watching paint dry was far more exciting.

Until 22 September 2011, that is. That day, researchers at the Italian end of the experiment were analysing the data from the incoming neutrino beam from CERN when they noticed something odd: the neutrinos were arriving slightly faster than expected. Now this may not sound alarming to anyone unfamiliar with nuclear physics. So what if these things are a little faster than usual? The problem is that neutrinos normally travel at the speed of light. And in spite of all those wonderful faster-than-light ways of travelling dreamt up by science fiction, Einstein's theory of

R. Rasker, *Mind, Make-Believe and Medicine*, https://doi.org/10.1007/978-3-031-29444-0_2

relativity is quite clear on the subject: absolutely nothing can move faster than light. To be honest, those speeding neutrinos were only a fraction of a percent too fast, but even that tiny amount was more than enough to make scientists scratch their head. Was Einstein wrong after all? Researchers of course immediately assumed that there had to be another explanation. Maybe there was an error somewhere in the recorded data, or maybe there was some fault in the equipment. However, finding the fault was like searching for the proverbial needle in a haystack, as these highly advanced physics experiments involve huge amounts of data as well as extremely large and complicated machinery. It's not like simply checking if the table lamp in the living room is properly plugged in (although this is quite close to what actually turned out to be wrong ...).

Painstaking analysis of the data so far revealed no clues as to what caused the anomaly. Recorded measurements consistently showed neutrinos clearly exceeding the light speed by a small but measurable fraction of a percent. The research team invited other scientists to look into the problem as well, and to repeat their measurements if possible. And even though the scientific community remained highly sceptical about the possibility of faster-than-light neutrinos,[1] the whole affair attracted a huge amount of attention, and generated a deluge of scientific articles on all possible aspects of this mystery. This included speculation as to how neutrinos could perhaps appear to travel faster than light after all. However, the most important of these articles supported the notion that some kind of error must have been made.

In the beginning of 2012, researchers finally found the culprit: a badly connected fibre-optic cable, causing a small extra delay in the signal from a GPS receiver used for timing the received neutrino beam. This was as close as you can get to a badly plugged-in table lamp ...

And sure enough, in June 2012, new measurements showed the incoming neutrinos behaving exactly as expected, arriving with the speed of light as they should. Einstein was once again vindicated, and the whole excitement gradually subsided. The measurement part of the OPERA project ended in December 2012, although data analysis still continued.

Superficially, this story confirms the view that many people have of science: nerdy people doing incomprehensible things with big, extremely expensive machinery, using esoteric language in the process, without producing anything useful for the ordinary person in the street. Which in this case is not even all that far off the mark: this type of 'big science' explores the limits of our current scientific knowledge, and for most people, those limits are far removed from everyday life. However, it also shows how scientists make

---

[1] As theoretical physicist Jim Al-Khalili put it: *'I'll eat my boxer shorts on live TV if the OPERA results hold up.'*

mistakes, and then leave no stone unturned until they understand exactly what they did wrong.

So let's explore what science is all about and how it works—and also how it fails or gets abused.

Science—What Is It Good for? Absolutely Everything!

This caption may sound overly pompous, especially in the light of the opening story, which involves esoteric science that doesn't appear to have any practical use. Yet there is a bit of truth to it: there is almost no material aspect of our life that has not been influenced by science in any way. Just look around you, and spend a few thoughts on the things you see: unless you are reading this book somewhere in pristine nature, almost everything in our daily environment has come into existence using science in one way or another.

Then there are also the non-material aspects of science: many of us would not even be alive today without science. Just think for a moment about the progress made in the past 150 years: up until the late nineteenth century, about one in every four children died before the age of five, and most people didn't live past sixty. Diseases were a constant threat, ranging from endemic, slow killers such as tuberculosis to epidemics such as cholera and typhoid fever, and of course mass murderers such as smallpox and the Black Death. And even without these diseases, everyday accidents such as a simple, superficial cut could easily result in life-threatening infections. All these things have improved dramatically in recent times: in our western world, less than 1 child in every 200 dies before the age of five, and the average person can expect to live up to the age of eighty—and in relative good health and comfort, at that. We also know much better than ever before what causes disease and how to prevent it, all thanks to science.

To be honest, this 'absolutely everything' in the headline includes some pretty bad things as well. Science may have contributed massively to our success as a living species, but this success is now turning into some of the worst thinkable threats to the natural world and to our own existence: our numbers and especially our insatiable consumption—also made possible by science—cause huge problems with pollution, global warming, loss of natural habitat and extinction of other species … It was also science that gave us the most horrible weapons, capable of setting off a truly global catastrophe, probably killing most of us in the process. Which, admittedly, is a bit of a sobering thought.

Still, science is by far the best tool that we have to understand our world, and to use that understanding to try and create a better world for both ourselves as well as all the other species that we share this planet with. There is not much of an alternative anyway, at least not an alternative in which we can maintain our modern-day standard of living. And because science plays a key role in discussing many other topics in this book, it deserves a chapter of its own.

What Exactly Is Science?

Simply said, science is the systematic effort to understand the universe and everything in it, including ourselves, in an objective manner. The important words here are 'systematic' and 'objective'. Just thinking about the world, asking questions and coming up with answers is not science. Most religions and philosophical systems also involve lots of thinking, asking questions and producing answers—but these answers often originate from human imagination, tend to depend on personal or shared beliefs, and as a result are not necessarily based in reality.

In a way, things were a lot easier earlier on in our history, when we had a far less detailed understanding of our world: we simply invented stories that explained things in more or less human terms, and that was all there was to it. Those explanations of course only worked up to a point, and most questions and lines of reasoning eventually led to the realm of human imagination and religion (and thus supernatural 'explanations'), where literally anything is possible.

As religion essentially ruled the world for most of that time, independent investigation into how the universe worked was also often discouraged or even forbidden. After all, religious leaders had all the definitive answers that anyone could ever need, and it was in their interest for this state of affairs to continue. This is also an important reason why it took until the sixteenth century for science to really get going, even though humanity had achieved a lot of great things in architecture, literature and arts for thousands of years already.

Scientific reasoning by definition cannot contain anything outside of reality. Everything that science works with must be observable and objectively proven to exist. This means that supernatural explanations are not part of science, and that for instance 'the evil eye' cannot be invoked to explain why people sometimes fall ill. One problem here is that we found that the real universe is insanely big and complex. Even today, with our highly sophisticated scientific tools, we can only comprehend parts of it by simplifying and generalizing things—which means that even with all progress so far, science can only give us provisional answers, not definitive truths.

Break It to Make It

This may sound strange, but scientists as a group absolutely love it when they turn out to be wrong—because that is often when the most exciting discoveries are made. Consequently, a lot of the effort invested by scientists is aimed at trying to find shortcomings and flaws in each other's and their own work. They are, in other words, advancing science by trying to break it.

Every scientist worth their salt should take into account the possibility that they might be wrong, and that all their hard work can be challenged, corrected and even overturned by others. This may happen when their work turns out to have errors, but also as a result of newer scientific insights. This provisional status of scientific work should not be taken lightly: Newton's law of gravity held up for well over two centuries, but it still turned out to be 'wrong' when Einstein came up with general relativity and his model of spacetime.[2]

Yes, individual scientists come up with new ideas, and yes, the goal of their research is to see if they are right about those ideas—and it can be very disappointing for these individual scientists if they turn out to be wrong after all their hard work. But science as a whole can benefit hugely when errors are found and corrected. The opening story provides us with a glimpse of this mindset. When those researchers of the OPERA project made what looked like a ground-breaking discovery, they did not simply jump to conclusions, but asked other scientists to help figure out what could be wrong. When it turned out that they indeed had messed up with their equipment, they readily admitted this.

Unfortunately, there are also examples where scientists are not so willing to admit that they were wrong. One such example is the 1989 claim by Stanley Pons and Martin Fleischmann that they had managed to achieve so-called *cold fusion*. This type of nuclear fusion could purportedly generate huge amounts

---

[2] Newton's law of gravity still gives excellent results under most circumstances, and is not wrong in the sense that it is completely useless, hence the quotation marks. Einstein's solution is just *better* at describing the movement of objects under the influence of gravity. And because Newton's gravity formula is much easier to work with than Einstein's calculations, it is still widely used, even by NASA and other space agencies. Only when very high precision is required or under otherwise extreme circumstances is it necessary to use Einstein's work.

of clean and cheap energy with relatively simple equipment. Even though their claims were eventually proven wrong by nuclear physicists, and their experimental energy production could never be replicated, they never actually admitted that they had failed.

All this shows us another important feature of science: it is a collaborative system. Even though discoveries are often attributed to individual scientists, their actual work usually depends on the work of others. Also, most scientific research involves many scientists working together, each individual contributing their special skills and knowledge to a project. Newton and Einstein may seem like excellent examples of solitary scientists completely overturning the world of science all by themselves, but even their work was based on (or at the very least inspired by) the work of earlier scientists. Einstein based his spectacular insights on the work of Maxwell, Lorentz and Poincaré, and Newton himself acknowledged much the same in a famous quote in a 1675 letter to fellow scientist Robert Hooke: '*If I have seen further it is by standing on the shoulders of Giants.*'

Branches of Science

There are literally hundreds of fields of science, some of which are quite accessible (e.g. Newtonian mechanics), while others are rather more difficult, such as a medical science or quantum physics. This book mostly deals with medicine, physics and chemistry. One should note that medicine is not one scientific field, but consists of many dozens of specialized fields, and is also closely linked to other sciences such as biology, chemistry, psychology and sociology, to name just a few.

The Scientific Method

Science is generally seen as the best way to understand and explain the physical universe that we live in, including our own existence. The reason for this is that science follows a set of rules named *the scientific method*, which aims to produce results that are as objective as possible. The scientific method comprises the following six steps:

- **Observation**: recognizing a particular phenomenon, pattern or question.
- **Hypothesizing**: thinking of a possible explanation for what is observed.
- **Prediction**: make predictions that are in line with the hypothesis.
- **Testing**: test the predictions (and thus the hypothesis) in a meaningful way.

- **Peer review**: have other scientists check the results.
- **Replication**: have the claimed results independently reproduced by others.

Well, that sounds simple, now doesn't it? Just follow these six simple steps, and hey, presto: you're doing science!

Unfortunately, and as always, it turns out that things aren't that simple, and that doing proper science is actually quite hard, for several reasons. In fact, a lot of this book is dedicated to exploring the many problems and pitfalls of both scientific and unscientific ways of thinking, and how our human traits more often than not get in the way of finding out how things *really* work. But first, we will take a closer look at the steps of the scientific method.

Observation

Most scientific research begins with a particular observation or idea. This may happen when people see a particular pattern, or when an event or phenomenon occurs, and people start wondering what caused it. Observation is a necessary part of the scientific method, but even the most painstaking observations are not scientific if they are not used to *explain* anything.

Hypothesizing

The next step is setting up a hypothesis. *Hypothesis* is basically just a fancy word for a story that offers a logical explanation for what is observed. A hypothesis is a line of reasoning, usually involving one or more steps. One essential thing here is that each of these reasoning steps must itself be scientifically and logically valid: you cannot skip steps or insert steps that are outside of science. If your hypothesis features a demon to explain why something bad happens, then you must either prove the existence of that demon (and also how it makes bad things happen), or else abandon your hypothesis.

Now hypothesizing about demons may sound a bit silly these days, but there are still quite a few types of alternative hypotheses out there that are based on equally implausible concepts. According to one such hypothesis, one can diagnose a person's state of health by just waving one's hands near their body, and even correct any health problems in the same manner (which is what several types of 'energy medicine' are all about, as discussed in the chapter on Energy Medicine).

When a hypothesis still appears to be correct after extensive research and testing, it can be accepted as a scientific *theory*, or as a part of an existing theory. Note that in this case the word 'theory' here does not have the common meaning of 'guess' or 'hunch', but is far stronger. A scientific theory is about as close as scientists will ever come to declaring something a truth or a fact.[3]

Prediction

The next essential step in any scientific endeavour is making predictions that are directly based on the hypothesis. There are two types of prediction:

* Predictions that *support* the hypothesis: 'When my hypothesis is true, and I do *this*, then *that* is what I expect to happen.'
* Predictions that can *falsify* the hypothesis: 'When I do *this*, and *that* happens, then my hypothesis can't be true.'

When a supporting prediction is confirmed, then this does *not* automatically mean that the hypothesis is definitively proven; it is just *more likely to be correct*. On the other hand, when a falsifying prediction is confirmed, then by definition this means that the hypothesis is wrong.

The concept of falsifiability is one of the most important principles in science. If it is not possible to come up with something that would falsify a hypothesis, it is usually not a good hypothesis to begin with.

Let's illustrate this with a simple example. Suppose you have a hypothesis saying that all crows are black. You can then make two predictions: (1) When I go looking for crows, I only expect to find black ones, and (2) When I go looking for crows, and I spot one with a different colour than black, then my hypothesis is wrong.

How this works out, is explained in the next step: testing.

Testing

After making one or more predictions, those predictions are tested to see if they are confirmed or not. Testing can essentially happen in two ways:

* **Experimenting**: this usually boils down to creating conditions that according to your hypothesis and predictions should produce a certain outcome, and then observing what happens.

---

[3] Good scientists will never officially call their knowledge 'truth' or 'fact', because there is always the possibility, no matter how small, that their knowledge is wrong in one way or another.

- **Exploring**: you go looking for evidence that is relevant to your hypothesis, and see if what you find supports or contradicts the predictions made.

To test our hypothesis that all crows are black, we can experiment by breeding crows and see what colour they have when they hatch. But this presents a problem: what if you need birds that are not black to begin with in order to find ones with a different colour? Because that is of course how breeding works: offspring normally inherit their properties from their parents, including plumage colour. So in this case, it is probably better to go out there and check the colour of the birds you can spot.

Then the next problem crops up: the supporting type of prediction can never give you a definitive answer. No matter how many black crows you find, it is always possible that somewhere out there is a white one that you missed. Yes, when you have been looking for years, and found thousands upon thousands of black crows and not a single white one, it becomes *increasingly plausible* that all crows are black—but it does not *prove* your hypothesis. You only have to find one white crow to conclude that it is wrong. This is the essence of falsifiability: you can point to a well-defined observation or experimental result that conclusively proves a hypothesis wrong.

Peer Review

Scientific study is never a one-person show, and every study is evaluated by fellow scientists before it is officially published. This so-called *peer review* is meant to find possible errors, shortcomings and other things that may detract from the scientific quality of the work. Scientists are, after all, only human, and just as prone to making mistakes as anyone else. Peer review also helps prevent less innocent kinds of mistakes such as scientific fraud.

Replication

The final step in the scientific method is *replication*, where other scientists try to reproduce the results that are found. Unfortunately, this replication step is often neglected or omitted, mainly because there is no glory in just repeating what others have done before—scientists much prefer to do new and exciting things, for which they can take full credit. Another reason is that original publications bring in not just fame, but also fortune: it is far easier to get funding for exciting new research than for replication studies.

As a result, quite a bit of scientific knowledge out there is based on one-off studies. This increases the chances that this knowledge is wrong, and there is indeed something that is called the *replication crisis*: it turns out that a lot of scientific studies upon replication fail to produce the original results, especially in fields such as psychology and medicine.

Probably the biggest replication crisis of all is found in homeopathy. Homeopaths and proponents of homeopathy claim that the effects of homeopathy are 'scientifically proven', pointing at hundreds of studies finding a positive effect. The problem is that literally none of those studies can be reliably replicated—they're all one-off studies, and almost certainly just statistical flukes. The fact is that there is not a single homeopathic preparation out there that shows consistent, repeatable effects in a scientific experiment.

Golden Milk

(free after *The Dragon in my Garage* from Carl Sagan)

'Hello *Daily Inquirer*? Hi, I'm John, the farmer on the old dirt road, and I have a sensational scoop for you! It turns out that my cows make gold in their milk!'

'Well, hello John, that certainly sounds interesting! Could we come over and see this happen?'

'Well, that's a bit tricky. These cows ain't really fond of strangers, if you catch my drift. They get upset, and then they won't give milk for a week. So I don't reckon you coming over here is a good idea.'

'OK, that sounds like bit of a problem. But maybe you can record a video of you milking a cow and show us the gold in it while you're at it?'

'No, sorry, that's no good. The gold can't stand light. It only works in the dark. As soon as you turn on any light, the gold dissolves again. All gone in a blink of the eye!'

'That does sound a bit odd. Does this mean that you haven't had any actual gold in your hands?'

'Oh yes, I've had it in my hands! But as I said, you have to be very careful with the light.'

'Then can you put some of this gold in a dark, closed container and send it to us? You should have quite a lot by now, don't you? And we can pay you for it if you like.'

'Well, yes, I could do that. But note that this gold is not very stable, and changes into dung at the drop of a hat.'

'OK, so what you're basically saying here is that you are willing to send us a load of bullsh... if we pay for it and pretend it's gold? Oh, he hung up ...'

The rather corny sidebar story is of course completely made up, but it is in fact inspired by a public statement from a high-ranking politician in India, who really claimed that Indian cows produce gold in their milk [1]. The story is relevant here because it illustrates how a hypothesis ('These cows produce gold in their milk') cannot be falsified, because every attempt to test the hypothesis is thwarted by new claims and provisions.

This endlessly adding of further restrictions and additional conditions (a technique known as 'Moving the goalposts') also happens quite a lot in pseudoscience. For instance, many practitioners of so-called energy medicine claim that the 'subtle energy' they work with can only be detected by themselves, using their special skills and sensitivities, but not by any conventional scientist. But as soon as real scientists think of ways to test the skills of these people, the energy medicine practitioners come up with new reasons why this will not work. One example is the claim that the purported effects are cancelled out by 'negative energy' or something similar as soon as scientists try to investigate the phenomenon. Needless to say that conventional science indeed never managed to replicate the claims and findings of these people.

Plausibility

Another important aspect of scientific research is *plausibility*. If someone comes up with a highly implausible claim or idea (e.g. that plain water is an effective medicine), then they should also come up with some very good evidence supporting that claim if they expect scientists to take an interest. Contrary to what many people think, scientists don't just start researching any wild idea—otherwise they would spend their entire careers on wild goose chases, and never get any serious work done. Or as Carl Sagan said it, 'Extraordinary claims require extraordinary evidence.'

This is also applied in a more formalized way to assess the results of research: when a particular result is found, *prior plausibility* is factored in to determine the probability that the result indeed reflects a real effect, instead of being just a statistical fluke. One problem with these so-called Bayesian statistics is that it is often very difficult to establish the prior plausibility for a given claim or phenomenon.

Why Science Is Hard

Doing proper science sounds easy enough ('Just stick to the scientific method'), but in reality, it is often very difficult indeed. There are two important reasons for this: the complexity of the scientific field itself, and human factors.

Reality Is Complex

As we became more successful in finding out how our world works, it turned out that our world was more complex than anyone ever imagined. Sure, Newton's mechanics are still relatively easy to comprehend, and that is also why this area of science was one of the first to be explored, and why it is still taught in schools. However, his work is superseded by Einstein's theory of relativity, which may provide a better model of reality, but this progress comes at a cost: it is also significantly more complicated.

When we turned our scientific curiosity to matters of life and death, things got even more difficult. It took hundreds of years before we even got a glimmer of understanding of how a single cell works, let alone how complete organisms function. The reason for this is that living creatures have evolved to stay alive, grow, reproduce, heal and ward off threats all by themselves. In the case of higher animals, this involves literally tens of thousands of proteins, enzymes, hormones and other substances, all working together seamlessly in a myriad of interconnected biochemical processes. To unravel this biochemical machinery is a gargantuan task, and even today, there are complex biological structures and processes that we will probably never truly understand. One example is our brain: it is made up of about a hundred billion nerve cells (*neurons*), each of which in fact isn't all that complicated. However, the real complexity of the brain stems from an even far greater number of *connections* between all those billions of cells. On average, each neuron is connected to 10,000 other neurons. It is this hugely complex network that enables our brain to function the way it does. It is however very doubtful if we will ever manage to understand exactly how this neural network produces consciousness, human drives and emotions, and does all the other things that our brain does.

For the same reasons, it can be very difficult to find out what the actual problem is if something goes wrong in our body and we fall ill. And even if we know what caused a problem, we still need to figure out what we can do to fix it. Sometimes, the best way to deal with it is to do nothing and let our body heal itself; lots of ailments and problems go away by themselves given just a bit of time and perhaps rest. However, lots of other conditions absolutely require some sort of intervention to prevent things from getting worse and even killing us. When treatment is necessary, one of the problems is that the body itself often gets in the way. Like all organisms, our body has evolved to keep itself alive and healthy as much as possible. One essential part of this is that our body actively tries to get rid of potentially harmful foreign substances—and that is a bit of a problem if this foreign substance is a medicine. This is one important reason why medicines that appear to work quite well in test tubes (in vitro) often don't work in actual living patients (in vivo). Furthermore, until about 150 years ago, it was generally impossible to actually take a look inside a patient to diagnose and hopefully fix a problem—because that would more often than not kill the patient, or at the very least cause horrible suffering. Routine operations have only become possible thanks to scientific progress in the fields of anatomy, anaesthesiology and bacteriology, among other things. And even better: science has given us several ways to look inside patients without harming them in any way.

To get an idea of how difficult medical science is: the average medical student spends at least eight years (equating to some 15,000 hours) on study and internships before they are deemed capable of diagnosing and treating patients. Add several more years to this when a student wants to specialize, e.g. in cardiology.

And even after all that hard study and work, gathering an immense amount of knowledge and skills in the process, *doctors still get it wrong on a regular basis*. However, this does not mean that modern medicine is no good—it merely means that modern medicine may well be one of the most difficult things we humans can do.

A completely different scientific field that is almost proverbially hard to understand is *quantum physics*, which attempts to describe how our world works on the smallest scale that we know of. The problem with this quantum world is that we can't properly describe it in normal human terms. In quantum physics, a 'thing' is not simply a well-defined object, but a constellation of countless so-called quantum wave functions, each of which can contribute to the macroscopic behaviour of what we humans think of as an object. Even quantum physicists themselves cannot give a fully accurate definition of even one elementary particle—the definition and description used depends on what aspects of a particle you are looking at. And this insane complexity gets even far worse when looking at all possible *interactions* between multiple particles. Another major problem we humans have with quantum physics is that its elements are described in terms of (un)certainties. When looking at quantum phenomena, even one particle (what we would call a 'thing') usually cannot be said to be in one place. Instead, it can be *in all places at the same time*,[4] with mathematical probability formulas telling you how likely it is that you find it in any specific place when you try to locate it.

---

[4] This weird sentence essentially says it all: that our human understanding and language are woefully inadequate to grasp and describe what is *really* going on in quantum physics …

It is probably safe to say that nobody on earth really *understands* quantum physics, not even quantum physicists who spent decades working in this field. Yet all their scientific work leads to the same conclusion: quantum physics still provides the best description of the building blocks of the real world that we live in. Quantum physics also made several predictions that were later confirmed in scientific experiments, and even produced some important applications. For instance MRI machines use a particular quantum phenomenon by the name of *nuclear spin* to create high-quality images of the inside of our body. This is just one example where esoteric scientific research such as in the opening story led to very useful practical applications.

Apart from being very hard to understand, quantum physics is also mentioned here because lots of practitioners of alternative medicine and pseudoscience invoke it to give a veneer of scientific credibility to what they are doing (and, in most cases, are trying to sell you). So if you stumble on the word 'quantum' in connection with products or services being offered for any type of healthcare application, then they almost certainly try to sell you useless pseudomedical or pseudoscientific nonsense.

The Brain Getting in the Way

The sheer complexity of the universe we live in is a very good reason why science can be hard, but it is not the only reason. Another important reason why we have so much difficulty investigating our world in an objective manner is that science requires a lot of Kahneman's laborious System 2 thinking, while our human brain generally prefers quick-and-easy System 1 solutions. In simpler terms: we are by nature pretty lazy and like to cut corners—and in science, cutting corners is a recipe for failure.

A general type of flaw in objective reasoning goes by the name *fallacy*. One fallacy that almost everyone of us commits has the Latin name Post hoc *ergo propter hoc*. This translates as 'After = Caused by': when two unusual things happen one after the other, we tend to assume that the first event caused the second event. You ate a piece of birthday cake an hour ago, and now your stomach hurts? Then there must have been something wrong with the cake! You take a few herbal drops, and sometime later, your stomach feels much better? Then those herbal drops cured your upset stomach!

In both cases, it is quite possible that the stomach pain had nothing to do with the cake, and also disappeared spontaneously, without the herbal drops having really cured anything.

Unfortunately, the Post hoc fallacy can sometimes have more serious consequences. Anti-vaccine groups keep spreading the myth that vaccines cause all sorts of serious health conditions. According to these people, many health problems occurring *after* vaccination are also *caused by* vaccination, prompting worried parents to decline vaccination of their children. At the time of this writing, they even attribute almost every sudden, natural death to Covid-19 vaccination. We'll get into more detail about this in the chapter on vaccines.

The Post hoc fallacy is also the main reason why alternative practitioners and their customers believe that alternative treatments really work, and even the most respectable scientists must be constantly wary not to fall into this trap.[5]

Another simple and very common fallacy is the *Popularity fallacy*: we are more inclined to believe things when a lot of other people believe those things as well. This fallacy too is used a lot in alternative medicine: 'Millions of people use acupuncture, so it must be effective'. There are lots of different fallacies, several of which are listed in the Appendix at the end of this book.

A different type of cognitive trait getting in the way of objectively gathering knowledge is more subtle, and is called *bias*. There are again many types of bias, and all of them have a negative impact on scientific results.

A very common example of bias is *confirmation bias*. This is a type of bias where researchers unconsciously or consciously favour data and results that support their hypothesis, while at the same time ignoring or playing down any information that may contradict or even falsify their hypothesis. This type of bias lies at the heart of a lot of bad science and pseudoscience, and even belief in conspiracies.

Another related and very common type of bias is *publication bias*, by which only studies with a positive result are published, while most studies with a negative outcome never see the light of day and end up in a drawer somewhere. The result is that the overall scientific landscape looks far more positive than it really is. And again, the main reasons for this are human weaknesses: positive results are what brings in fame and fortune, not only for the scientists involved, but also for the institutions they're affiliated with. Studies with a negative or inconclusive outcome, on the other hand, are seen as a mistake or a blemish on someone's career, something that should be forgotten as soon as possible. After all, negative outcomes often happen when scientists turn out to be wrong about something. No matter how science as a whole may benefit from finding and correcting errors, individual scientists do not like to be wrong—one would almost think they're human.

---

[5] In case you wonder why this Post hoc fallacy is so common: it is in fact just another manifestation of our overly active pattern recognition instinct already described in Chapter 1.

Publication bias is a major problem for several reasons. One problem is that different scientists may spend money, time and effort on researching the same thing without knowing each other's work, unaware that the underlying hypothesis has already been researched and proven wrong. Had they known this, they might have decided to conduct their study in a different way, or to abandon the subject altogether.

There are many other types of bias, some obvious, other quite subtle. Several of these are also listed in the Appendix.

Nobel Disease

One remarkable phenomenon involving scientists taking a wrong turn in their career is known as *Nobel disease*. This happens when highly respected scientists start working outside their field of expertise, sometimes with disastrous results. This has even happened to several Nobel laureates, hence the name. One well-known example is Linus Pauling, whose brilliant work in the field of quantum chemistry and X-ray crystallography advanced the fields of chemistry and biochemistry in no small way. In 1954, he received the Nobel Prize for chemistry, and in 1962, he received another Nobel Peace Prize for his peace activism. In the 1960s, he became convinced that huge doses of vitamins, especially vitamin C, could effectively treat all sorts of physical and even psychiatric disorders, up to and including cancer and schizophrenia. He based his ideas on personal experience—a well-known pitfall that has caused many people, scientists and laypeople alike, to start believing things that are not true. Pauling's pursuit of his wild megavitamin ideas eventually led to a new branch of alternative medicine he coined *orthomolecular medicine*. Up until this day, there is no scientific evidence that orthomolecular medicine is good for treating any condition—apart from actual vitamin and mineral deficiencies of course.

Anti-scientific Views and Sentiments

Not everyone is convinced that science is the best way to gather knowledge and improve human well-being. Some people and groups are distrustful of science, or have an outright negative view of science. Many people view science as 'cold' and 'inhuman', and they are not even completely wrong: science indeed tries to gather knowledge in an objective way, explicitly minimizing the influence of human emotions and other cognitive traits in the process. This 'dehumanized', scientific way of dealing with reality is in apparent contrast with the notion that science often has a profound impact on the lives of actual humans, real people with emotions and beliefs. This is certainly something that scientists should not ignore. Scientists in many fields such as medicine and technology should always keep in mind that they are ultimately trying to change the lives of people—hopefully for the better.

Other anti-scientific sentiments often emphasize the bad things that science has caused, such as pollution, ever more destructive weapons, and science pandering to corporate greed, to name just a few. This view is however overly negative because it ignores the many good things that science has brought us. Life certainly was not better in pre-scientific times.

One of the focal points of anti-science and distrust in science is human health: lots of people do not trust pharmaceutical companies and their products. They often think that scientists are being paid to produce favourable research outcomes for newly developed medicines, and that 'Big Pharma' in general lets profits prevail over human health. These ideas (and whether or not they are true) will be discussed in Chapter 6.

Then there are proponents and practitioners of alternative medicine who reject medical science, or even only part of medical science, favouring whatever type of alternative medicine they personally believe in. Alternative medicine is also home to some peculiar examples of cognitive dissonance: it often rejects regular medical science, but at the same time comes up with lots of 'scientific research' that supposedly supports its tenets. This mindset is often tightly interwoven with *pseudoscience*, something that is described further on.

The interesting thing here is that these people do not reject all of science and its products, but only a small part. They happily make use of the products of high-tech science, such as smartphones and computers, to spread the notion that other (medical) science is invalid or should not be trusted.

Lastly, one particularly interesting reason for distrust in science is in fact one of its strongest points: the notion that scientific knowledge is always provisional, and should be updated or even abandoned whenever new information becomes available. This is aptly expressed in the following quote, apparently from an anonymous American politician:

Why trust scientists? Just give them new data and they change their mind!

The point here of course is that in politics, changing one's mind is often seen as a sign of weakness and untrustworthiness, and not as a sign of intelligent, rational behaviour.

Bad Science

The biases, fallacies and other pitfalls mentioned so far were mostly assumed to occur by accident, often as a result of our very human tendency to use 'lazy' System 1 thinking.

Other human traits that can interfere with a scientist's intention to deliver good scientific work range from relatively benign character flaws, such as unwarranted overconfidence and overstepping the boundaries of one's field of competence, to more serious problems such as 'fudging' data, and even outright fraud. This is often motivated by the desire to get positive results with associated fame and fortune. Other scientists 'just know' that their hypothesis is right, and then proceed to make up the expected positive results even if their research turns out negative. One major problem is that dodgy science and fraud often remain unnoticed, at least until other scientists try to replicate the results, or notice anomalies in the research data—things that usually only happen when a scientist comes up with claims or results that are remarkable enough to raise an eyebrow or two. Microbiologist Elisabeth Bik is one of the very few scientists spending their time systematically checking scientific publications for signs of manipulation and fraud. She is especially adept at spotting manipulated, duplicated or otherwise suspicious images, and has identified hundreds of papers where things were not quite right.

Another example of bad science—or rather: bad scientists—emerged during the recent Covid-19 pandemic. Dozens of scientists and doctors let their beliefs prevail over good science, and started spreading dubious or even outright false information about Covid-19 itself and the best way to treat and prevent it. They often opposed measures to curb the spread of the disease, and suggested that we should basically let it rip through society unchecked, while only protecting the most vulnerable—an impossible proposition. Some kept promoting medicines such as hydroxychloroquine and ivermectin even after these had been proven ineffective, and some opposed Covid-19 vaccination, falsely claiming that the vaccine caused lots of injuries and even deaths. All without proper scientific evidence.

The big problem here is not just the contrarian position of these doctors and scientists, but the fact that they tried to suggest that they represented 'science'—while the real scientific consensus was completely different from what these rogue scientists claimed. The important point here is that we should never just accept the point of view and arguments of one individual scientist, but always consider the *totality* of the scientific evidence.

Note that *Bad Science* is also the title of a highly recommended book by British physician Ben Goldacre, in which he deals with much the same subjects that are discussed in this book. Not only does he address the usually poor science in alternative medicine, he is just as critical of any faults and shortcomings in regular medicine in general and Big Pharma in particular.

Scientists Are only Human …

It has been mentioned several times that science explicitly welcomes criticism and corrections, in order to improve the scientific body of knowledge. When scientists are confronted with flaws or shortcomings in their work, they are expected to correct the flaws or even retract their work. This is why we have this whole peer review process in the first place, and why science should be transparent.

Now this is all nice and dandy for science as a whole, but individual scientists unfortunately are not always keen on criticism, even if that criticism is well-founded. After all, nobody likes to be wrong, and especially highly respected and well-known scientists sometimes see criticism as a public humiliation or even as an attack on their person. That this sometimes leads to really unsavoury developments is something that the aforementioned Elisabeth Bik can testify to: after she criticised a paper by a French physician and microbiologist who claimed that hydroxychloroquine was effective in treating Covid-19, this microbiologist did not address her scientific concerns, but instead threatened to sue her for defamation. In response Bik, stating that she feels seriously intimidated, has received pledges of support from the scientific community in general and sceptical organizations in particular. At the time of this writing, no actual legal proceedings have taken place, but the threat alone is a clear sign that some scientists tend to let their (hurt) pride prevail over scientific objectivity.

Corporate Influence and Financial Interests

Science is often expensive. Correction: science can be *insanely* expensive. Even relatively small-scale studies can cost upwards of a hundred thousand dollars, developing a single medicine costs on average a billion dollars, and really big physics and astronomical projects can cost billions of dollars.

And alas, everywhere there is money to be spent or earned, corruption lurks, from the lowest to the highest level. Science is no exception to this rule. When financial success depends on scientific success, there will always be individuals as well as organizations that try to achieve this success by less than honest means. Individual researchers may fudge scientific data in order to get more funding, and for instance pharmaceutical companies may present their research in a more favourable light than what is warranted by the actual scientific results. After spending hundreds of millions of dollars on the development of a promising new medicine, it can be very hard to abandon the whole thing when in the end, it doesn't perform as well as expected.

Even though deliberate scientific fraud seems pretty rare, an anonymous survey showed that about two percent of scientists admitted to have falsified or modified data at least once in their career in order to get a 'better' outcome [2]. Almost one in three has used dubious research practices at one time or other.

Getting caught usually has severe consequences: individual scientists publicly lose the respect of their colleagues, and often their scientific career as well. Corporations don't get away with this either: if caught, they can expect very serious fines, sometimes amounting to hundreds of millions of dollars or more. In addition, they may also be banned from selling products that were at the core of any fraud.

Politicized Science

Another problem is politically motivated bad science, where a government tolerates or even encourages bad scientific research. One such example is research in the field of Traditional Chinese Medicine (TCM). The Chinese government considers this type of alternative medicine as a highly prestigious part of their cultural heritage. As a result, the vast majority of Chinese papers on acupuncture (a part of TCM) claims strong positive results. For comparison: most high-quality western scientific studies find that acupuncture has no effect beyond placebo. Something very similar is happening in India, where Ayurveda and homeopathy have now gained recognition as official systems of medicine, even though both have been thoroughly discredited by proper scientific research.

Pseudoscience

Pseudoscience is where things really fly off the rails. *Pseudoscience* is something that resembles science to a certain degree and often even uses scientific jargon, but has little or nothing to do with real, established science. Just take a look at the following:

Colorivitreous Nasal Therapy

Colorivitreous nasal therapy is a new development for treating a broad range of ailments that result from modern-day stress, bad lifestyle habits, food sensitivities, toxins, harmful radiation, and a lot more. It usually takes only five or six sessions for the patient to clearly experience beneficial effects and regain their positive energy.

In the first session, the patient's ailments and mood are charted to produce a spectral map, combining ancient knowledge about the influences of colours on human health and emotions with the latest insights in Colour Theory.

Then, a carefully selected globular translucent element with precisely matching spectral properties is introduced into the nasal passage; this location is chosen for its proximity to the brain's frontal lobe. Here, it exerts its beneficial effects, its spectral profile resonating with the body's energy field, damping out the negative frequencies through effective interference. During this process, biophotons are exchanged with the surrounding tissues in accordance with Feynman diagrams, which are of course well known from quantum mechanics. The resulting collapse of the multipath quantum state to a single, well-defined optical path guarantees the precision required for optimal efficacy.

Does this sound crazy to you? It should—not only because I just made it up from A to Z, but also because what it basically says is that you can effectively treat lots of ailments by shoving a marble ('globular translucent element') up your nose. Which of course is nonsense. Yet you can find literally hundreds if not thousands of 'treatments' with similar claims on the internet, with the only difference that to the best of my knowledge, they don't involve marbles. People fall for these things because they sound scientific, even though in reality, this 'explanation' is a meaningless word salad. The body has no 'energy field', and certainly no 'negative frequency'. Other terms such as 'interference' and 'Feynman diagram' are pilfered from legitimate science, but have no meaning here.

The problem is that only people who have some knowledge of proper science are capable of recognizing this nonsense for what it is. Most other people vaguely understand the health claims, and take the rest of the text for granted as something they can't (and don't need to) understand anyway.

Other well-known examples of pseudoscience are astrology, parapsychology and energy medicine. The common denominator of all these things is that they consist of a loosely defined collection of phenomena and rules describing the effects of those phenomena, without being rooted in real science in any way. This means that they are more accurately described as systems of belief. Pseudoscientific claims and jargon are also often used in fraudulent schemes to sell people treatments and devices that do not work at all, analogous to my *Colorivitreous Nasal Therapy*.

A rather sinister example of profit-driven pseudoscience was the ADE-651 bomb detector scandal. In 2008, a British company by the name of ATSC sold hand-held devices that could supposedly detect bombs and explosives at distances up to several kilometres away. These devices were based on 'electrostatic ion attraction' and contained a 'detector card preprogrammed with chemical fingerprints of explosives', causing a telescopic antenna to swivel and point in the direction of any explosive in the vicinity. Priced at a hefty £40,000 each, these devices were sold in significant numbers to Middle East countries, where they were used to prevent bombings.

In 2010, it turned out that these devices contained no functional parts whatsoever, and were in fact a complete scam. The 'detector card' was just a generic anti-theft tag, and in actual tests, the device consistently failed to detect any explosives placed nearby. By that time, several Middle East countries had already spent dozens of millions of dollars on these fake detectors, and several large bombings in Iraq had claimed dozens of lives because the Iraqi military had relied on these useless devices for their safety. In 2013, James McCormick, ATSC's director and developer of the ADE-651, was convicted of fraud, and sentenced to 10 years in prison [3].

This just goes to show that even governments can be taken in by a sales pitch based on pseudoscientific babble. The big mistake that those governments of course made is that they completely failed to independently test the device before spending millions of dollars on them; they simply believed what McCormick told them.

But even the hilarious pseudoscientific claim from that politician in India about desi cows producing gold in their milk when the sun shines on their hump is not completely harmless. It is not unthinkable that poorly educated people will believe this, and decide to spend what little money they have on a desi cow. And there will of course always be less scrupulous people willing to sell them such cows—at a premium price, as goes without saying.

How to Recognize Pseudoscience

The problem with pseudoscience is that it looks and sounds just like real science to a non-scientist: it appears to have a consistent and systematic logic, with its own 'laws' and of course its own jargon. A lot of practitioners and proponents take it completely seriously, and often even have their own 'academies' and do their own 'research'. Also, impressive-looking devices are regularly involved as well, especially in the field of so-called energy medicine.

At first glance, pseudoscience seems to be indistinguishable from real science for most people. There are, however, a few simple checks by which pseudoscience can be recognized as such.

The first check is amazingly simple: just try to look up the name of the particular alternative practice on Wikipedia, and see if it is called a pseudoscience. For instance, Wikipedia's article on astrology opens like this: '**Astrology** is a *pseudoscience* …' This statement is then further supported by a wealth of information on the subject, complete with scientific and other sources. Now of course you do not have to believe that first sentence right away. It is, after all just a simple statement that may well be wrong. However, further on in the article, this statement is supported by lots of evidence and background information, and it becomes increasingly difficult to claim that all those supporting things are wrong as well.

But maybe you don't trust the judgement of other people, scientists or not. Well, you can do a lot of thinking yourself—so go ahead, and engage your own System 2 thinking. Try to see through all the jargon and sciencey-sounding text, and look at what actual claims are made. Do these claims sound plausible? In the case of astrology, the central claim is that events in the life of people here on earth are closely intertwined with the exact positions of planets in our solar system against the background of some groups of stars. However, those planets in our own solar system are already hundreds of millions of kilometres away from us, so how can they have any influence on us? And the star groups that form the signs of the zodiac—an essential element of astrology—are even much further away. It is hugely implausible that astronomical objects on those distances have even the smallest effect on things happening on our earth. Then think about another astrological claim: the effects are not simply physical (like our moon causing tides), but usually have to do with individual emotional and psychological issues, such as success in love, or decisions about friendships and our career. How can exquisitely human things like this be controlled by lifeless globes of rock and gas, millions and millions of kilometres away? And even more unlikely, how can the position of those globes of rock and gas at our time of birth have any predictive power for what happens in the rest of our life?

Even our own personal therapists or counsellors or life coaches already have a hard time figuring out what it is that we want, what we need, and how we can achieve it—and they are sitting right across the table, doing their very best to help us. And then some planets and stars at truly astronomical distances can do better than that? It just does not make sense. You would have to abandon most of what we know about the planets, the stars and the universe (and humans, for that matter) in order to believe that there really is something to astrology.

Another example stems from 'energy medicine', where practitioners sometimes make highly detailed diagnoses using impressive-looking devices named VEGA-Test or BioScan or the likes. You just have to hold two metal rods in both hands, and within mere minutes, you get a huge list detailing the state of health of every organ in your body. This is amazing! And, when you stop and think about it for just a second, it is not just amazing, but unbelievable—literally so. If these machines work as claimed, then why doesn't every doctor have one in their office? Why do they still refer patients for extensive lab testing? Why do hospitals still use huge, multi-million-dollar machines for making scans of our body, when a far better device is small enough to sit right on the practitioner's desk—at only a fraction of the cost? The answer of course is that these machines used by alternative practitioners simply don't work.[6]

The Pseudoscientific Mindset

In our opening story we saw that when confronted with an unexpected result, scientists left no stone unturned in trying to find out what was going on. They did not simply accept what they observed with their own eyes, because that would mean that almost all progress in physics over the past century had to be thrown out the window. This is how Good Science is done: when observing something unexpected, don't just take it at face value, but try to explain it. And as already said earlier on: scientists love these moments, because this often means that they stumbled upon something completely new. Or in the words of a scientist and hugely prolific science-fiction writer:

> *The most exciting phrase to hear in science, the one that heralds new discoveries, is not 'Eureka' but 'That's funny...'*
>
> *Isaac Asimov (1920–1992)*

The observed anomaly in the OPERA project not only drew a lot of attention, but also made scientists drop whatever they were doing up until then, and start digging away at this puzzle, not relenting until every aspect of the mystery was solved. The fact that it turned out to be just a simple error did

---

[6] As of the writing of this book, two Germans who made millions of dollars manufacturing and selling completely useless 'bioresonance' devices were sentenced to several years in prison for fraud, because their machines indeed did not work as claimed at all. Additionally, they were sentenced to pay back several million dollars of their fraudulent earnings. Also see the chapter on Energy Medicine.

not so much cause disappointment, but rather provided a kind of satisfied relief that once again, our current scientific knowledge was confirmed.

Let's compare this to, say, Reiki. Just like Einstein's theory of relativity, Reiki is relatively recent, having been contrived in 1922 by one Mikao Usui. The basic concept of Reiki is that our universe is permeated by a kind of life energy ('chi' or 'qi'), and that Reiki practitioners can not just detect this energy, but also manipulate it, in order to treat and possibly heal a wide variety of physical and mental conditions. Also, these people use scientific-sounding words and phrases such as positive and negative energy, flow, blockades, balancing, and a lot more.

You have to admit: this sounds an awful lot like those quantum physicists, who also claim that they can detect exotic forms of energy, and even manipulate and use it, and also use scientific jargon in the process.

As a result, we would expect that just like in quantum physics, Reiki too has a huge body of scientific literature describing and defining this *qi* in detail, and that there are also a lot of scientists working with qi, researching it, making new discoveries, expanding our knowledge about qi …

Except that this is not what we see. There isn't any proper scientific literature describing qi *at all*, and there aren't any scientists working with qi *at all*. Why is this? Simple: it appears that qi *does not exist at all*. Nobody has ever succeeded in detecting or measuring qi in any objective, reliable way, for instance with measuring equipment or even a hugely sensitive machine like the one used in Gran Sasso. All that we have is some specially trained people who claim that they can feel this qi and even manipulate it, but they can't demonstrate its existence either—and when tested to see if they can really feel the qi in a living person, they all fail. Reiki is, in other words, pseudoscience.

As with all forms of pseudoscience and implausible alternative medicine, it comes down to its adherents telling us that we should have an 'open mind' and also 'do our own thinking' (meaning that we should be willing to reject well-established science and logical reasoning)—but what they really are saying is, 'Hey, listen to what we have dreamed up, and if you start believing it too, you can join our club and become our friend!'

The irony here is that these people claim to have an open mind, but somehow, this openness never includes the possibility that they may be quite wrong.

We will revisit Reiki and several other related phenomena in Chapter 10.

Conclusion

This concludes the chapter about science, and even this rather long exposé only barely scratches the surface. There is a lot more to science, and even one whole book would not nearly be enough to describe it all. Still, the most important principles are hopefully clear by now, and in the chapters to come, a more complete picture of what is science and what is not will emerge.

So it's on to the next chapter: back to nature!

3

Our Daily Bread, All-Natural

All Natural!

'Natural Mineral Water'

'Nourish Your Skin Naturally!'

'Relieve Stress through Natural Relaxation Massage'

'90% Natural Ingredients(*)
*: Including water'

'100% Natural Cleaning Products'

'Our Naturopathy Clinic for Natural Healing'

'Reveal your Natural Beauty'

'Better Health through Natural Health and Fitness'

'Natural Laminate Flooring'

The first chapter presented a simplified, bird's eye view of how our human brain developed from simple animal instincts and instant responses to rather more sophisticated ways of thinking and reacting. In the process, we increasingly started living in a world of our own human making, with the natural world gradually relegated to the background of our life.

Science, the subject of the second chapter, goes even one step further by also minimizing the influence of our human brain as much as possible in our quest for objective knowledge.

© The Author(s), under exclusive license to Springer Nature Switzerland AG 2023
R. Rasker, *Mind, Make-Believe and Medicine*,
https://doi.org/10.1007/978-3-031-29444-0_3

In spite of those remarkable cognitive developments and our hugely increased understanding of the world around us, we are constantly reminded of our past, in the form of the evolved traits that brought us here. This is especially the case when those traits have us barking (or climbing) up the wrong tree. We often see patterns and signs that aren't real, we tend to listen to our emotions rather than to reason, and we trust people from our own group more than anonymous outsiders—even if these outsiders know far better what is best for us than the people in our own social group.

Our bigger brains made it possible to change our environment to suit our own needs and preferences. Our modern, mostly human-made environment is safer than ever before, with abundant food, with tools and possessions to make our life easier and more comfortable, and of course with lots of other people around us to help make all this possible. However, it seems that both our brain as well as our physical body are struggling to keep up with developments. One major health threat is no longer a potential lack of food, but the exact opposite: our modern-day abundance of food. We literally eat ourselves sick. Historically, food was often scarce, so we evolved to eat every bite we could get our hands on, taking advantage of rare occasions of abundance by storing food as body fat. This essential survival trait is now turning against us.

By the same token, we get sick from a lack of physical exercise because we are inherently lazy. Or to put it in more friendly words: we only physically exert ourselves when necessary, and tend to conserve energy otherwise. In the past, we had to spend a lot of time and energy roaming the land in search of food, so we all got plenty of exercise. Nowadays, we could live a lifetime with no more exercise than walking maybe a few dozen paces a day. For all the rest, we can spend our life just sitting at our desk, in our car, or on our couch. This kind of sedentary lifestyle may be optimal if you're a limpet, but it is considerably less healthy for humans, both from a physical and a cognitive point of view.

Talking about mental stress: compared to our ancestors, we face a huge increase in cognitive challenges in our daily life. Instead of seeing at most a couple of dozen members of our family or tribe on a daily basis, our brain now has to cope with the presence of hundreds or even thousands of people in our direct vicinity, most of whom are strangers to us. Activities that are considered essential for our survival have also shifted from physical work to mostly brain tasks, with complex cognitive capabilities being valued more than physical strength. As these capabilities generally involve quite a bit of Kahneman's System 2 thinking, this means that our modern life is rather taxing from a cognitive point of view. Recent developments in digital technology have only made this worse: our daily environment no longer comprises just an already complex physical and social world, but has expanded into a digital realm, where almost anything is possible and constant social interaction is more or less the norm.

It therefore comes as no surprise that our 'unnatural' lifestyle is blamed for many of our most common health problems, up to and including a lot of mental problems. One of the culprits often blamed for this is our modern diet, full of processed products, additives, GMO's and other unnatural things.

It is also not surprising that in contrast, nature is depicted as an idyllic environment where we should be perfectly at home, without all the stress and hassle of modern life, providing us with everything we need to stay happy and healthy. As a result, 'natural' has become synonymous with 'healthy' and 'good', and nowhere does this show more clearly than in commerce: all sorts of products are being advertised as natural in one way or another, even if they have little or nothing to do with actual nature. So before we explore the main topic of this chapter, the world of (un)natural food, we first take a broader look at nature and everything natural.

The Real Nature of Nature

Let's bust the illusion right here: real nature doesn't do 'nice'. At best, nature is indifferent to us, and often it is plain hostile. We evolved to survive in nature, with the emphasis on *survive*: there are lots of things in nature that try to harm us or kill us. Remember those highly sensitive pattern-recognition instincts from the first chapter? We evolved those instincts for a very good reason: keeping us alive in a rather less-than-idyllic natural habitat. All kinds of creatures big and small try to eat us, or take advantage of us in other ways. Predators and infectious diseases are just some of the threats to our existence. Scientists estimate that about half of all living species are parasites, and even today, a significant proportion of people in underdeveloped rural areas suffer from one or more parasitic diseases. In fact, one of the biggest killer diseases on our planet is a parasitic disease: malaria kills hundreds of thousands of people every year.

Then there are countless creatures, both plants and animals, that protect their own existence by being poisonous or possessing spikes and spines. Their survival strategy is simple: 'Eat me or even just touch me, and you will regret it.'

What is more, natural living doesn't come natural to us at all. Surviving in nature requires knowledge, skills and training that most of us do not have.

When suddenly stranded in a truly natural environment, many people would perish within days or weeks, depending on conditions, and almost no-one who would actually enjoy the experience.[1] There is even a Discovery TV series named *Naked and Afraid* based on the premise that surviving in nature (and in a completely natural state, i.e. with no clothes and virtually no equipment) is quite a challenge.

On a personal note: as an avid cyclist, I love to go out on my bicycle and ride around the countryside, often for hours on end. Especially during quieter moments, I can experience an exhilarating feeling of freedom and relaxation, and enjoy the idea that I have it all to myself—the fields, the woodlands, the occasional buzzard, or a roe deer or hare that I spot … Oh yes, I really enjoy nature[2]! Well … for a couple of hours that is, until I get tired and hungry, and start longing for a cool drink, a shower, a change of clothes and a comfortable place to relax and get a bite to eat. Then the charm of all that wonderful nature quickly pales, and I happily return to my distinctly unnatural home, have a couple of glasses of unnaturally clean water, take an unnatural hot shower, change into some unnaturally clean clothes largely made of unnatural substances, and have an unnatural cooked dinner, often with distinctly unnatural ingredients, conveniently bought in a supermarket (which are pretty scarce in nature as well …).

Nature is nice to visit, but you wouldn't want to live there.

What Is 'Natural' Anyway?

One simple definition of 'natural' is something as it exists in wild nature. The more extended version of this definition is that this something should also be completely untouched by humans.

However, this second definition, which firmly sets us humans apart from nature, is a bit silly when you think about it: we humans are very much part of the natural world. And even though we brought much of that natural world under our own control, we still rely on it for our survival, for instance in the form of insects pollinating our food crops or microbes helping us in countless ways.

The final, commercial definition has little to do with either of these, and is better regarded as a sort of false synonym for qualifications such as good, pure, and healthy—often in contrast to 'artificial' and man-made, which is

---

[1] Which of course also goes for many animals raised in captivity: their chances of survival are slim, would they be released in the wild without special care and training.

[2] And that nature is better described as 'Nature Light', with nice paved bike paths, no big predators or other natural hazards, and always people nearby to turn to for help.

deemed less good, less healthy, and even plain bad. Ironically, many of the products that are advertised as being 'natural' have nothing to do with nature at all.

This one, found on a Web site offering laminate flooring, is a good example:

Natural Laminate Flooring

Evidently, laminate flooring is not a natural product. It is in fact about as unnatural as it gets, as all the ingredients of this product are themselves highly processed products from the chemical industry and the oil industry (although the raw ingredients of those processed materials *are* in fact natural, as I'll explain further on). Even the natural-looking wood or stone structure of laminate is just a photographic print on a paper layer. So what we have here is a gratuitous *appeal to nature*, only meant to give the product a positive connotation.

Let's dissect another one:

Reveal your Natural Beauty

As you may already have guessed, this wording was found on a Web site selling cosmetics. Now please stop and think for a moment. What do you think of as 'natural beauty'? One would say that this means that someone is good-looking in their natural state, i.e. *without* cosmetics. Cosmetic products basically cover up things instead of revealing them (and yes, using cosmetics to highlight certain features still covers up the *natural* look). Then again, this company probably wouldn't sell much if they were to advertise their products with the slogan *Paint Over your Natural Ugliness*. As a side note: in the world of cosmetics it is apparently not only the beauty that is deemed natural, but of course a lot of the products as well. Never mind that all those 'natural cosmetics' in reality are highly processed products from the chemical industry.

Next there is this one, prominently printed on a bottle of shampoo I found in my own home:

90% Natural Ingredients(*)
*: Including water

So 90% of the ingredients in this shampoo are supposedly 'natural'. Sounds pretty good, doesn't it? Until you realize that (a) this includes the water that is present in the shampoo, and (b) shampoo typically *is* 90% water. So it is in fact water that makes up virtually all of the natural ingredients. Which is just silly, because all water is natural; there is no artificial or synthetic water. Yes, you can create 'unnatural' water by burning hydrogen with oxygen, but this way of obtaining water would be insanely expensive as well as a huge waste of energy.[3] All water is just plain old H_2O, regardless of its origin. In the end, maybe a fraction of a percent of this shampoo's ingredients stems from truly natural sources such as plants.

But even the whole notion of 'natural ingredients' is in fact meaningless. In the end, *all* ingredients of *all* products are natural. Just think about it: the base ingredient of that plastic shampoo bottle is crude oil. Which is as natural an ingredient as you can get, as it comes from decomposed plants that lived several hundred million years ago, long before the first human-like creatures walked the earth. Yet almost nobody would associate the oil industry and its huge range of products with 'natural'.

The message is clear: nowadays, the word 'natural' is more often than not meaningless. This goes for commercial messages in particular, where the *natural* label is often slapped on regardless of the actual natural origins of products and services.

The rest of this chapter is dedicated to one of the most important as well as most hotly debated things in human life: our food, and in particular the notion that our food should be 'natural'.

Natural Food

Historically, we got all our sustenance straight from nature: water, vegetable plants, nuts and fruits, meat, and sometimes special treats such as honey. Assuming that our apelike ancestors in Africa had a diet resembling that of modern-day apes, we started out as omnivores with a mostly vegetarian diet, with animal-based food being only occasionally on the menu. Later on in our development towards hunter-gatherers, meat and fish became a more important food source. Researchers found that there were periods in history when the human diet was mostly animal-based, with relatively few vegetable ingredients. Especially large animals (known as *megafauna*) were hunted for food, often leading to the extinction of those animals wherever humans turned up.

With the invention of agriculture, our diet once again changed to be more plant-based, although the concurrent development of livestock breeding also provided easy access to meat. In addition, several groups of humans evolved

---

[3] Still, homeopaths have done just that—and then they even diluted this *New Water* ('Aqua Nova') with normal water until there was no molecule of this 'New Water' left, claiming that this diluted water(!) had very special medicinal properties. Also see [4].

the capability to digest milk after infancy, unlocking yet another source of animal-based nutrients in the form of dairy products.

So there is in fact not one 'natural' diet. We have spent long periods being largely vegetarian (sorry, *paleo diet* fans), then switched to a rather carnivorous lifestyle (sorry, vegan fans), and ended up being the omnivores most of us are today.

Nowadays, it seems that there are as many food hypes and diet fads as there are stars in the sky, and that everyone has a distinct opinion on the subject—or rather: Opinion, with a capital O. Which is not all that strange: in our modern world, food is often more than just stuff that we need to stay alive. For many people, what they eat and drink is a significant part of their lifestyle, or even of their spiritual or political conviction. A lot of these diets demonstrate once again the 'natural' hype, emphasizing health, well-being and natural origins, and rejecting industrialized production and processing of food.

Eat What You Need

However, before we get into the (un)savoury details of (un)natural nutrition, let's take a more down-to-earth look at what we eat and why. Basically, we need six distinct types of nutrition to keep us alive and healthy, often referred to as the six *essential nutrients*. In this context, the word 'essential' not only means that we absolutely need to eat or drink it, but also that it is something that our body cannot make by itself.

Proteins are the building blocks of our body. Almost all of the cells and structures in our body are made up of proteins. We get these proteins from our food, albeit in a roundabout way. First, our digestive system breaks down most of the proteins from the plants and animals that we eat into so-called *amino acids*. Then, these amino acids are absorbed into our body, and only then can they be used to make not just our own proteins, but also many other substances such as enzymes and even our DNA.

Carbohydrates are an important energy source for our body. Most carbohydrates we eat come in the form of sugars and starches, a large proportion of which is again broken down by our digestion into *glucose*, a universal source of energy in all living creatures—including us, humans. Especially our brain is highly dependent on a constant supply of glucose.

Because we cannot function without energy, we have evolved the ability to store any surplus of carbohydrates and fat in our food as fat tissue. These fat reserves can be converted back into glucose in lean times, so that a couple of days without food does not automatically mean a death sentence. And because high-energy food was not exactly abundant in most of our history, we also evolved a natural preference for sweet and fatty foods, as well as a tendency to keep eating it as long as it is available, plus an almost unlimited capacity to grow fat. Which makes that tub of ice cream lurking in the freezer almost irresistible …

Fats are another essential type of nutrient that we absolutely can't do without. Contrary to carbohydrates, which are almost exclusively used to supply energy, fat comes in lots of different varieties with lots of different functions. Many types of fat are simply a source of energy, but some types of so-called *fatty acids* are essential for making cell membranes and functional structures of our nervous system such as *myelin*, the insulation material of our nerves. Other functions of fats and fatty acids in the body include regulating hormone secretion, modulating immune functions, stabilizing and transporting all sorts of chemicals in the body, and much more.

Vitamins are chemicals that we need in small amounts to keep our metabolic processes going and thus to keep us healthy. Our body can only make vitamin D by itself, and vitamin K can be made by gut bacteria. All other vitamins must be present in our food.

Minerals are needed in relatively small amounts, just like vitamins, but they are chemically simpler. Minerals can have lots of different functions. Iron, for instance, is an essential element in *haemoglobin*, the oxygen-carrying molecule in our blood. Calcium is necessary for bone development, but it is also involved in muscle function and nerve signal transmission. Sodium and potassium are essential for the functioning of the nervous system and for regulating hydration, among (many) other things. Magnesium is involved in literally hundreds of biochemical reactions. In fact, one could write a complete book on just the roles and functions of all the different minerals in the body.

Minerals and vitamins are also known as *essential micronutrients*, because they are necessary for good health, but only in small amounts.

Water can be considered as the most important helper substance of all, as it is absolutely crucial for supporting and enabling almost every other process going on in our body.

The main problem in western societies is not so much a shortage of any of these nutrients, but an excess intake of carbohydrates and fat, which can be blamed on evolution. Commercial forces only make things worse: food producers want to sell more food, and the best way to do this is to make their food as tasty as possible—which unfortunately often means adding sugar and fat. Add to this that these 'bad' foods are often also significantly cheaper than fruit and vegetables, and the result is a huge obesity problem, especially among lower income groups.

Do-It-Yourself or Take-out?

Our body is amazing at processing food, and it is capable of creating many of the tens of thousands of proteins, enzymes and other substances we need all by itself. It does this by breaking down the things we eat into smaller, simpler chemical compounds, and then using these smaller chemical building blocks as raw material for whatever is necessary.

However, as the above list already showed, this does not go for all the things we need. What's more, some of those essential nutrients we can only get from particular sources. Which is where this whole 'natural' thing comes in again, together with healthy and unhealthy diets.

Vitamin C is an interesting example: almost all plants and most animals can make their own vitamin C from glucose. However, this DIY does not work for humans and most other monkeys and apes. Some 61 million years ago, our proto-primate ancestors lost the ability to synthesize their own vitamin C as a result of one particular genetic mutation. This mutation probably happened by chance, and because the mostly vegetarian diet of those animals provided plenty of vitamin C already, this was no problem at all. And it remained no problem over the course of millions of years—until the sixteenth century, when sailors were unwittingly placed on a diet containing no vitamin C, causing a condition called scurvy, with all sorts of nasty symptoms and even killing them in the end.

So we definitely have to eat our fruits and veggies in order to stay healthy.

Then there is this other vitamin, B12. In a natural diet, vitamin B12 can only come from eating animals or animal products such as eggs and dairy. Which means that we also need animal products in our diet.

So there you have it: just based on these two vitamins, we can safely assume that we humans are indeed omnivores, and that a healthy, natural diet contains both plant-sourced and animal-sourced foods. This is of course no surprise, as it is a well-known fact that people with a vegan diet, with no animal-sourced components at all, need to take vitamin B12 supplements or so-called fortified foods in order to stay healthy. In other words: a strictly vegan diet is neither natural nor healthy, at least without taking additional vitamin B12.

On the opposite side there are some exceptions, with for instance the Inuit doing just fine on a diet of mostly meat and animal fat, with virtually no plant matter at all. They get their vitamin C mostly from animal sources—as most animals make their own vitamin C. The only catch here is that the vitamin C content of meat is generally quite low, so you would need to consume a lot of it in order to get the daily recommended intake. In addition, this meat needs to be fresh and uncooked: not only does vitamin C degrade with heat, it also leaches out of food during cooking because it is soluble in water. Another catch is that this diet must contain lots of fat as a source of energy; lean meat alone will cause so-called *protein poisoning*, because converting proteins into energy produces toxic waste products that take a heavy toll on the liver and kidneys. This is also known as *rabbit starvation* or *mal de caribou*, where people on a diet of only lean meat (such as rabbit or caribou meat) become very sick and eventually even die.

So if you hate vegetables and fruits, it is possible to live on a predominantly carnivorous diet. It just has to be raw meat, preferably including raw liver, which contains quite a bit of vitamin C (and lots of other healthy nutrients), and lots of fat. But for some strange reason, this kind of raw-liver-and-blubber diet has not become popular in our western world at all …

Summarized, the message is simple and clear: there is indeed something to say for a 'natural' diet, defined as a diet containing all the foods that our ancestors probably ate: fruits, vegetables, combined with proteins, fats and additional carbohydrates, both from plants and animals. Yes, this sounds an awful lot like the food groups recommended by almost all national institutes of health worldwide, and yes, it really is this simple: just eat varied and not too much. There are some 'superfoods' that contain more essential nutrients such as antioxidants and vitamins than other food types—but none of those magically improve your health if you have a healthy overall diet already. You can get the same amount of healthy nutrients by eating more of those other healthy foods, or even by taking a multivitamin supplement. No need to spend $10 per day on a bowl of açaí berries.

Also, there are no foods to avoid at all cost, at least what is normally considered food. Even highly vilified substances such as refined sugar (sometimes even called 'white poison') are not bad per se. Sugar is a source of energy, present in honey, fruit and lots of plants. It's just a matter of consuming it sparingly. As explained before, the problem is not so much the inherent nutritional quality of the food available to us, but the amount we eat, especially the disproportionate amount of energy-bearing nutrients. We all know that candy or doughnuts or sugar-laden soft drinks are unhealthy, so these should be reserved as a special treat, not taken as a daily snack. Other foods with a high glycaemic index such as rice, white bread and potato products should be eaten in moderation. As for fruit (which is healthy, right?): eat the whole fruit instead of fruit juice. The latter contains significantly more sugar by weight, because you don't get the fibres and other solid ingredients from the fruit itself. Also, it is far easier to tip cups of e.g. orange juice down the hatch (each containing the sugar from 4 oranges) than it is to eat the same number oranges.

Having said this, it is time to take a more in-depth look at some of the common trends, myths and misconceptions about food, especially in the light of what is considered natural and unnatural. We start out with what may well be the most well-known natural food trend: organic food.

Organic Food

First off, note that 'organic' is not necessarily the same as 'natural', but that again depends on the definition of what one considers natural and what isn't. For the sake of the argument, we'll just assume that organic farming at least strives to be more 'natural' than its industrial counterpart, especially when it comes to keeping the soil fertile and controlling pests.

In the context of food and farming, the adjective 'organic' does not have a precise scientific definition,[4] but it generally refers to farming in a way that is sustainable, causing as little environmental damage as possible. This mostly entails using compost and animal manure instead of synthetic fertilizers, pest control through other means than pesticides whenever possible (see the sidebar for a novel example), and techniques that upset the soil and biodiversity as little as possible, while still giving a fair yield per unit area of land.

The concept organic farming and natural food is not exactly new. Already in the early twentieth century, Rudolf Steiner came up with the idea of *biodynamic agriculture* as an important element of his anthroposophic philosophy. This particular type of farming not only forbids the use of any artificial substances, but also mixes in a generous scoop of pseudoscience in the form of astrology and mysticism. The idea was that the produce from biodynamic farming could only be truly holistic and thus wholesome if it involved not just the right resources, fully natural soil treatment and natural farming practices, but also a matching mindset of farmers themselves.

---

[4] This is not to be confused with *organic chemistry*, which is defined as chemistry involving molecules containing multiple carbon atoms linked together with so-called covalent bonds.

Even tough biodynamic farming is still practised in some places, modern organic farming has all but done away with the more spiritual elements. It simply tries to be productive like any normal agricultural business, albeit with a bigger emphasis on sustainability and respect for the environment than regular farming.

The big question is of course whether organic food is actually better than non-organic food. It turns out that the answer largely depends on which aspects you look at.

As far as consumer health goes, the answer is simple: no, organic food is not significantly better for us than non-organic food; both have roughly the same composition, the same nutritional value and the same taste. This even goes for aspects such as pesticide residues. Organic agriculture also uses pesticides, and even though these pesticides have natural origins, they are often no less harmful than many of the modern synthetic pesticides used in regular agriculture. Also, strict rules about pesticide usage and residue levels apply in most countries; regular sampling of products on supermarket and the greengrocers' shelves turns up either no detectable pesticides at all, or levels far below what is considered safe for human consumption. Organic agriculture even comes with its own health risk: using raw manure from animals and especially human waste as a fertilizer can contaminate produce with parasites and pathogens such as *E. coli* bacteria. This risk can, however, be minimized by composting and properly taking care of soil life.

For farmers, the answer is less clear-cut. Anyone who uses pesticides is inevitably exposed to far higher levels of the stuff than consumers, so regular farmers are more at risk than their organic brethren. But here too, the difference between organic and regular farmers is not as big as one would expect. In regular farming, many of the really hazardous and environmentally unfriendly pesticides have been phased out over the last decades, and organic pesticides are not by definition harmless either. They are after all still supposed to kill or at least repel organisms, and it is quite hard to come up with a pesticide that targets exactly the critters that we want to get rid of, without affecting any other organisms. Nevertheless, organic farming appears to be doing better when it comes to using more natural, non-chemical pest control methods, thus reducing the risk to farmers.

Now if organic farming has no clear benefits for the consumer, and only limited benefits for the farmers, then perhaps it is at least better for nature and the environment?

Well, yes—to a certain extent. The environmental goals of organic farming are very laudable, but it should come as no surprise that the dream of a localized, fully circular and thus sustainable way of farming is still a far cry from reality. The main problem is that strictly avoiding pesticides and using only locally produced natural fertilizers would make organic farming so labour intensive and require so much land that its products would become prohibitively expensive. Even though organic farming already uses compost and manure instead of industrial fertilizer, most of these organic fertilizers still have to come from outside sources in order to get sufficient yield, which merely displaces the environmental effects of obtaining fertilizer instead of eliminating it.

Another thing is protecting crops against pests. There are lots of ways to control specific pests without chemical pesticides, but then again, there are also lots of pests. Even when you succeed in eliminating one particular beetle or fungus or caterpillar by non-chemical means, there are often several other species happy to take their place.

Chemical pesticides have several advantages from a farmer's point of view: they're easy to use, and often take out several species of pest all in one go. But unfortunately, these advantages are also serious drawbacks from an ecological point of view: they cause collateral damage by spreading into the environment and killing off other, often beneficial organisms. As it turns out, many of the pesticides in use in organic farming are not superior to modern industrial pesticides in any way. Still, as organic farming actively strives to reduce the use of pesticides, this is still a point in their favour.

Another problem is that at the moment, organic farming generally still has a lower yield than industrial farming techniques, so it requires more land and more labour to produce the same amount of food. This increased land use offsets some of the benefits. Some critics even claim that it would simply be impossible to feed our current world population using only organic farming methods, just because of lower efficiency alone.

Whack-a-Beetle Instead of Spraying Poison

The Colorado potato beetle has been a serious problem for potato farmers for the past 150 years. The traditional way to try and control this particular pest was the use of chemical pesticides, some of which were pretty nasty substances such as copper arsenate, lead arsenate and mercury compounds, to name just a few. Yes, you read that right: as early as the 1860s, people were spraying compounds containing lead, arsenic and mercury on their potato fields. And what's even worse: the beetles eventually grew resistant to these chemicals, often prompting farmers to use even more of these poisons. Modern insecticides may be less harmful, but still have the drawback that the beetles eventually develop resistance, and keep happily munching away at our potato plants, largely unharmed by the noxious concoctions released over their heads.

A group of Dutch farmers has come up with a completely different approach, based on the beetles' natural behaviour: when disturbed, they drop from the leaves of their host plant and keep still for several minutes, pretending to be dead. Based on this, these farmers have developed the Colorado Beetle Catcher, a machine with rotating flaps gently whacking the leaves of potato plants while running collection troughs underneath, catching the beetles as they drop from the plants. Instead of crawling out of those troughs right back onto the potato plants, the beetles keep perfectly still, meeting their demise when the troughs are filled with water later on, simply drowning the insects instead of poisoning them.

Apart from the mechanization, turning the beetles' natural behaviour against themselves is certainly a novel (and natural!) approach.

Maybe one of the most positive effects of buying organic food as a consumer is as a kind of political statement. By buying organic products, we implicitly say that we want agriculture to move away from the current highly industrialized practices that are destroying our natural environment. Our modern-day ever larger mono-cultures can only exist through extensive use of pesticides and industrial fertilizers, often causing vast areas of land to become completely devoid of life apart from the planted crops. Even worse: more often than not, these profit-driven large-scale farming operations are not even producing food for direct human consumption, but for our livestock, to satisfy our taste for cheap meat.

Summarized: eating organic food is not better for our personal health. However, organic farming does have some benefits for nature and the environment, indirectly affecting the health and well-being of our children and grandchildren. This is why organic farming and especially the development of environmentally sustainable farming methods should be further encouraged.

Next, we move on to some other interesting topics in the realm of natural food, and see how these measure up in terms of natural versus unnatural.

GMOs

Another pet peeve of adherents of 'natural food' are GMOs, short for Genetically Modified Organisms. The basic concept of GMOs is simple: you change the genes of a plant or animal so that it gets a new, desired trait. You do this by looking for an organism that already has this trait, and finding out which genes of that organism are responsible for this trait. You then simply copy these genes in the plant of your choice, and almost as by magic, your plant has this new trait. Easy-peasy!

Well … not exactly. This 'simple' procedure requires a *lot* of expertise in genetics, and often takes even a well-funded laboratory several years and anything between one million up to a hundred million dollars or more before success can be claimed—if any. Then again, potential profits can also be huge.

As a result, GM (genetic modification) of food crops has become the domain of a small number of wealthy organisations, and this is an important point of criticism against GM: that the world's food supply ends up in the hands of just a few powerful corporations that let profits prevail over access to food. This may be a legitimate fear, but this problem is not unique for GM. A large part of the regular agriculture market is already controlled by just a dozen or so large corporations.

Also, there are several non-profit initiatives developing GMOs for humanitarian purposes. One example is Golden Rice, which has been genetically modified to produce beta-carotene, an important vitamin A precursor. Every year, half a million children in poor countries go blind because their diet consists of just plain rice, without enough vitamin A and other nutrients. Golden Rice can prevent blindness caused by vitamin A deficiency.

Another claim of many GM opponents is that GM 'goes against nature', and that it is akin to playing God. It also does not really help that Hollywood often depicts genetic manipulation as something that always ends in disaster. No wonder that GM food plants are often referred to as 'Frankenfood', and that opponents of GM keep warning us for all kinds of dangers of this completely unnatural process. In 2012, one researcher by the name of Gilles-Éric Séralini even published a study that purportedly showed that rats on a diet of GM maize developed cancer more often than rats fed with non-GM maize. The study turned out to be seriously flawed. One of its many problems was that Séralini used rats that already had an 80% chance of developing cancer in their lifetime on a completely normal diet. Also, the biggest increase in cancer was found in male rats, and then only in those who got the *lowest* amount of GM food. The study was unanimously criticized by other scientists, and subsequently retracted by the publisher [5].

Still, is seems that GM goes against nature in the worst possible way, creating genetic cross-overs between two or more completely unrelated organisms. This kind of thing never happens in nature, or does it?

Well, yes, it does. In fact, it happens *all the time*. So-called retroviruses, for instance, insert their genetic code into the DNA of host cells—including human cells—infected by the virus. When this DNA is later read back by the cell, this foreign viral DNA is treated just like the cell's own DNA, and is ultimately translated into new virus particles. The most well-known type of retrovirus is the HIV virus that causes AIDS, but there are many more viruses that use this trick, most of which are more benign than HIV.

When these retroviruses happen to infect reproductive cells such as female egg cells, then those viral changes in our DNA can even get carried over to the next generation, becoming a permanent part of that genetic lineage. To give you an idea how often this happens: between 5 and 8% of our own human DNA is in fact genetic material from viruses (so-called endogenous retroviruses) that infected our ancient ancestors over the course of millions of years. That is a LOT of manipulation of our DNA, all by viruses that use this method to procreate. We are truly a cross-breed between humans and lots of different viruses. There is even increasing evidence that some of these ancient retroviruses were essential for the evolution of placental mammals (including us), by modulating the mother's immune response in the placenta [6].

What this show us, is that 'genetic manipulation' is a completely natural process, and probably as old as the very first life forms on earth. What this also shows us, is that DNA modification generally does not have disastrous results.

There are even many more ways in which the genetic code of organisms can get altered, usually in a completely random fashion. One of these is selective cross-breeding of food crops in the traditional way. When we plant for instance apple trees, the individual trees will have random mutations in their DNA. These mutations sometimes cause particular changes that we appreciate, such as bigger or sweeter apples. When breeding the next generation, we select only the plants with those desired new traits. The end result is a plant with changed DNA, and all its descendants will have the desired trait as well. In other words: we genetically modified an apple tree to produce bigger and sweeter apples.

The main difference between selective breeding and GM is that with GM, we can make changes that would be impossible to achieve through cross-breeding, because we can use genes from completely different species. Another advantage of GM is that it is extremely efficient from a genetic point of view: we only add or change the genes that we want, and leave the rest untouched. With selective breeding, you just have to wait and see if any of the vast amount of mutations that are taking place have the desired effect. So the natural method of genetic modification is largely an arduous, lengthy process of trial-and-error, whereas direct GM is a highly targeted process, changing exactly what you want to change and nothing else. There is nothing inherently dangerous or even 'unnatural' about it.

Food Additives

Another thing often considered 'unnatural' are food additives. As the name already suggests, *food additives* are substances that are added to food for a specific purpose.

As with any aspect of food, this too has attracted the attention of lots of self-proclaimed health experts, making all sorts of mostly unfounded claims about potential health hazards of these additives. Most of these claims are merely an expression of *chemophobia*, where people are scared of anything that is (or even just sounds) 'chemical'.

Why Add Chemicals to Food?

There are lots of reasons to add particular substances to food. Some additives are colouring substances to make food more attractive. Without colouring, for instance cheese would often have a rather unattractive off-white colour, depending on the diet of the dairy cattle. To make sure that cheese has the yellow colour that we expect, cheese makers often add something called *beta carotene*. Now this may sound rather artificial, but it is in fact the exact same chemical that is responsible for the natural yellow colour of cheese. The only difference is that natural beta carotene passed from the grass that the cattle ate into the milk from which the cheese was made. The end result is exactly the same: yellow cheese with a bit of beta carotene. Then there's this: beta carotene is not just a naturally occurring chemical, it is in fact quite healthy, as it is converted into vitamin A inside our body.

Colouring may be considered a rather frivolous reason for adding substances to food, and nowadays, lots of foodstuffs are explicitly advertised as having no artificial colouring and other additives (although ironically, these are often the most unhealthy and unnatural foods thinkable, such as candy and popsicles).

Lots of food additives are added for far more important reasons: our health and safety. For instance preservatives are added to prevent food from spoiling, and thus protect us from food poisoning. One example is the addition of nitrite to sausage and other meat products to prevent the growth of a rather nasty bacterium by the name Clostridium botulinum, which produces the most potent toxin known to man: botulinum toxin. Without this nitrite additive, food poisoning as a result of *botulism* would kill lots of people every year. Fun fact: *botulus* is the Latin word for sausage, and already in the late Middle Ages, people knew that adding potassium nitrate (which gets converted into potassium nitrite) to sausage meat would make it safer to eat and preserve it for longer. As an added bonus, the meat also kept a nice pink-red colour.

Yet another reason for using food additives is to restore food to a more 'natural' state. For instance fruit juice is transported from the countries of origin in a highly concentrated form, which is made by boiling off the water. This water is added again in the destination country. This makes transport far more efficient, because you no longer have to haul 95% water across the globe. The only problem is that this boiling also destroys any vitamin C that was originally present—which is why this vitamin is added again to restore the vitamin C content of the original juice. So even though the act of adding the vitamin C is unnatural (which is also the reason why by law, it must be listed as an additive), both the vitamin C itself as the resulting fruit juice are virtually indistinguishable from fully 'natural' juice.

The only way to get more natural than this is to go out and buy oranges, and squeeze the juice yourself. Or, even better, eat the oranges, because that way, you also get other important nutrients such as fibres.

E Numbers

Companies selling food products are not allowed to just put anything in their products; they can only use ingredients and additives that have been tested and are proven safe for consumption. Also, they are bound by law to list *all* ingredients on the label, so secret ingredients are not allowed.

Most countries have official lists of approved food additives; in the European Union, this list is known as the *E number* list. Every additive on this list is identified by a capital 'E' (for 'Europe') followed by a unique three- or four-digit number, followed by its chemical name and sometimes its common name, plus additional information [7]. For instance the additive E300 has the chemical name ascorbic acid, better known to us mortals as vitamin C.

The advantage of using these E numbers is that product labels no longer have to feature scary-looking and often quite long chemical names for any additives, but merely a couple of short E numbers. This also prevents errors and ambiguity that often crops up in chemical names, as well as problems across different languages. For instance the French chemical name of ascorbic acid is *acide ascorbique*.

But alas, if the obligatory mentioning of all those 'chemicals' on food labels was already causing a fair amount of chemophobia, these even more cryptic E numbers often only made things worse: 'There's secret code chemical stuff in our food!' Some people even felt prompted to write complete books detailing the horrors of E numbers. In one of these books, for instance E508 is described as follows:

> E508: synthetic technical additive and seasoning. Although some sources consider this additive as harmless, the majority [of sources] mention the following **risks**: intestinal disorders, intestinal ulcers, vomiting, diarrhoea, weakness, shock and internal bleeding. **Avoid!** [original emphasis]

So what is this poison that we find in lots of food products? This is in fact potassium chloride, or potassium salt. Not only is this salt present in significant amounts in unrefined sea salt (often praised for its 'natural' origins), but it is even an essential mineral in our food. Without potassium, our nerves and brain cannot function, and we would quickly die. It is as simple as that. So no, E508 is certainly not something to **Avoid!**

Unfortunately, there are many more people out there who spend a great deal of their time telling the world about all those 'chemical' and 'toxic' things that we should avoid, and should make certain that we only buy pure food without additives. One lady called Vani Hari who runs a blog under the moniker *The Food Babe* famously made the following quote:

If you can't pronounce it, don't eat it!

She basically claims that anything with a long and hard to pronounce chemical name is automatically bad for your health. According to this principle, the substance going by the tongue-twisting name of 4-(4-Hydroxyphenyl)butan-2-one should be avoided like the plague. In reality, this is raspberry ketone, the chemical that gives raspberries their distinctive flavour. In another gaffe, Hari posted a scary article on her blog about an 'unnatural' food additive that could purportedly cause cancer—right next to a picture of herself raising a glass of organic white wine for a toast. It can be said with absolute certainty that the alcohol in the wine is thousands of times more carcinogenic than even the most vilified food additives. To her credit, she has removed the picture since, and posted several blog items about the dangers of drinking alcohol—albeit again with other largely unproven and quite scary claims.

Over the course of the years, misleading information like this prompted several manufacturers of food products to switch back to listing the full chemical names on their labels again, because for many people, E numbers had become synonymous with poison. Some of these critics even went as far as to demand 'banning of all E numbers'. I for one would certainly be curious to see how they would like the banning of, for instance, E948.

The bottom line:

* Most additives/E numbers are substances that are also found in nature. They are not 'unnatural'.
* Many additives/E numbers make our food safer, e.g. by preventing spoilage.
* All additives/E numbers have been tested extensively for safety, which is why they are explicitly allowed in our food in the first place.
* Some additives are unhealthy in larger doses, such as nitrites. However, these additives are used to prevent far greater risks, such as botulism in meat products.

Supplements

Dietary supplements, or supplements for short, are micronutrients that people take in addition to their normal diet. They come in the form of pills, capsules, powders or liquids. They are generally made up of the same vitamins, minerals, fatty acids and other micronutrients that are naturally present in food already, and as such, they are promoted as a 'natural' part of a healthy lifestyle. This of course raises a question: why take supplements if we get the same vitamins, minerals and other nutrients through our diet?

Do We Need Supplements?

For the majority of us, the answer is a simple no. Most people get everything they need from a normal, varied diet. There are however some exceptions:

* Pregnant women are advised to take extra folic acid (which is converted in the body into folate, or vitamin B9), as research shows that this significantly reduces the chances of the child developing *spina bifida* and other neurological birth defects.
* Supplemental vitamin D is advised for young children throughout the year, and for everyone else during the winter season. Our body can make its own vitamin D, but requires sunlight with sufficient ultraviolet light type B (UV-B) to do so. Especially at higher latitudes, the winter sun provides insufficient UV-B.
* Anyone with a particular deficiency or malnutrition problem may benefit from taking supplements—but it must be noted that nutritional deficiencies are quite rare in our western world with its abundance of high-quality

food. Still, people with conditions that interfere with the intake of normal nutrients may need supplements. Examples are people who follow a very strict diet (e.g. for weight loss), or people with a vegan diet, who would otherwise not get enough vitamin B12 (which is normally only obtained through eating animal-sourced food). Other common causes of malnutrition are cancer and addiction problems.

If only relatively few people need to take supplements, then why do so many people insist on taking them? Recent statistics show that in western countries, between 60 and 80% of people regularly take vitamins, minerals and other supplements, many even daily.

One important reason is that vitamins and minerals are essential natural nutrients, so they are considered Good with a capital G—and you can't have too much of a Good Thing, now can you? (Well, actually you can, as explained a bit further on.)

As supplements are generally considered harmless, many people take them 'just to make sure' that they get enough vitamins, minerals, etcetera, even if they don't have reason to believe that they actually need them. For similar reasons, people with minor but annoying ailments such as night-time leg cramps or fatigue complaints tend to take certain supplements that are associated with deficiency diseases with similar symptoms. E.g. many people who experience recurring muscle cramps will start taking magnesium tablets, as cramps and twitching may be symptoms of magnesium deficiency [8]. If those cramps subsequently disappear, these people *will continue taking these supplements* in the strong belief that they indeed had magnesium deficiency, so they should take magnesium supplements indefinitely (in other words: the Post hoc fallacy).

As a result, supplements are Big Business, with pharmaceutical companies that make them raking in an estimated annual revenue of well over 150 billion dollars worldwide. And contrary to medicines, supplements are an almost risk-free product group: they're considered healthy and natural, and people use them voluntarily, often for a considerable length of time, without any prescription. To top it off, supplements are generally regulated far less tightly than medicines, lowering production and quality control costs.

Truth be told, most supplements are indeed quite harmless, especially when taken in recommended dosages. Some supplements such as vitamin C can even be taken in very high doses (one gram per day or more) without any harm. There are, however, no indications that these high doses are good for anything, and scientific research into vitamin C shows that an intake over 200 mg does not increase the vitamin C blood level any further—it only increases the amount of vitamin C in the urine, which means that it is almost immediately excreted by the body instead of being used [9]. In other words: taking so-called megadoses of vitamin C only produces expensive pee, and nothing else.

Still, there are lots of alternative practitioners such as naturopaths, ortho-molecular therapists and (often self-proclaimed) nutritional advisers out there who claim all sorts of health benefits for megadoses of vitamins. Note that many of them do not just sell health advice, but also the supplements they recommend, which usually means that they will sell you things that you don't need (and often at hugely inflated prices, at that). There is in other words a definite conflict of interest there.

If you want good nutritional advice, the best start is to look for a dietitian, or else a properly educated nutritionist who is not associated with product sales. In most countries, the title of 'dietitian' is protected by law, and ensures that the person in question is well-educated and works in accordance with the highest scientific and medical standards.

Too Much of a Good Thing

As already mentioned, the general belief is that even if they don't work as intended, taking vitamins, minerals and other supplements at least can't hurt. Unfortunately, this is not always true, and for some vitamins and minerals, overdosing is a very real risk.

- Iron supplements can quickly become toxic in larger doses. In severe cases, an iron overdose can be lethal.
- Calcium is another essential nutrient that can become toxic if taken in large doses.
- Vitamin A toxicity can occur naturally when eating too much liver, especially from certain animals such as polar bears, seals and fish, which store vitamin A in their livers. Note that taking too much beta-carotene (a so-called vitamin A precursor) does not cause problems, apart perhaps from an orange-coloured skin, because the conversion of beta-carotene into vitamin A is tightly regulated by the body.
- High doses of vitamin B6 can cause nerve problems, especially in the limbs, with symptoms such as tingling sensations ('pins-and-needles'), numbness and lack of motor control. One Dutch speed skating champion has experienced this to his detriment, when he took high doses of (among other

things) vitamin B6 as recommended by his personal orthomolecular therapist. He probably missed at least one important sporting season as a result
of neurological symptoms.

⁕ High doses of vitamin D can become toxic by causing hypercalcaemia,
which is an excess blood level of calcium, associated with all sorts of symptoms. A well-known alternative medicine proponent by the name of Gary
Null suffered from vitamin D poisoning when his own vitamin D supplement product line was erroneously manufactured with a thousand times
the intended dose of vitamin D.

This is by no means an exhaustive list, and even a relatively harmless
supplement such as vitamin C can cause symptoms such as diarrhoea and
nausea in large enough doses. Or as the old saying goes: The dose makes the
poison.

One should be especially careful when children are around; many vitamin
pills look and often even taste like candy. This means that you should safely
lock away vitamins and other supplements in the same way that you lock
away medication, and that children should never be allowed to take even the
most innocent vitamins without your supervision.

Raw Foodism

A somewhat peculiar diet fad is known as *raw foodism*, which says that
uncooked food is by definition healthier than cooked food. The main ratio-
nale for this belief is that uncooked food is more natural, and that it contains
more and healthier nutrients than cooked food.

It is certainly true that cooking food is unnatural (barring accidental bush
fires providing naturally cooked meals to survivors). No animals except us
humans have ever been observed cooking their food. However, the reasoning
that it must be healthier because it is uncooked is seriously flawed, and not
supported by scientific evidence. In fact, the opposite applies: uncooked food
comes with several extra problems and health risks compared to cooked food:

⁕ It is much harder to extract nutrients from uncooked food. Cooking
destroys the cell walls of plants, making all those wonderful nutrients easier
accessible to our digestive system. Cooking also breaks down collagen (i.e.
the chewy bits) in meat, making it far easier to digest. Without cooking,
we would have to spend a lot more time and effort chewing our food—
something that would also impact our dental health through extra wear

and tear of our teeth. Research even suggests that cooking food was what really enabled us to develop into modern humans, by providing us with much more energy and other nutrients than we could otherwise obtain from raw food [10].

* Uncooked plant foods can be contaminated with pathogens and parasites, especially if manure and/or human waste is used as a fertilizer. Many a case of *E. coli* food poisoning can be traced back to lettuce and other uncooked vegetables that were grown and served under less than hygienic conditions.
* Uncooked meat, poultry and fish are an even bigger microbial health hazard, and should only be consumed when fresh and prepared under hygienic circumstances—and even then, there is always the risk of parasites.
* Raw milk and raw milk cheese can harbour a host of nasty bacteria such as listeria, salmonella, campylobacter and many more.
* Raw eggs are often contaminated with *E. coli* and salmonella, as are raw chicken and other poultry. Especially the weak and elderly are at risk, and the careless use of raw eggs in recipes such as Bavarian cream has been known to decimate populations in elderly care homes.
* Several foodstuffs are in fact poisonous when uncooked. Wheat, potatoes and leguminous vegetables such as beans naturally contain so-called lectins, which can really ruin your day.[5] Cooking destroys these lectins, making these foods safe to eat.
* And of course lots of foods taste way better when cooked—which, incidentally, is often caused by the increased amount of nutrients that are released by cooking.

Note that all these drawbacks and risks of uncooked food have one hundred percent natural causes. As said before: the fact that something is natural does not automatically mean that it is good for us.

Then there is also another fallacy at play: surviving on a raw food diet is significantly easier today than it was in the past. This is because our modern-day fruits, vegetables and other foodstuffs have been selectively bred to contain more nutrients than their ancestors. If we could go back for instance 20,000 years in time, there would be only few plants that we would recognize as food plants; and those that we could identify as such would provide less nutrients, especially energy. Even as recent as 500 years ago, apple varieties were generally not the big, sweet-and-sour sugar-laden fruits that we know

---

[5] Which in fact is exactly *why* many plants evolved to produce these substances in the first place: to deter animals from eating them.

today, but more like crab-apples: small, hard, and pretty sour. These apples were often only palatable when cooked(!).

Life on earth has survived for well over a billion years without cooked food, but the invention of cooking has had far more advantages than drawbacks, and certainly contributed to the survival of our ancestors.

There is, however, one major health hazard linked to cooking: the fire that is used to cook the food, especially when this cooking takes place indoors. Smoke from open cooking fires is a well-known cause of all sorts of health problems—problems that are very much like the health damage associated with tobacco smoking.

Nuke It!

Some people have no objections to cooking food in general, but believe that cooking food in a microwave oven is somehow 'unnatural', and changes or even ruins the food. It is claimed that using a microwave somehow 'kills' food (or at least the vitamins). Some even believe that microwaved food can cause cancer and other health issues.

None of this is true. Microwaves are simply radio waves of a particular frequency that increase the vibration of water molecules in the food. This increased vibration of molecules has a name: heat. And yes, this heat induced by radio waves is exactly the same as heat from fire or induction cooking or any other source. The radio waves do not do anything else. The do not change the composition of food, nor do they leave anything behind—and they certainly do not make the food radioactive; they just heat it.

Heating food with microwaves can even be healthier compared to traditional ways of cooking. When boiling vegetables in water, vitamins and minerals leach out of the food and are discarded with the water. When cooking vegetables in a microwave, this can be done with far less or even no extra water, often just using the water naturally present in the vegetables. This means that no water and thus no nutrients are lost. As an added bonus, it also saves quite a bit of energy, because it only heats what you eat, and not the water that is thrown away.

Raw Water

This must be really healthy water! How else can so many small critters survive in it?

One recent and particularly silly fad related to natural food and raw foodism is so-called 'raw water' or 'living water'. This is where at least one company sells untreated and unfiltered spring water, complete with everything that may or may not be naturally present. This means that their water may contain not just minerals, but also bacteria, algae, viruses and other microbes—and, notably, animal poo (or do you think that e.g. waterfowl and fish leave the water to relieve themselves?). When present, those algae and bacteria of course multiply, causing the water to go greenish and cloudy within days. Which, according to the company, is completely normal and nothing to worry about. As they say, 'Just keep it in a cool place, consume it within one lunar cycle, and you will be fine'. The reference to 'one lunar cycle' as the product expiration period is a neat touch, and no doubt serves as an effective way to exclusively appeal to people with a more spiritual mindset, to put it politely.

Things become even more puzzling when reading claims that this untreated spring water is ostensibly 'the purest substance on the planet'. Now we were always told that 'pure water' is supposed to mean just water, with no contaminants in it. Apparently we were wrong.

Every self-respecting country goes out of their way trying to provide its citizens with clean drinking water *without* microbes and contaminants. In fact, many municipal water supplies would be shut down immediately and warnings would be issued to the community if their water would have the same amount of microbial contamination as this 'raw water'.

Yet these people turn one of the cornerstones of public health completely upside down, claiming that community water treatment somehow 'kills' the water, robbing it of many of its wholesome properties. Admittedly, this raw water probably contains more minerals than ordinary tap water, but this does not make it significantly healthier. The brunt of the daily dose of minerals that we need comes from the food we eat, not from water. And yes, when we look at the microbes that may be present, we may find some beneficial strains—but then again, we almost certainly have these beneficial microbes in our gut in huge numbers already, so just like with the minerals, the 'good bacteria' in that raw water won't make any difference. The problem is that this water may also contain less friendly microbes, as in: the ones that make you sick. You simply can't tell.

So no, drinking this microbial contaminated 'raw water' has no benefits at all, and may even cause health problems. At a hefty $1,50 per litre, it just serves to line the pockets of the ones selling it.

The Best Food Is No Food?

One last curious food fad that deserves to be mentioned goes by the name *breatharianism*. The most striking premise of this cult-like philosophy is that we humans can live *without any food whatsoever*. Its practitioners claim that they can live off a mystical form of energy called 'pranic light', which ostensibly is absorbed into the body by gazing into the sun. Some of these people claim that they have not eaten in years.

This is utterly untrue.

In 1999, one of this cult's practitioners calling herself Jasmuheen (born Ellen Greve) claimed that she could live on a diet of nothing more than a biscuit and a cup of tea two or three times a week. The interesting thing here was that she was willing to demonstrate for Australia's *60 Minutes* TV cameras that she could stay perfectly healthy and happy without any food or water for as long as she wanted. Arrangements were made that during her demonstration, she would be supervised 24 hours a day, and that a doctor would continuously monitor her state of health. However after four days, her health had deteriorated to such an extent that the doctor found it irresponsible to continue the trial. In just that short time span, Greve had lost six kilograms of weight, and developed a dangerously low blood pressure combined with a very high resting heart rate. Yet in spite of these clear signs of life-threatening dehydration, Greve said that she would be happy to continue, blaming her condition on air pollution and noise from traffic in the place where the trial took place. When Greve's condition kept getting worse even after moving to a quiet, clean mountain location on day three, the trial was stopped nonetheless. There is nothing wrong with a bit of sensational TV, but the makers of *60 Minutes* did not want an actual death on their hands. Despite all of this, Greve still maintains to this day that she could have continued indefinitely.

Many other practitioners of breatharianism were caught (ch)eating, with the excuse that 'they just liked the taste every now and then'. Yes, there have been a few believers who really did manage to abstain from eating and drinking for an extended period of time. They all died.

What the Science Says About Breatharianism

A YouTube vlogger and woo-debunking scientist going by the alias Thunderf00t (real name: Phil Mason) has dedicated a video to breatharianism and its practitioners [11]. In his video, he explains the science behind eating, drinking and breathing, and why it is physically impossible to live without eating any food. He even explains how you can prove that someone is not telling the truth if they claim to live without eating: take a carbon dioxide meter, and simply measure if there is any carbon dioxide in the air they breathe out.

Carbon dioxide (CO_2) is a gas that is made up of carbon and oxygen atoms, and it is created in our body when energy is produced in our cells. The oxygen comes from the air that we breathe in, but the carbon does not come from the air—it comes from our food. And because the air we breathe out contains far more (about 5%) carbon dioxide than the air we breathe in (some 0.4%), we literally lose carbon and thus weight with every breath. Which means that we regularly have to eat carbon-containing foods (mostly carbohydrates and fats) to stay alive. Especially our brain cannot survive for very long without glucose, the carbohydrate that is the main source of energy in our body.

If we don't eat, the body will first use its stored reserves of carbohydrates and fat in order to maintain a healthy blood glucose level. Once those reserves are exhausted, the body will start breaking down its own tissues and convert these to glucose to keep the brain going for as long as possible. This is why people who do not eat will not only lose all their fat, but eventually a lot of their muscle tissue as well. When there is nothing left to convert into glucose, their brain shuts down, at which point the person dies. But long before that, many internal organs will already have suffered serious and sometimes fatal damage. And this is what happens when someone is still drinking water. Without water, most people die from dehydration within a few days.

Mason's video also contains an experiment with himself as a guinea pig. In his experiment, he used an accurate scale to weigh himself several times per hour between meals. It turned out that he lost up to 100 g of weight per hour when awake, and still some 35 g per hour when asleep.

This means that he needed to consume some $16 \text{ h} \times 0.1 \text{ kg} + 8 \text{ h} \times 0.035 \text{ kg} \simeq 1.9 \text{ kg}$ of water and food per day to maintain a fixed weight. Now his weight loss was relatively high because he was also on a diet at the time, but even normal adults will lose some 1.5 kg of weight every day—which is of course replenished all the time through eating and drinking. This also closely matches Ellen Greve's recorded weight loss of 6 kg over 4 days of not eating and drinking at all. So what do you think? Would Greve have survived her demonstration if she had continued? Would her weight loss have stopped eventually? I don't think so.

Then there is the ethical side of breatharians' claims. Even today, millions of people suffer from serious malnutrition. It is hugely insulting to these people to suggest that they could get by just fine without any food whatsoever, if only they would adopt the right mindset.

Certainly, not eating at all can be quite natural—it is called 'starvation', and it is not particularly conducive to survival.

Conclusion

We have taken a good, critical look at nature and all things natural, and it turns out that these days, 'natural' is often just a label that is slapped on willy-nilly to increase sales of almost any thinkable sort of product.

Real nature is not particularly friendly, and contains lots of things that are pretty unhealthy for us, and sometimes even deadly. This is also an important reason why most of us prefer to live in environments of our own making, and not in pristine nature.

Then we turned our attention to food, especially in relation to nature and our diet in (pre)historical times. We have survived on many different diets, but it seems that a semi-vegetarian diet with at least some animal-sourced foods is the most wholesome, as it contains everything we need. This is in fact close to what many people consider a 'natural' diet. And for those who want to forego animal-sourced foods altogether, there is now the option to add vitamin B12 and other essential nutrients to an otherwise completely vegan diet. The main problem with our modern-day food is that we eat way too much carbohydrates and fats—because we have evolved to really like sweet and fatty foods, and because we have managed to create an abundance of these foods never seen before in history.

Next came several other aspects of our modern-day food, including how it is grown and what is in it. It turns out that as far as our health is concerned, it doesn't make much of a difference if food is grown organically or not, or if genetic manipulation is involved. The same goes for food additives: they're all safe for human consumption, and they are often added to make our food safer. Interestingly enough, many of the same people who are wary of food additives will happily swallow *the exact same products* if sold to them separately, as supplements—even if they don't need those supplements at all.

After all those (un?)natural chemicals it was time to go back to the very basics of natural food, and saw that raw food may sound nice, but has some drawbacks, to put it mildly. To end this seemingly endless natural food saga, we took a look at the concept of eating no food at all. As already expected, this is Not A Good Idea.

In the next chapter, we will see how we stay healthy, and what we can do when our health fails us: we'll learn about medicine, both the 'alternative' ('natural') and the regular kind.

4

Get Well Soon

Back Quartet in Ache Minor

For some time now, Barry had been having this dull pain in his back, making life pretty uncomfortable. Also, a constant state of fatigue wasn't making things any better. When attempts to take some rest and relaxation didn't improve things, Barry consulted a chiropractor, who opined that things should definitely get better after chiropractic adjustment. This at first seemed to bring some relief, but it was only short-lasting, so after six sessions, Barry decided that this was no good. Then he stumbled upon a Web site of an orthomolecular practitioner who described his exact problems, and offered a solution: a special supplement combination aimed at restoring muscular health. It contained several vitamins, magnesium, calcium, turmeric, several essential amino acids and a couple of enzymes. It did not immediately improve things, but after a while, Barry began feeling better. Even though the supplement regimen costs several dollars per day, he continues using it, and apart from some minor episodes, his back pain has mostly gone. The best thing is that his remedy is 100% natural, supported by the body's own healing powers!

—

Keisha, 32, felt like almost twice her age: a stiff back when getting up in the morning, brain fog, grumpy temper. Things got slightly better after the first few cups of coffee, but she still had to drag herself through the day, and she was glad if she could finally plop down on the couch after making dinner and putting the children to bed. After some tests for common conditions that all came up negative, her doctor attributed her condition to chronic stress combined with excess weight and a poor physical condition. He suggested she start on a workout program focused on weight

© The Author(s), under exclusive license to Springer Nature Switzerland AG 2023
R. Rasker, *Mind, Make-Believe and Medicine*,
https://doi.org/10.1007/978-3-031-29444-0_4

loss. This didn't really work, she simply could not get herself to take the exercise. As her conventional doctor could not offer any other solution except painkillers for her back, she decided to consult a naturopath instead. This naturopath found that Keisha probably had adrenal fatigue, and prescribed high doses of vitamin C and B5, plus several flavonoid supplements, and magnesium to top it off. When after several weeks, this still had only resulted in minor improvement, the naturopath suggested that additional Reiki sessions might give the energy boost needed. This appeared to have been the key to recovery: slowly, her energy returned, and she started feeling better. And whenever friends or family members now mention back problems or vague complaints of fatigue, Keisha can wholeheartedly recommend her naturopath and Reiki. This holistic and completely natural approach was much better than any painkiller!

—

Britney was having serious back pain, causing sleep problems, bad moods and general malaise. Her doctor could not find anything seriously wrong, and told her that prolonged lower back pain was very common, affecting up to 30% of people. What he advised was pain-guided activity, or in other words: no real treatment. Britney should just go about her routine as usual, taking it easy when symptoms got worse. Painkillers should only be used as a last resort, for instance when she desperately needed a good night's sleep. At first, Britney found this decidedly unsatisfactory, and even thought that her doctor was being rather lazy. Surely there was more that could be done? On the Internet, she found dozens of treatments based on just as many causes, many of which sounded quite plausible. It seemed that almost every alternative practitioner had more success in treating lower back pain than the average doctor. Still, she decided to give it more time, also because those alternative treatments were not exactly cheap, and she had to keep a tight budget. Nothing changed for several months, and she was getting increasingly frustrated. Then, after three months, she realized that things had in fact improved – almost imperceptibly at first, but her back pain was definitely less prominent. Since then, things steadily got better, although she still has residual stiffness, some days worse than others. But according to her doctor, this might be a good moment to take up regular exercise. So maybe next week she should go take that introductory gym workout? Anyway, she was quite pleased: her back got much better all by itself!

—

The pain had been bothering him for quite a while, and Luke was growing more desperate for a definitive solution. Yes, painkillers helped a little, but he didn't really want to use them, certainly not on a daily basis. The pain itself wasn't so much excruciating as it was exhausting: this nagging discomfort, always there, draining his energy. He'd made some half-hearted attempts at doing exercises he found on the Internet, but he had no idea if he was doing things right or not, and it didn't appear to do much good anyway. Then his daughter brought up the suggestion that he might try acupuncture; one of her friends had quite good experiences with it. Luke was sceptical, but after yet another week in dull agony, he decided to try it anyway. The experience was quite different from what he expected: the practitioner turned out to be a very friendly woman who obviously knew what she was doing, and was quite understanding of his doubts. She explained everything she did, and also asked a lot of questions about his work and his family, and how a stressful life could give rise to all sorts of complaints. After some initial uneasiness about being poked with needles, the treatment itself was surprisingly relaxing. More importantly, his back pain, if not gone completely, was far more easily ignored the following days. And although the pain did return, and subsequent acupuncture sessions did not always provide relief, he definitely felt a lot more energetic. Several months later, things had improved significantly, no doubt thanks to the intervention of this acupuncture professional!

—

The first part of this chapter picks up where we left off in the previous chapter: our love of all things natural. We shall explore the wonderful world of natural medicine, starting out with what is in fact the alpha and omega of medicine: our self-healing capabilities, enhanced by some essential human traits. Then we will see how medicine developed through the ages, and at what point science became the leading principle for what we now call conventional or regular medicine. We will also see how at the same time alternative medicine diverged from regular medicine. Finally, we try to establish how well the various forms of medicine work, or if they work at all.

But before that, here is an important disclaimer and warning:

The information given here is NOT medical advice or medical information; it is for entertainment purposes only.

If you suspect that you have a medical problem, always consult a regular doctor first, even if you would prefer to consult an alternative practitioner.

Now let's dive into the wonderful world of medicine!

True Natural Medicine

Life has existed on this planet for several billion years, and throughout that time, disease and death have been an unavoidable aspect of this life. Yet organisms managed to survive, thrive and develop in ever more complex forms, even when suffering disease and damage. One important reason for this is that from the very beginning, organisms evolved a capability for healing themselves in various ways. Natural healing is an amazing phenomenon, and involves lots of different aspects and mechanisms.

The most obvious mechanism is restoring parts of the body by replacing damaged or diseased tissues. This can range from the healing of relatively minor wounds and broken bones to regrowing complete limbs—at least in some animals. This literal self-healing mechanism is also the most easily explained: it is basically the same mechanism that directs growth and development of the whole organism from its origin as a single fertilized egg cell. If something gets damaged or lost, 'simply' reactivate the growth system for that part, and stop growing once everything is back to normal again. Easy!

And yes, for us as a person, the whole process is often pretty easy, and boils down to just waiting for the injured part to repair itself. This goes for the majority of ailments and conditions: they resolve on their own. Kudos for natural healing!

But even the healing of a small wound involves a hugely complex interplay of chemical, genetic and even electrical signalling mechanisms, regulating itself by producing specific concentrations of chemicals, turning genes on and off, and attracting special cells from within the body. One of the first things to happen is the clotting of blood at the damaged site to stop the bleeding—and blood clotting itself is already an amazingly fast but also delicate and complex process. At the same time, the tissue damage causes special signalling proteins to be released, which activate several more repair mechanisms.

While these various 'repair crews' start their work, trying to restore the tissue to its original state, those signals activate still other mechanisms to keep out bacteria and other organisms. Those infectious organisms would otherwise take advantage of this unhindered access to the inside of our body, where they would find plenty of food and ideal conditions to multiply, and cause far worse problems than just that minor initial wound—read: serious infections.

This latter mechanism is of course the immune system, which, together with our skin barrier and to a lesser extent our personal bacterial gut and skin flora, is our main defence against infections. The immune system is another hugely complex yet delicate system that, just like blood clotting, must work fast and thorough to prevent potentially deadly problems, but should also be tightly regulated to keep it from causing damage itself. If the latter happens, we get conditions such as allergies and auto-immune diseases. We will revisit the immune system more extensively in the Chapter 8.

There are still other, less obvious mechanisms that can be considered part of our self-healing capabilities. One hugely important complex of self-regulatory and self-healing mechanisms is collectively called *homeostasis*, which basically describes the normal state of our body when we're healthy and well. Homeostasis is mostly about chemical processes and the optimal balance of chemical compounds such as minerals, proteins and hormones in the body, but also involves other things such as body temperature and blood pressure. Homeostasis is not regulated by one central system, but instead by the combined actions of many semi-independent interacting systems. Some systems work via the brain, while others are purely chemical mechanisms.

Some parameters need to be extremely tightly controlled, while others can vary considerably. For instance the blood pH level (acidity of the blood) must lie between 7.35 and 7.45; any value outside this small range will very quickly lead to critical health problems and death. As a result, the blood has several chemical mechanisms (so-called *buffers*) to maintain a healthy pH level. In contrast, the pH level in the stomach not only is much lower due to the presence of stomach acid (hydrochloric acid), it also has a much wider range, and can vary between 1.5 and 4. In other words: even a single homeostatic parameter such as pH has not one optimal value for the body as a whole, but multiple values and ranges, depending on the location inside the body.

Some homeostatic mechanisms work almost instantaneous; for instance so-called chemoreceptors in the carotid arteries and the aorta monitor the concentration of carbon dioxide and oxygen in the blood. When carbon dioxide blood levels rise even a little bit, these chemoreceptors immediately send a signal to the part of the brainstem that regulates breathing, prompting us to breathe deeper and faster. We experience this situation as feeling out of breath, perhaps even as suffocating, at which point we start panting to get rid of the excess carbon dioxide, and things hopefully normalize again.

Somewhat slower chemical mechanisms maintain healthy concentrations of mineral ions such as sodium, potassium and calcium in the blood. This is mostly done by stimulating or inhibiting excretion of these minerals through the kidneys, depending on whether concentrations are too high or too low, respectively.

In short: almost every parameter and substance found in the body has an associated homeostatic regulating system, and it is the hugely complex inter-action of all these systems that keeps us alive and healthy. In this respect, 'natural healing' means that those automatic mechanisms successfully correct any parameters that have gone out of whack, so to speak.

Why We Still Need Medicine

It should be abundantly clear by now that we are equipped with lots of wonderful mechanisms to keep us healthy and even heal us in case of disease or damage. In many cases, we can indeed just lie back and wait for our ailments and discomforts to go away all by themselves. And make no mistake: even our modern, highly advanced medicine still relies heavily on the body itself to do a lot of the healing.

But as we all know, those self-healing mechanisms are unfortunately not perfect: we all experience health problems sooner or later. This only gets worse the older we get. The biggest cause of age-related problems is that our homeostasis and repair mechanisms start to falter. But even at a young age, our body can't handle each and every problem by itself. An infectious disease may spread too fast through the body for the immune system to keep up with, or we eat something toxic, upsetting our body chemistry. Genetic faults are another cause of health problems big and small. We also have inherent weak points—our back being one of them, as the opening anecdotes show. Evolving to walk upright may have freed our hands to achieve the most wonderful things, it came at the cost of putting extra strain on our back, pelvis, knees and feet.

And then there's this: evolution generally does not produce perfectly built organisms; evolution may in fact be considered 'lazy', as it tends to produce organisms that are 'just good enough'. Regardless whether an organism has all sorts of defects or physical drawbacks, as long as it reproduces in sufficient numbers, then that is good enough for long-term survival. Evolution and nature don't care about the well-being of organisms. Yes, feeling sick and miserable can of course be bad for survival, especially if it means that the organism can't feed or breed any more. But as long as it procreates in larger numbers than it dies off, it doesn't matter if it suffers from whatever condition.

For us humans all this basically means that being healthy and vigorous is not something we should take for granted. Health depends largely on luck, and falling ill is for a large part simply a matter of bad luck—so it is advisable to enjoy our health as long as we have it. We can of course increase the chances of a long and healthy life through all sorts of lifestyle choices. But even the healthiest people can get serious and even deadly ailments.

Now good health may at best be a temporary state of being—sooner or later we all die—but as humans, we can't just ignore or accept the suffering and death of fellow human beings; we want to *do* something about it. The main reason for this is that we are not just social creatures, but also quite emphatic: when we see other people suffering, we feel a lot of the same distress that they experience.[1]

This brings us to the *raison d'être* of medicine: to cure ailments if possible, or, if a cure is not possible, at least relieve suffering as much as possible.

Let's see how this is done, and what difficulties are encountered when trying to help someone who is sick or injured. We start out with one of the

---

[1] Research shows that we very much experience the same emotional component of this distress, but not the sensory component (pain) [12].

oldest but still very important 'medicines' we all received as a child: mummy's kiss.

Mummy's Kiss

For the most part of human history, the only available medicine was natural medicine as described earlier, meaning the self-healing capabilities of our body. The only additional 'medical' intervention that we prehistoric humans had available was 'mummy's kiss', in other words: empathy, soothing, and making the patient as comfortable as possible. Apart from this, it was up to the body itself to get rid of the disease, heal the broken arm or close that nasty gash in the leg. But even though effective medical intervention did not exist, this emphatic, caring approach was (and still is) very important. Not only did it keep predators away from a weakened patient, it also helped patients to relax and save their energy, which is important to overcome disease and trauma.

There is also quite good archaeological evidence that those ancient humans not just cared *about* each other, but also cared *for* each other: lots of prehistoric skeletons have been found showing all kinds of healed trauma, clear signs of old age and chronic disabilities [13]. Without permanent aid and care from other humans, those conditions would normally be a swift and certain death sentence out in the wild. So these people must have been supported by their tribe, even though their condition made it difficult for them to make a useful contribution; in fact, more often than not, they must have been an outright burden to the tribe. Yes, especially older people can be of great value, possessing things that younger ones don't have: a lifetime of experiences, memories and survival skills, which are invaluable assets in any natural environment. But evidence shows that children with injuries and disabilities were also cared for and kept alive.

Even today, with our modern medicine and hugely improved understanding of what causes medical problems and how to solve them, loving care and empathy is still one of the cornerstones of successful medicine. It certainly is an important part of alternative medicine: many successful alternative practitioners take the time to listen to people's life stories, show lots of empathy, and emphasize that the healing process is a collaborative, holistic effort, in which the patient plays an active role (even when this 'active role' turns out to be lying on one's back with the practitioner performing their healing art…). This highly empathic and social approach is further enhanced by a calm and soothing environment, and a strong suggestion that a cure is always possible—more often than not a mild, 'natural' cure that does not involve anything invasive, scary or painful.

This personal approach and really taking the time to listen to patients is one important area where conventional medicine may still learn something from the alternative world: most regular doctors are on a tight schedule, and a GP consultation is often limited to just a couple of minutes. As a result, patients may feel more as if they're being processed as a number instead of receiving care and attention as (and from) a human being. The problem here of course is money. Spending an hour or more to patiently listen to every patient, even those with harmless ailments, would make the cost of healthcare skyrocket—so after a short but thorough check that indeed nothing serious seems to be wrong, conventional medicine will more likely than not send the patient on their way with the advice to wait and see if the problem resolves by itself. If in pain, take an aspirin. Duh.

Let Food Be Thy Medicine …

As we saw in the previous chapter, all sorts of health claims are connected with food. And yes, good nutrition is important for good health, but mostly in preventing diseases. In this context, the well-known quote '*Let Food be Thy Medicine, and let Medicine be Thy Food*' is often attributed to the ancient Greek physician Hippocrates, but these literal words are nowhere to be found in his writings. The quote itself most probably stems from the 1920s, and only became widely popular in the 1970s. However, Hippocrates *did* say in his famous eponymous oath that he would administer the best dietary treatment he could think of to benefit his patients, and this is indeed a sensible thing to do, especially if you consider that Hippocrates came up with this wisdom almost 2500 years ago—long before our modern-day obesity epidemic and all those diet fads and misconceptions that we talked about in the previous chapter.

In fact, Hippocrates' pledge about the use and benefits of food is rather more sensible than the more modern made-up quote: while good nutrition is of course essential to stay alive and healthy, it does not cure any disease,[2] and as such, it does not make sense to say that food is a medicine. Perhaps the closest thing is not eating certain foods, e.g. to cure obesity. The reverse '*Let Medicine be Thy Food*' is even sillier: medicines are not food. Medicines are administered to bring about certain effects in the body's chemistry, and don't normally provide any nutrition.

---

[2] Except malnutrition, of course.

However, in line with Hippocrates' wisdom, a proper diet can certainly benefit patients. E.g. people with kidney problems should generally take it easy with salt and other minerals, diabetics must be careful with carbohydrates, and cancer patients should make certain that they maintain a healthy diet overall, especially because their disease as well as its treatments can often cause significant malnutrition.

Traditional Medicine

Until about 200 years ago, medicine and its views on how to deal with disease were loosely based on ancient *humoral* and *miasma* theories,[3] but in practice were mostly determined by local tradition and the ideas and experiences of individual doctors. There was no large, uniform body of scientific medical literature, and nobody had yet had the idea to actually test the effectiveness (the *efficacy*) of treatments. Some treatments were universal across cultures, such as bloodletting and herbal medicine. Other treatments were only used locally.

Medical theory and practice were also closely intertwined with local religious and cultural philosophy, and rituals were often a standard part of a medical treatment.

Starting at the end of the eighteenth century, things began to change. Science had already achieved great successes in the field of physics, and was slowly beginning to make inroads in the fields of chemistry, biology, and medicine. In 1796, Edward Jenner had just discovered the principle of vaccination, and in the very same year, a man by the name of Samuel Hahnemann had come up with homeopathy as a far more benign alternative to the traditional forms of medicine of the day, which quite often did more harm than good. One might consider his invention as the birth of the first true 'alternative medicine'.

The Perkins Patent Tractors

The desire for non-invasive, painless and risk-free healing of disease and discomfort is universal throughout human history, but must have been be particularly strong in the 1700s and 1800s. The age of Enlightenment and

---

[3] *Humoral theory* is based on the concept that the balance of four types of bodily fluid (blood, yellow bile, black bile and phlegm) defines a person's physical as well as mental constitution, including their health. *Miasma theory* says that diseases are caused and spread by unhealthy air, produced by (among other things) rotting materials.

the emergence of humanism placed a strong emphasis on reason, freedom, and the innate nobility of the human mind; suffering and disease were no longer considered inevitable events to be humbly endured in expectation of a far more glorious afterlife. Yet in contrast, medical treatments of the day still were nothing short of brutal, and quite often it was the treatment and not the disease that killed patients.

In 1796 (again!), Elisha Perkins, until then a respectable American doctor, patented a new medical device he claimed to have invented: two tapered rods, made from (in his own words) 'unusual metal alloys', that could supposedly 'draw out the noxious electrical fluid that caused suffering'. Perkins claimed to have successfully cured thousands of patients, often with grave conditions, and he convinced dozens of doctors, professors and other citizens in high standing that his patented treatment was quite effective. Any criticism from more sceptical doctors and academics was brushed off as jealousy and elitism. Perkins sold thousands of sets of tractors at 25 dollars per set (well over 400 dollars in current-day money), and became quite wealthy.

Encouraged by this success, he then claimed that he had found a cure for yellow fever, a disease that his tractors apparently could not cure. This yellow fever cure consisted of a mixture of table salt and vinegar. Unfortunately, it did not work at all—and during a yellow fever outbreak in New York in 1799, Perkins contracted the disease himself and died only days later.

Only after his death did people take a more sceptical look at his tractors, performing comparative tests with tractors made from completely different materials such as wood and ivory. It turned out that these fake tractors performed just as well (or poorly) as the 'real' ones. Examination of the tractors also showed that the purportedly 'unusual metal alloys' were just brass and iron, and the final verdict was that Perkins had descended into quackery and fraud. So it turned out that the Perkins Patent Tractors were useless, and that any successes could be attributed to what we now know as the placebo effect, together with some human traits that will be discussed in more detail later on in this chapter.

The Emergence of Science-Based Medicine

From the 1850s onwards, medical science really took off, especially after Robert Koch and Louis Pasteur made groundbreaking discoveries about the role of microbes as a major cause of infectious disease. Anatomical knowledge increased quickly, and treatments were subjected to scientific study. Also, knowledge in the fields of chemistry and biology grew by leaps and bounds.

In the decades to follow, medicine progressed to become ever more successful, with some huge milestones marking this progress. The work of Pasteur and Koch led to important public health improvements such as clean drinking water and sanitation. As a result, outbreaks of cholera, yellow fever and typhoid fever became increasingly rare. Smallpox, another scourge of humanity, was driven back (and eventually eradicated) by smallpox vaccination, literally saving hundreds of millions of lives.

Improved hygiene also turned hospitals from veritable death traps into places where people could actually be cured of their ailments. Together with the discovery of effective anaesthetics, this meant that surgery was no longer a patient's nightmare. For the first time in history, surgeons could start paying close attention to what they were doing, instead of just getting the job over with as quickly as possible. Half a century later, the arrival of antibiotics meant that infections were no longer a major cause of death, further diminishing the risks of accidental injuries, infectious diseases and again surgery.

The success of science-based medicine and related public health measures is perhaps best reflected in a rapidly decreasing child mortality: up until 1870, between 20 and 40% of children in western countries did not make it to the age of five. By 1920, this figure had fallen to 10%, and now, a century later, less that 0.5% of children in developed countries die before the age of five. However, the progress of science-based medicine also shows in other metrics, such as an average life expectancy that is higher than ever before in history, as well as the number of conditions that can be successfully treated. Then there is the fact that we now know the cause of most conditions—although to be honest, knowing the cause of something does not always mean that there is also a cure. And there are still a lot of conditions that we don't know the cause of, such as Alzheimer's disease, ALS, and Multiple Sclerosis, to name just a few serious ones. But even lower back pain such as in our opening anecdotes often occurs with no clear cause or reason.

What's in a Name?

In this book, I consistently use the term 'alternative medicine', as this is the original and most well-known designation used for treatments and diagnostic practises that are not part of conventional, science-based medicine. However, over the past few decades, alternative medicine has gone through a succession of different names, mostly because of negative connotations with earlier names.

Alternative medicine has the problem that it strongly suggests that it is a viable alternative to conventional medicine. It is not, if only because conventional medicine can successfully diagnose and treat lots of medical conditions that alternative medicine cannot diagnose or treat at all. For this reason, and because the term 'alternative medicine' became increasingly associated with quackery, its proponents decided to come up with a new name, *CAM*.

Complementary and alternative medicine, usually abbreviated to the more neutral-sounding acronym CAM, suggests that alternative treatments are *complementary* to conventional medicine, in other words that those alternative treatments offer something extra that conventional medicine doesn't. There is a little bit of truth to this: most alternative treatments indeed offer one thing to patients that is often lacking from conventional medicine: more attention for patients, and time to listen to their stories, as also described earlier. Notwithstanding this rebranding, CAM is exactly the same old alternative medicine that it always was. As CAM also suffered from the same reputation problem that plagued alternative medicine (after all, the 'AM' part still means 'alternative medicine'), yet another name was coined: *Integrative Medicine*.

Integrative medicine, or IM for short, is the latest name change in the alternative world. This term has done away with the unfavourable 'alternative' connotation, and 'integrative' suggests even stronger than 'complementary' that alternative medicine should be integrated into and thus become a legitimate part of conventional medicine. Unfortunately, this strategy seems to work: alternative treatments such as therapeutic touch and acupuncture increasingly find their way into hospitals and other regular healthcare institutions, even though scientific research finds them completely ineffective.

Holistic medicine is also often used as a synonym for alternative medicine, suggesting that alternative practitioners treat the 'whole person', and not just a condition. We will return to this later.

SCAM is the acronym of *So-Called Alternative Medicine*, and it is the only term that is not used by alternative practitioners themselves—for obvious reasons. However, the designation 'so-called alternative medicine' was first used by Great Britain's Prince (now King) Charles, a great proponent of alternative medicine. Edzard Ernst, the world's first (and so far only) professor of alternative medicine, seized the opportunity to introduce the acronym as the best descriptive term for alternative medicine: it often deceives people, patients and practitioners alike.

Medicine Diverging

As already mentioned, homeopathy, invented in 1796 by Samuel Hahnemann, can be considered one of the first true forms of alternative medicine, departing from what was then mainstream medicine. Just a few decades later, when science-based medicine was just in its very infancy, homeopathy had already attracted a decent following, with homeopathic doctors, home-opathic schools and even homeopathic hospitals. Initially, those hospitals achieved some remarkable successes compared to regular hospitals, especially with regard to patient death rates during outbreaks of infectious diseases. Yet already then, regular doctors and scientists questioned and criticized homeopathy, for a very simple reason: when studied closely, homeopathy's therapeutic effects seemed to evaporate; it did not appear to actually *do* anything. And as time passed and medical science progressed, homeopathy did not develop at all—quite the contrary: in the years to follow, all of home-opathy's founding principles were proven wrong by science, time and again. So maybe homeopathy's most remarkable feat is that in spite of this lack of scientific evidence, it still has practitioners and followers up to this day, being practised in very much the same way as in Hahnemann's day. As homeopathy has a full chapter of its own, we will leave this particular form of alternative medicine for now.

By the end of the nineteenth century, the rapid expansion and popular-ization of science in general and medical science in particular also attracted the attention of opportunists who had little interest in science, but all the more in money and fame as a healer. Discoveries in the field of electricity and magnetism led to countless grifters touting the benefits of electrical and magnetic 'treatments' they made up on the spot. The same happened again when radioactivity was discovered in the early 1900s: lots of health products containing radioactive ingredients such as radium were advertised, sometimes even supported by doctors and other academics. And history repeated again rather more recently, when the term 'quantum physics' became more widely known among the general public—as evidenced by a simple Internet search for the phrase 'quantum healing', turning up millions of hits.[4]

People also invented completely new forms of treatment that were not directly inspired by science. One example is chiropractic, dreamed up by a greengrocer and 'magnetic healer' by the name of Daniel David ('D.D.') Palmer in 1895. According to Palmer, almost all thinkable conditions are caused by so-called *subluxations* (partial bone dislocations), and could be cured by 'adjusting' those subluxations. There is no evidence at all that these subluxations exist, or that chiropractic manipulation has any effect on other conditions except musculoskeletal problems. Yet even today, a significant proportion of chiropractors still subscribe to the myth of subluxations, and claim that their 'adjustments' can help alleviate many problems that have

---

[4] Quite remarkably, there appear to be no alternative medicine proponents claiming Einstein's relativity theory as the basis of their favoured type of alternative medicine. Then again, maybe this too is just a matter of time …

nothing whatsoever to bones, joints or muscles. There is no evidence at all for these claims.

Around the same time as chiropractic, yet another form of alternative medicine by the name of Reiki saw the light of day. Reiki supposedly works with a universal life energy (*qi* or *chi*, which is also reflected in the second syllable of the name) that can be tapped into for purposes of personal development as well as healing; more about this in the chapter on Energy Medicine. In the early 1900s, Rudolf Steiner came up with what he called anthroposophical medicine, based on his personal philosophy, mysticism, and all things natural.

In the 1950s, China's leader Mao turned China's traditional medicine into a new source of national pride, touting its ancient origins as well as its beneficial properties. Mao himself did not think that Traditional Chinese Medicine (TCM) was any good (he exclusively relied on western medicine), but he saw it as a way to unify the Chinese people. Also, there were only very few western-trained doctors in China at the time, as the country had only just outgrown its agricultural roots in order to become a more modern, industrialized nation. For much the same reasons, a similar process took place in India, where nationalist forces embraced both Ayurveda and homeopathy, even going so far as to award these systems of alternative medicine an official status in healthcare.

In post-war decades, alternative medicine drifted more or less to the background, probably as a result of the great successes of medical science, such as the invention of penicillin and other effective antibiotics, and the success of vaccination programs against diphtheria and later polio.

From 1970 onwards however, the popularity of alternative medicine increased again, after Western news reports about remarkable successes of Traditional Chinese Medicine, especially acupuncture. At the same time, the emergence of the New Age movement sparked fresh interest in 'energy medicine' and other esoteric, mostly oriental life philosophies and systems of medicine. The early 1970s also saw the birth of orthomolecular medicine, devised by Nobel laureate Linus Pauling, and based on the concept that many conditions can be cured with high doses of vitamins.

In addition, some bad incidents with conventional medicine (most notably the thalidomide scandal in the early 1960s) provided a harsh reality check: science-based medicine wasn't all roses, and could absolutely harm lots of people. And, of course, notwithstanding its great successes and general optimism about scientific progress around the 1950s, it turned out that conventional medicine could not cure each and every ailment. Alternative medicine jumped in the gap, suggesting it could help with problems that regular medicine could not solve, especially vague and/or chronic complaints.

'Just Treating Symptoms'

One common criticism from the alternative world is that conventional medicine 'just treats symptoms'. And yes, this claim is often true: a lot of the time, doctors only treat symptoms without fixing the underlying cause of a medical problem. The reason for this is simple: in many cases, a doctor can't address the underlying problem, simply because there is no known cure, or because fixing the underlying cause does not cure the main problem. For example smoking is the cause of many serious conditions such as cancer, COPD and strokes. None of these conditions, once manifest, can be cured by stopping smoking. But doctors can treat the conditions and their symptoms caused by smoking.

Whatever the case may be, treating 'just' the symptoms of a condition can help patients tremendously, for instance by reducing pain or discomfort, increasing the patient's quality of life in no small way.

Stimulating Self-healing?

Quite often, alternative practitioners claim that their treatments 'stimulate the body's self-healing'. This raises a question: exactly what part of the self-healing capabilities of the body are stimulated? The body does not have one generic self-healing mechanism that can be turned up and down like a heater thermostat, but lots of different systems, as also discussed at the beginning of this chapter. The same goes for claims about 'stimulating the immune system', or simply 'helping with' an arbitrary list of conditions.

It is very simple: there are no known substances or treatments that actively stimulate the body's self-healing capabilities, and there are also no substances that can stimulate the body's immune system.[5] Stimulating the immune system as a whole would be quite undesirable in any case, because that would quickly lead to problems such as allergies and auto-immune disorders. There is also not a single scientific study supporting any claims about stimulating self-healing.

---

[5] Well, actually there *are* substances that can stimulate the body's immune system—and in a highly targeted way, at that. These substances are called *vaccines*.

These vague claims of 'stimulating self-healing' only serve to obfuscate the fact that most alternative practitioners can't tell us exactly how their treatments are supposed to work, let alone *if* they work at all.

But Does It Work?

So here we are today: medicine has quite a history, and for the past 150 years, we have two distinct kinds of medicine: conventional or science-based medicine, which is what we usually get when visiting a scientifically trained, licensed doctor, and alternative medicine, which is practised by a variety of people.

The essential purpose of any kind of medical intervention, regardless whether it is conventional or alternative, is of course that it should work: does it do anything beneficial for a patient with a particular condition? To answer this question, we need to take a more scientific look at things.

What the Science Says

It is finally time to take another look at our opening anecdotes. If you took the trouble to read all four, you probably wondered about those repetitive and frankly rather dull stories. People have almost identical problems with their back, get treated in a variety of ways, and get almost identical outcomes: after several weeks, the problems are gone, or at least much better. So all treatments worked, thank you very much, and we all get to go home early. Case closed.

Well … not so fast. Did those treatments actually work? Maybe you should take another look at those stories, and look at the different treatments. Yes, you spotted it: one 'treatment' was not really a treatment, but consisted of simply waiting to see if the pain would go away by itself. And it did.

So if the problem spontaneously resolved in one case, did the *other* treatments actually do anything? The answer seems to be yes when reading each individual case—and each individual practitioner will assure us that their intervention was successful.

Even ignoring that those four cases are made up by yours truly, it is in fact impossible to draw any conclusions based on these anecdotes. The story about the Perkins Patent Tractors shows us that popularity is not a good measure to judge the effectiveness of a treatment either.

The best scientific approach would be to look for trials with dozens or even hundreds of patients—for each type of treatment, that is—and to evaluate each of those trials for quality and outcomes.[6] Trials like this have indeed been carried out for countless treatments in both conventional and alternative medicine, and results have been combined in so-called *literature reviews*. But instead of boring you with heaps and heaps of paperwork, we will look at things from a slightly different perfective: we will be looking at the basic *categories* of treatments, what mechanisms underlie those categories, and what scientific evidence exists for those mechanisms.

What Makes Medicine Tick

Medicine, both the regular and the alternative kind, boasts an arsenal of literally thousands of different treatments. However, all these treatments can be placed into just a handful of main categories, and it is those basic categories that we will inspect more closely. First, let's take a look at what constitutes regular medicine. The following table shows the main types of interventions used by regular doctors, more or less in order of invasiveness.

Regular Medicine

Category	Explanation and examples
Do nothing	Simply wait and see if the problem goes away by itself
Manual therapies	Physiotherapy, massage and other therapies dealing with mostly musculoskeletal conditions
Lifestyle interventions	Advice, coaching and therapy with regard to nutrition, exercise, addictions etcetera
Psychological interventions	Psychological therapy, psychiatry
Pharmaceutical interventions	Pills 'n potions—basically everything that alters the body's chemistry in a way that is (hopefully) beneficial to the patient
Radiological interventions	A non-invasive way to destroy tissues; mostly used as cancer therapy
Surgical interventions	The 'hands-on' approach, where doctors physically repair things inside the body or remove for instance cancer tissue

There are some particular treatments that do not fall into one of these categories, but those are relatively uncommon, to the point that most people

---

[6] For an overview of more than two hundred types of alternative treatment, see Edzard Ernst's book *Alternative Medicine—A critical assessment of 202 modalities*, ISBN: 9783031107092.

never heard of them (can you say *lithotripsy*?)—so for the big picture, those can be safely ignored. By the same token, some novel treatments such as immune therapy are ignored or lumped in with pharmaceutical interventions for now.

Now let's see what kinds of alternative treatments we have.

Alternative Medicine

Category	Explanation and examples
Manual therapies	Chiropractic, massage therapy, reflexology
Lifestyle interventions	Advice, coaching and therapy with regard to nutrition, exercise, addictions etcetera; mostly practised by naturopaths and sometimes orthomolecular practitioners
Herbal and nutritional interventions, natural remedies	Mostly natural products (herbs, supplements and other preparations) that alter the body's functioning in a way that is (hopefully) beneficial to the patient; examples are herbal and orthomolecular therapies, but homeopathy also falls into this category
Energy medicine	Therapies that aim to change a patient's state of health by manipulating special 'life energy'; examples are reiki and therapeutic touch (non-invasive) and acupuncture (semi-invasive)
Mind–body therapies	Therapies based on the concept that the state of mind can influence what happens in the body; examples are yoga, meditation and other similar therapies

So in all, we have just 10 different categories of interventions that cover most of the treatments that regular and alternative medicine have to offer. Now let's look at how well each of these is supported by scientific evidence. As we're talking about not just individual treatment forms but complete categories, this evidence must be pretty strong, as in: there must be a clear consensus among scientists and doctors that a particular form of medicine indeed works. Anecdotes or even a couple of positive studies are not strong enough (we will look at what makes good evidence in the chapter on medicines).

The **wait-and-see** approach is in fact pretty successful, simply because the vast majority of common medical complaints eventually resolve by themselves—thanks to the body's self-healing capabilities discussed earlier on in this chapter. While regular doctors quite often take this approach, especially in case of less serious conditions, it is rarely advised by alternative practitioners. Wait-and-see also has some drawbacks: because no treatment takes place, the *placebo effect* (which often makes patients feel better) is less likely to occur. Also, patients may feel that their doctor is not taking them seriously if they're just sent home with no actual treatment. This means that the doctor must take the time to explain matters, and make the patient understand why wait-and-see is a good strategy.

Manual therapies are moderately effective for problems with muscles, tendons and joints. They can relieve stiffness and mild pain, and mobilize the affected parts. In regular medicine, this category of treatments is mostly the domain of physiotherapy. In alternative medicine, chiropractors and osteopaths provide these treatments, and as such, they are about equally effective as their regular counterparts. However, the alternative world also offers quite a lot of manual interventions that are not supported by good scientific evidence. Examples are the use of chiropractic or osteopathy for other conditions than musculoskeletal complaints.

Reflexology is another manual therapy that is not supported by good science; it is based on the idea that the feet, ears and hands have special points that are somehow directly connected to other parts of the body, and that massaging these points can cure problems with those other body parts. There is no evidence that these points and connections exist, and there is also no evidence that massaging those points is good for any condition.

So overall, regular medicine does somewhat better here than alternative medicine, mostly because alternative medicine offers several types of manual therapy that don't work at all.

Lifestyle interventions can be very effective for numerous conditions, and both regular and alternative practitioners can really help their patients with this. The reason for this is simple: we all know what is generally healthy and what isn't. Ideally, we eat sufficient vegetables and avoid an excess of sugars and fat, we take regular exercise, and we avoid chronic stress. And of course we don't smoke, and we avoid alcohol and other addictive drugs. The problem is that we live in a world with an excess of cheap, tasty but often unhealthy food, and are surrounded by things to make us comfortable (read: lazy). All this can cause a host of problems including obesity, cardiovascular disease and diabetes type 2, but also depression, sleeping disorders and general malaise. It's safe to say that both regular and alternative practitioners can achieve success here, although it is advisable to get a health check with a regular doctor before embarking on an exercise or slimming program.

Psychological interventions have mixed efficacy in regular medicine. Relatively simple, well-defined problems such as phobias can be treated successfully most of the time. Success rates are distinctly lower for more complex problems, and many psychological or psychiatric issues are never resolved, even with years of therapy. Scientific research in this field also suffers from the so-called *replication crisis*: it turns out that many studies with originally positive outcomes show completely different outcomes when repeated. This means that for lots of treatments, there is no high-quality scientific evidence of efficacy.

However, even though this particular area of regular medicine has its problems, it is still doing much better than its alternative counterpart. Therefore, one should always consult a properly educated regular professional in case of mental issues. Yes, there are lots of alternative practitioners out there who claim that they can help with mental problems, but these people usually have no proper training in the field of psychology or psychiatry, and can often make things worse.

Pharmaceutical interventions are medicines, so pills and other therapeutic products made by pharmaceutical companies a.k.a. *Big Pharma*. These products work by altering the body's chemistry. As already hinted at in the paragraphs on self-healing and homeostasis, this biochemistry is insanely complicated, and that means that developing effective medicines is *very* difficult. It may involve staggering amounts of money and time, sometimes billions of dollars and years of hard work. Because pharmaceutical companies are required by law to provide scientific evidence that their products are both safe and effective, many medicines work as claimed. Still, there are still lots of ineffective medicines out there as well.[7]

Herbs and supplements are the alternative world's counterpart of Big Pharma's products. The main product groups here are herbal products and supplements (vitamins and minerals), but also homeopathic products. While there are dozens of herbal products that indeed have proven efficacy, many others don't do anything at all, or are even harmful. Barring a few exceptions, the herbs and supplements prescribed by alternative practitioners are significantly less effective than prescription medicines in regular medicine.

---

[7] See Chapter 6 for reasons why ineffective medicines can appear on the market.

More about this in Chapter 6, dedicated to medicines both regular and alternative, and Chapter 7, which deals with the curious system of medicine called homeopathy.

Radiological interventions are the exclusive domain of regular medicine, for one main reason: radiation treatments are very dangerous—so dangerous, in fact, that there is a whole specialized body of legislation dealing with radiological hazards, detailing exactly when, where and how radiation sources may be used, and by whom.

Radiation therapy is quite effective in doing what it is supposed to do: destroy living tissue. Which is why it is almost exclusively used for treating malignant conditions, and why it often comes with very serious side effects, even when administered by highly trained experts.

Energy medicine could be considered the 'radiological intervention' of the alternative world, but for the fact that it is the exact opposite of radiation treatment in literally every respect: its 'energy' is claimed heal instead of destroy, and its practitioners insist that it is always one hundred percent safe to administer. And, completely contrary to nuclear and physical radiation, this energy is completely undetectable by any scientific method. It has no objectively measurable effect on the body, and even energy medicine practitioners themselves fail to detect this energy when tested under laboratory conditions.

Acupuncture, which is also based on energy that ostensibly flows through special paths called *meridians*, has similar problems: no trace has ever been found of this energy or those meridians, and it turns out that it doesn't matter at all where an acupuncturist sticks the needles (or even if they actually stick needles in at all).

We will explore the mysterious world of energy medicine in Chapter 10.

Surgical interventions are the exclusive domain of regular doctors, for the very obvious reason that cutting into people comes with major risks, especially if you don't know what you're doing. So one would expect that the vast majority of surgical interventions has been proven effective, right? Well, not quite. In recent years, studies have been done with 'placebo surgery' or *sham surgery*. To the surprise of many, lots of patients who had received sham treatments did just as well as those who got the full procedure [14].

So it appears that a significant percentage of surgical interventions is rather less effective than always assumed. These examples emphasize the importance of studying the actual efficacy of every intervention, even if common sense says that a treatment should absolutely work. Common sense (also involving Kahneman's System 1 thinking) has been wrong too often to rely on …

Still, there is no doubt that surgery is very effective in treating many conditions and medical problems. Every year, cancer and heart surgery saves hundreds of thousands of lives worldwide, broken limbs wouldn't heal so well without surgeons fixing the bones, and most people with a 'simple' appendicitis would quickly die without surgery, to name just a few examples.

Mind–body therapies are again part of the alternative world. The most well-known and popular interventions in this category are meditation and yoga. Proponents claim that relaxing and focusing the mind can influence the state of health of the body. There is little scientific evidence for this theory, but people can certainly benefit from the relaxing effects of these therapies, especially when suffering from stress-related complaints. As chronic stress can have serious negative effects on the state of health, relieving this stress through meditation and similar techniques may indeed improve overall health and well-being.

Alternative Cancer Treatments

One special category of alternative treatments not mentioned so far are alternative cancer treatments.

All alternative cancer treatments have one thing in common: *they do not work*. In fact, multiple studies show that cancer patients who opt for an alternative treatment instead of a regular treatment die significantly sooner than those who choose regular healthcare [15].

Many alternative cancer treatments are offered by unscrupulous opportunists who have no qualms about robbing desperate patients of not just large sums of money, but also the last months of their life—as these treatments often demand full commitment from the patient. If the treatment fails (which it usually does), it is often the patient who is blamed for not strictly adhering to the treatment regimen. Many desperate cancer patients have lost all their money and their home this way, and some have even racked up huge debts, hoping that it would work for them. It never does, and most testimonials from happy 'cured patients' are either made up, or come from people who later died of their disease after all. Cancer can be very unpredictable, and the only glowing testimonials that we will see are from people who survived longer than expected—not from the far greater number of people who were not so lucky (an effect known as *survivorship bias*).

One of the things that contributes to the false impression that these treatments work is the fact that most cancer patients also receive conventional treatments—and then attribute any recovery to the alternative treatment.

False cancer diagnoses are yet another problem. People mistake an innocuous skin blemish for skin cancer, then treat it with for instance cannabis oil, and claim that this cured their cancer when the spot disappears. Less common but far more reprehensible are false cancer diagnoses from alternative practitioners, who then sell the patient a treatment, and later claim success when the patient is 'cured' from a cancer they never had in the first place.

Lastly, there is this thing called spontaneous remission, where cancer disappears all by itself. This can happen when the immune system starts recognizing and destroying cancer cells. When this remission coincides with a treatment, this can again create a strong illusion that the treatment was what cured the patient. However, spontaneous remission is quite rare, and happens in less than one percent of all cancer cases overall.

The Patient Got Better—But Was It the Treatment?

I mentioned several times now that there must be high-quality scientific evidence that a treatment (or category of treatments) indeed has real, beneficial effects before we can conclude that it works. Just observing that a patient gets better after a treatment is not particularly good evidence, as there are several alternative (pun intended) explanations for such an observation.

The best known mechanism is the placebo effect, but there is also regression to the mean (when symptoms are particularly bad, they usually tend to get better shortly thereafter), and of course the fact that the majority of medical problems eventually go away by themselves. Each of these things, combined with human traits such as our overactive pattern recognition skills, can contribute to a strong illusion that the treatment actually worked, even if it didn't work at all.

Then again, it is quite possible that the treatment *did* work.

So how can we tell the difference? The rather unsatisfactory answer is that we can't—at least not based on just one case, or even a couple of cases. And the thing here is that most patients who had just one experience like this would like to scream it from the rooftops '*Of Course it Worked! I got better, didn't I?*'

I will explain the mechanisms mentioned in more detail in the science part of the next chapter.

Testing Treatments

The best way to find out if a treatment really works is by conducting so-called randomized controlled trials (RCTs). In an RCT, a group of patients with the same condition is randomly divided into two groups: the treatment group and what is called the *control group*. As the name already suggests, the treatment group receives the actual treatment that is being studied, while the control group receives a fake treatment called *placebo*. In the ideal case, both patients and researchers should be *blinded*, so that nobody knows who receives the real treatment and who receives the placebo.

(Giving the control group no treatment at all has the problem that the treatment group will often show better results due to the placebo effect.)

At the end of the trial, the blinding is lifted, and the outcomes are compared. If the treatment group shows a significantly better outcome than the control group, then this means that the treatment seems to work. Or more precisely: it seems to works *better than placebo*—because patients in both groups will likely show placebo effects, including the ones in the control group who did not receive a real treatment.

Unfortunately, alternative treatments are rarely tested in high-quality RCTs, and rely mostly on the observation of people getting better after treatment. Most properly designed RCTs for alternative treatments show no effect, and trials showing positive effects are usually the ones with a lower quality and/or only a small number of patients. As a rule, these positive outcomes can't be reliably replicated.

This being said, there are some alternative treatments that have been found to work. Examples are herbal treatments, manual therapy and lifestyle interventions. I shall revisit clinical trials and the placebo effect in more detail in Chapter 6.

Conclusion

In this chapter, we have seen that in general, alternative medicine does not work nearly as well as regular medicine, even though regular medicine certainly has its own shortcomings, drawbacks and risks. Yes, some types of alternative medicine work—to a degree. Herbal treatments and lifestyle interventions are examples of things that may actually help patients. But these are only a minor part of alternative medicine, which brings us to the following quote from comedian Tim Minchin:

Do you know what alternative medicine is called when it has been proven to work?
Medicine.

The next chapter focuses on another big problem in both regular and alternative medicine: diagnostics. This part of medicine is at least as important as the various treatments. Curiously, diagnostics are very often overlooked in the discussion about regular versus alternative healthcare, as this discussion usually only looks at the efficacy of treatments.

The next chapter also looks at the less favourable aspects of medicine: risks, errors and shortcomings of medicine, once again both from an alternative and conventional medicine perspective. Finally, we will address the question why almost all interventions appear to work, even the ones that don't do anything.

5

What Is Wrong with You?

Rotten Apple

Liz got called to the ER, where a kid was just brought in with what was most likely a broken wrist. The boy was sitting on a table, sobbing and holding his limp left arm, with a man standing next to him.

'Hello, I'm Dan, Elroy's dad', the man introduced himself. Then, nodding to his son, 'Damn kid, getting into trouble all the time. And now he broke something. Fell out of a tree, he says.'

Liz found the man's gruff demeanour distinctly unsympathetic. She nodded curtly at the man, introduced herself, and then shifted her attention to the boy.

'Hi Elroy, I'm Liz, and I'm going to look at your arm. Can you tell me what happened?'

'I fell out of a tree …', the boy said timidly.

'OK, where was this? And can you tell me how high up you were?', Liz asked. 'And does it hurt anywhere else? Or is it just your arm? Can I have a look at you?' She almost had to drag the answers out of the kid, and he seemed quite intimidated. She also noticed the boy nervously glancing at his father, who felt prompted to interrupt.

'When I was a kid I fell out of trees a lot, never broke a thing. Playing Rotten Apple we called it when that happened, huh.' His almost disdainful chuckle didn't make things any better, and Liz was getting the uneasy feeling that something wasn't quite right.

'Sir, could you please step out for a moment? We really need to examine your boy, take X-rays and see what exactly is wrong.' The man looked taken aback for a

© The Author(s), under exclusive license to Springer Nature
Switzerland AG 2023
R. Rasker, *Mind, Make-Believe and Medicine*,
https://doi.org/10.1007/978-3-031-29444-0_5

moment, then said, 'Oh, sorry, of course, you must do your job … Hey kid, be a man, alright? Do what the doctor says, and you'll be fine again soon.'

After the man had left the room, Liz asked the boy again. 'Now, can you tell me what happened?'

'I don't want to get into trouble …', the boy said.

'Now why would you say that?', Liz said. 'Is there something you need to tell me? Don't worry, I'm a doctor, and you can tell doctors everything. Even bad things, because we're not allowed to tell anyone what you tell us. Did you fall out of a tree? Or did someone hurt you?'

'No … but we … I … did something wrong. I didn't fall out of a tree. We went into this place where they're building new houses, even though dad told me never to go in there. There's all sorts of neat stuff to play with, tubes, planks, everything, it's really awesome!' The boy's eyes lit up for a moment. 'That's where I got hurt, when I fell in a hole. And now I'm afraid that dad will be really mad when he finds out.'

'And when your dad is mad, then what happens?' Liz asked.

'Well, he shouts at me that I'm stupid, and then I don't get pocket money for a week, when it's really bad,' Elroy said. 'Are you going to tell my dad?'

Liz drew a relieved breath. Yes, her hunch was correct, there was something not quite right, but it wasn't as bad as she had feared. 'No, I won't tell your dad if you don't want me to. But I think that you should tell him. And yes, he may be a bit angry, but I think he'll understand. After all, he just said that he got into trouble too when he was a kid. I'll help you talk to him if you like. But first let's get that arm of yours sorted out.'

After the boy got his arm set, with a 'wow, awesome!' plaster cast as a witness to his ordeal (isn't pain medication a great thing …), Elroy's dad unexpectedly stepped up to Liz. 'Hello doctor, I want to say sorry for being rude just then, and thank you for your help. We were all a bit shaken up when he came running in screaming, with his broken arm and all. And Elroy also told me what really happened. Damn kid, just like me when I was his age!' But this time, the man looked down at his son with a broad smile, and Elroy smiling back to his dad. Liz graciously accepted the apology, wished them good luck as they left the hospital, and basked in the feeling of having helped a hurt, frightened boy and his angry dad – but only for one short moment, as the next call required her attention once again …

The discussion of regular versus alternative medicine almost always focuses on *treatments*: is it effective or not? Is it safe? Does it have side effects? The previous chapter presented a bird's eye view of the major categories of treatments, and tried to establish whether those treatments worked or not. This emphasis on treatments is actually a bit strange. Shouldn't you first know what condition a patient is actually suffering from *before* any treatment takes place? And what exactly causes a particular condition?

In this chapter, we will take a look at how health problems are diagnosed, comparing regular and alternative medicine over the years—and, importantly, where and how doctors and practitioners developed their diagnostic skills. In other words: what education they received before they started diagnosing (and treating) patients. This is also where we will take a closer look at the not-so-sunny side of healthcare: risks, errors and even abuse.

Diagnostics

The importance of diagnostics should not be underestimated. Knowing what is and what isn't wrong with a patient is often essential before deciding on a treatment. Correctly diagnosing patients is one the most difficult parts of being a doctor—and the hugely popular TV series *House, MD* revolved around this premise: at the beginning of each episode, a patient was brought in with certain symptoms. Sometimes these were simple symptoms suggesting a simple cause—which of course turned out to be something completely different. More often than not the symptoms were quite puzzling, and our protagonist Dr. House and his team left no stone unturned to arrive at the correct diagnosis. Once the main mystery was solved, the actual treatment that followed was usually just a formality.

House is pretty realistic in that it shows how doctors start out by first looking for red flags[1]: does any of the patient's symptoms suggest that something serious may be wrong? That persistent dry cough may seem innocent, but it can be a sign of lung cancer in an elderly patient with a smoking habit. However, it is probably something completely different (and far less serious) in a teenage girl.

Once serious conditions have been ruled out, doctors will usually check for conditions in order of likelihood. For this, they try to gather as much relevant information as possible. Is that girl with her cough familiar with any previous allergies? Does she live in an environment with dry or polluted air? Has she secretly taken up smoking? When the most likely causes have been ruled out, less likely causes are considered. Quite often, this process can take quite a while.

---

[1] Although it is quite unrealistic in many other respects.

Experience and Intuition

Now all this would suggest that doctors always painstakingly investigate and weigh all symptoms in a more or less rational process, resulting in the best imaginable diagnosis. However, this is not how medicine works, except maybe in the case of medical students (and of course Dr. House). All doctors have more or less automated the diagnostic process through years of training, with possible conditions already popping up in their head as they listen to and look at a patient, trying to fit everything they see and hear into one or more likely patterns. This works on both the conscious and the unconscious level; consciously, they're actively collating all the information, and trying to assemble a diagnosis. Unconsciously, checks take place and warnings may be raised if something somehow 'doesn't fit' the familiar pattern. This was also what happened in this chapter's opening story, where the doctor got an uneasy feeling about the interaction between the boy and his father.

Maybe this process is best illustrated by comparing how beginners and champion chess players think: beginners look at the board and the individual pieces, apply the rules to each of those pieces, and try to evaluate possible future moves to determine the best choice for the next move. A chess champion, on the other hand, hardly bothers with individual pieces or moves any more, but considers complete board positions (read: patterns). They recognize stronger and weaker positions, based on having encountered countless of those positions, and choose their moves in order to realize a stronger position. They often even have developed an intuition that tells them which position offers the best chances if they're uncertain, or which position may hold a trap that is not yet manifest.

Still, experience and intuition in medicine are controversial topics,[2] and for good reason: until science got into the act some 150 years ago, doctors throughout the ages exclusively relied on tradition and their own experience—with tradition basically being the experiences of doctors before them. As we all know, this did not exactly result in very effective medicine. The main problem here is that experience is only as good as the body of knowledge that it is built upon. An untrained or badly trained doctor or practitioner will not get better by building personal experience—if anything, they will get worse, because their growing experience will also increase their self-confidence, even if this is unwarranted.

It's even worse for intuition: without knowledge and training, intuition is no better than random guesses from our sloppy System 1 thinking. Only

---

[2] Infectious disease specialist Mark Crislip formulated this as follows '*The three most dangerous words in medicine: 'In My Experience*'.

through internalizing lots of knowledge and seeing lots of real cases can a doctor build useful intuitive capabilities. And even then, any hunches should always be critically scrutinized, because they can still be wrong in one or more ways. Just look at the opening story: the doctor correctly felt that there was something not quite right—but luckily, she did not jump to the conclusion that it was the boy's father who did something wrong.

Getting It Wrong

Even though medical doctors literally spend years in medical school and internships before they are allowed to treat patients, diagnosing patients still involves a fair amount of trial-and-error, and they still get it wrong on a regular basis. Research estimates that at least one in every twenty diagnoses in regular healthcare is incorrect, and that half of these misdiagnoses could even result in harm [16]. There are two important reasons for this:

* Many diseases and disorders have similar symptoms. This is because many organs and systems in the body have just one general response to, for instance, infection[3]: most tissues will show swelling, redness and tenderness; the intestine will fight infections by getting rid of its presumably noxious contents as fast as possible (i.e. diarrhoea and vomiting), and the nose and lungs respond in a more or less similar way by producing copious amounts of mucus. Fever is another general symptom of infection.
* However, one condition can also cause completely different symptoms in different patients. Just look at Covid-19 infections: lots of people had no symptoms at all; others experienced symptoms ranging from just a runny nose and a cough to severe flu-like symptoms, pneumonia, inflammation of the heart, blood clots and internal organ damage. About one percent of people died. Similar things happened after people recovered from the infection itself: while most people were fine, still a significant percentage ended up with long Covid, with various, often debilitating symptoms.

The underlying cause of this large variety in symptoms is the great complexity as well as variety in living organisms, and of course external factors, such as lifestyle. Conditions and symptoms may also vary with age, sex, genetic make-up or ethnicity. So there are *lots* of things that doctors must

---

[3] Please note that this 'one response' is by no means a simple response. As already explained in the previous chapter, lots of very complicated things happen with even a 'simple' local injury.

take into account before reaching a diagnosis. It is almost a miracle that they still get it right most of the time …

Alternative Diagnostics

So how do alternative practitioners do when it comes to diagnostic skills? Well, unfortunately, and in one word: poorly.

The first reason for this is that alternative practitioners do not nearly get the same amount and depth of medical training that regular medical doctors receive. A significant percentage of alternative practitioners has no medical training at all, and most others received only a fraction of what medical students get. As a result, their diagnoses are incorrect a lot of the time, and any treatments based on those diagnoses are then of course also not effective.

The second reason is that many alternative practitioners do not subscribe to scientific standards, including generally accepted scientific principles of health and disease. This goes for treatments as well as diagnostics. Their diagnoses involve unscientific phenomena such as 'blocked energy' or other pseudoscientific concepts. And no, 'traditional' diagnostic methods are no good either—just look at how utterly ineffective as well as brutal medicine was throughout history, before science got in on the act. As a patient, you really don't want to be diagnosed and treated in the way that it was done even 150 years ago. Yet countless alternative practitioners make an appeal to tradition when asked how they know what to do when diagnosing and treating patients.

'Live Blood Analysis'

One example of a pseudoscientific diagnostic method is called *live blood analysis*, often used by orthomolecular practitioners and naturopaths. A small drop of blood is obtained from a patient's fingertip and examined under a microscope for a couple of minutes. Practitioners claim that this way, they can diagnose countless health problems: vitamin and mineral deficiencies, poisoning with heavy metals or other unspecified 'toxins', infectious diseases ('chronic Lyme' is a particularly popular diagnosis), parasites, allergies, immune system problems, weak or failing organs and lots more. All by looking at just one tiny drop of blood under a microscope.

Now just take a moment to think about this. Normally when you need a full panel blood test, a nurse draws several vials of blood and sends these off to a lab. This lab, usually equipped with millions of dollars worth of state-of-the-art analytic equipment, then needs anything up to a week to process and analyse the blood, and compile the results. A full metabolic test panel can quickly cost over a 1000 dollars, increasing to several thousand dollars if tests for heavy metals and infectious agents are included.

Yet an alternative practitioner can get *better* results within mere minutes by just looking at one small drop of blood with a simple microscope? If this actually works as claimed, then why doesn't every doctor use this diagnostic procedure by now? It would save *billions* of dollars in healthcare—not only in diagnostic costs, but also in treatments that are much better targeted. No more wasting money on all those expensive labs, wrong diagnoses and unnecessary treatments!

There is, unfortunately, one tiny problem: live blood analysis does not work *at all*. It is not suitable for diagnosing any condition whatsoever, and this in turn means that any treatment based on this fake diagnosis is of course also no good. People pay for a bogus 'diagnosis', and pay again for a 'treatment' based on this diagnosis. And more often than not, they keep on paying indefinitely for rather pricey supplements, to treat 'deficiencies' and other conditions that they do not actually have.

This lack of proper diagnostic and medical skills is one of the biggest problems of alternative medicine. Practitioners will almost invariably diagnose and subsequently treat conditions in ways that are in line with the type of alternative medicine they practise, not with scientific insights. Someone complaining of, for instance, pain in the lower abdomen will most likely receive completely different diagnoses and treatments, depending on the practitioner they consult:

- A chiropractor may diagnose for instance 'irritable bowel syndrome' or (in case of 'old-school' chiros) 'subluxations', and treat it by manipulation and mobilization of the pelvis, lower back and abdomen.
- An acupuncturist may diagnose an energy problem in the intestinal organs by looking at the tongue and feeling the pulse, and suggest (surprise surprise) acupuncture to correct this issue.
- A homeopath will in fact not even try to diagnose the problem, but instead record an extended history of the patient's life, previous conditions, mood and anything out of the ordinary as 'symptoms'. After which a 'remedy' is selected that is associated with this highly detailed, unique collection of symptoms. More about this in Chapter 7.

- An orthomolecular practitioner may use live blood analysis or a bioresonance device to diagnose things such as deficiencies, organ weakness or toxins, and offer for instance supplement-based treatments to fix this.
- A Reiki practitioner will most likely detect a problem with the body's energy field, and suggest a Reiki treatment consisting of balancing and restoring the proper flow of energy.

And then, a couple of days after any of these treatments, in the bathroom, it turns out that the problem was just a bad case of constipation—which was not diagnosed by *any* of the alternative practitioners. Yet many patients and practitioners will *still* claim that the diagnosis and the treatment were successful. After all, the problem went away, now didn't it? That's what counts! Who cares if these practitioners were not exactly on the mark …

Now this example is perhaps a bit silly, as constipation is so common as well as obvious that even completely untrained people will probably recognize it. However, the point is that many alternative practitioners are incapable of diagnosing even fairly common medical problems—either because of a serious lack of training, or because their training is seriously disconnected from medical and scientific reality.

Another thing to note here is that most of these alternative 'specialisms' strictly stick to their own field of alternative medicine: if you consult an acupuncturist, then this acupuncturist will never refer you to, for instance, an orthomolecular practitioner. A homeopath will not send a patient on to a chiropractor. One exception is naturopaths, who are trained to treat patients in many different ways, both alternative and regular. Another exception applies when practitioners recognize or suspect a serious health problem that they can't deal with—in those cases, the patient is usually referred to a regular doctor or to hospital.

(Strange enough there *is* a sort of solidarity across all forms of alternative medicine, where no alternative practitioner will ever disparage or chastise any other alternative practitioner, no matter how egregiously incompetent the latter is. Yet they will all attack regular medicine at the drop of a hat.)

Getting It Right After All

In all fairness, alternative practitioners do not get it wrong all of the time:

- Common, easily recognizable conditions are often correctly diagnosed, even by practitioners with no or very limited training.

* A non-negligible fraction of alternative practitioners received at least basic medical training, and should be able to reach a correct diagnosis more often than a completely uneducated practitioner.
* Many patients consulting alternative practitioners already know what is wrong, because they first consulted a regular doctor who diagnosed the problem. When the regular doctor could not offer an effective treatment, they then decided to try their luck in the alternative circuit.

However, even a correct diagnosis is of course no guarantee that any subsequent treatment will fix the problem. The reason for this is that an alternative practitioner will often decide on a treatment that is not science-based and thus not (proven) effective. Also, even science-based regular treatments are not always effective, or there simply is no effective treatment. Also see the previous chapter.

The Root Cause of Disease

Many alternative practitioners admit that they don't diagnose patients in the same way that regular doctors do. In fact, they often claim that their diagnoses are *better* because they will find and treat the 'root cause' of the problem, whereas in their view, regular medicine 'only looks at symptoms'.

Nothing could be further from the truth. This alternative *root cause* is usually some kind of vague unscientific or pseudoscientific 'energy' problem, imaginary (and usually unnamed) 'toxins', a fictitious problem with one or more organs ('adrenal fatigue' seems in vogue right now), or the by now classic 'chronic Lyme disease'. All these 'root cause' diagnoses are completely made up, and many are not even based on real conditions or phenomena.

It is in fact science-based medicine, not the alternative world, that is working tirelessly to find the *real* root causes of diseases and conditions— and with tremendous success over the past 150 years. Just look at the history of medicine: *every single time* the cause of a particular ailment was identified, it was science-based medical research that found it, not the alternative world.

As mentioned before, there are still numerous conditions that we don't know the cause of, and especially vague health complaints often defy diagnosis—but that does not mean that we can just make up something and call that the 'root cause', as many proponents of alternative medicine do.

The Holistic Approach

Another often-heard claim in the alternative world is that they work in a *holistic* manner, examining and treating 'the whole person', as opposed to regular doctors who purportedly only look at the condition and then 'just treat the symptoms'. This too is a fallacious claim. Every doctor worth their salt uses a holistic approach when needed: if a patient complains of, for instance, sleeplessness and general fatigue, a good doctor will not just prescribe sleeping pills, but instead ask questions to find the most likely (root) cause of the problem: does the patient experience stress in their work or personal life? Does the patient consume coffee, and if so, how much? How about alcohol or other drugs? How long have the symptoms been going on? Did the patient experience any other symptoms such as panic attacks or feelings of depression? Or perhaps occasional pain or discomfort? Etcetera. Yes, prescribing sleeping pills may be *part* of the treatment to improve the patient's condition, but only after getting a more complete picture of the situation, and addressing the underlying problem. It really doesn't get any more holistic than this.

Of course there are also medical problems that are *not* diagnosed or treated in a holistic manner. If someone turns up with a nasty cut in their hand because they slipped with a knife when cooking, then the wound gets cleaned, stitched and bandaged, and that's it. No need to get into the cook's life story or any other details.

Just as with 'root cause', alternative practitioners in fact often use the pretence of 'holistic treatment' to obfuscate their lack of medical knowledge to correctly identify the real cause and provide an appropriate treatment. Which in fact is pretty clever: simply diagnosing and treating 'the whole person' automatically includes diagnosing and treating anything that may be wrong with this person, now doesn't it?

One Cause, One Cure

Some alternative practitioners go one further, and claim to have discovered One Cause and/or One Cure. These claims are most often made with regard to cancer, but some practitioners extend this to virtually every disease known to man.

For instance the Italian alternative practitioner Tullio Simoncini claims that all forms of cancer are in fact nothing more than a common yeast named *Candida albicans* growing out of control, and can be treated by injecting sodium bicarbonate. His claims are demonstrably wrong. Candida is not involved in any cancer, and bicarbonate injections are not only ineffective against cancer, but also quite dangerous. At least one of Simoncini's patients died as a result of this treatment, and Simoncini was sentenced to 5 years in jail for culpable manslaughter.

Another example is a man named Jim Humble, who claims that drinking a chloride dioxide solution (which he calls *Miracle Mineral Solution* or MMS) can prevent as well as cure virtually all diseases, including serious conditions such as Alzheimer, cancer, ALS, malaria, and hundreds more. There is no evidence for this at all. Chlorine dioxide is used as an industrial bleach and a disinfectant. As such, it kills microbes and cells—*all* microbes and cells. If you drink it, it damages and kills the cells in your intestinal tract, often resulting in nausea and diarrhoea (which its advocates say is a *good* sign …). In the most egregious cases, it is administered as an enema to autistic children in an attempt to 'cure' their autism, which is supposedly caused by parasites inside the body. This treatment seriously damages the intestine, sometimes to the point where the inside layer of the bowel sloughs off—which, when excreted, is then falsely identified as 'killed parasites'. This is nothing short of criminal child abuse.

Maybe the most sweeping claim ever was made by a Canadian naturopath called Hulda Clark. She maintained that all diseases were caused by one type of parasitic worm, and that these parasites (and thus all diseases) could be eliminated by using a small device (a 'zapper') she sold to people. If only things were that simple … No, not all diseases are caused by parasites, and no, her zappers do not treat or cure anything (also see Chapter 9). All apart from the fact that most people in western countries do not harbour any pathogenic parasites.

It is quite simple really: whenever someone claims that lots of completely different conditions all have one common cause, or that one particular treatment can cure lots and lots of different conditions (a so-called *panacea*), then they are wrong, period. Unfortunately, these people are often quite convincing and even charismatic, and tend to raise smoke screens of sciencey-sounding (i.e. pseudoscientific) jargon in support of their claims. Laypeople usually lack the knowledge to see through these false claims and are an easy victim for whatever product or service is peddled. Remember: panaceas simply don't exist; there are literally thousands of different causes for at least as many diseases and conditions, and again thousands of different treatments, many of which are highly specific for a particular condition.

Risks and Medical Errors

So far, I talked about the effectiveness of various types of treatments and about the difficulty of diagnosing medical problems. Risks were mentioned in the passing, and the picture emerged that hazardous treatments were almost exclusively found in conventional medicine, not alternative medicine. It is time to take a closer look at possible negative effects of both types of medicine.

First, Do No Harm

In the previous chapter, I already mentioned the ancient Greek physician Hippocrates and his oath to treat patients in the best possible way. One famous quote attributed to Hippocrates is the phrase '*First, do no harm*'. As with the quote about food being a medicine, this one too is not literally part of the Hippocratic oath, although the original text comes pretty close: 'I will do no harm or injustice to them [my patients].'

Many alternative practitioners maintain this adage as a literal first rule of conduct, and interpret it in such a way that they should never hurt and/or damage a patient, under any circumstances. Consequently, they quite often disapprove of conventional medicine because it does harm to patients as a matter of medical routine, e.g. in the form of medicines that may have side effects, or surgery which, by definition, involves cutting people.

This seems like a reasonable position at a first glance. Conventional medicine involves a lot of things that may or even will cause harm to patients. And just look at how many people die when in hospital or in the care of a regular doctor! We never hear of alternative practitioners having to deal with life-or-death situations, and their treatments are almost always gentle, risk-free and of course universally beneficial.

Now please pause and ponder this for a second. And maybe a hint is in order here: what to do when a patient has, for instance, appendicitis? This is a fairly common medical problem, and hundreds of years of case reports show that without the right treatment, most cases of appendicitis develop into life-threatening abdominal infections, killing patients within days. The only 'right treatment' here is surgery,[4] meaning cutting into patients, harming them.

The problem here is of course a far too literal interpretation of this Hippocratic rule: if causing a certain amount of harm to a patient will save their life,

---

[4] Recent research suggests that antibiotics can sometimes cure an appendicitis, but that surgical intervention is usually more successful [17].

then this harm is what doctors must do. In fact, *anything a doctor or practitioner does or does not do* has the potential to cause harm. Even the mildest and most 'natural' of treatments—up to and including doing nothing at all—can absolutely be harmful if this means that a patient suffers serious damage or death that could have been prevented by a suitable treatment, regardless whether that treatment also involved some degree of harm.

A far better principle is that any treatment should have **a positive benefit/risk balance**: the potential benefits of a treatment should outweigh the potential risks. This means that a simple cold can be 'treated' by simply doing nothing, but that an acute appendicitis as described above absolutely justifies emergency surgery to remove the inflamed part of the intestine. Yes, the latter involves cutting into patients and seriously upsetting and harming them—but the alternative is that they will most likely die.

So when we assess the pros and cons of alternative medicine vs. conventional medicine, we can't just look at potential benefits of treatments and diagnostics, but we must also assess the risks involved. So far, conventional medicine seems rather more effective than alternative medicine, and regular doctors certainly seem to do a far better job at diagnosing conditions than their alternative brethren. But does this outweigh the generally greater risks of conventional medicine? Many proponents of alternative medicine defend their beliefs by pointing at the dangers, real and perceived, of conventional medicine: many pharmaceutical products may have serious side effects, and things like surgery and radiation therapy are inherently dangerous and harmful. This means that even small mistakes can cost lives—and, as doctors and other healthcare workers are only human too, mistakes can and will happen, sometimes with deadly consequences.

In comparison, alternative medicine seems a lot safer: only very rarely do we hear about patients of alternative practitioners getting harmed, and scandals with for instance drugs are also quite rare. One logical explanation for this is that alternative treatments are inherently milder. Yes, they may be less effective than conventional medicine, but that also means that they have less side effects and less risks. And maybe 'less effective' and 'less risk' cancel each other out, so that overall, alternative treatments have more or less the same benefit/risk balance as regular treatments?

If only things were that simple.

It is a fact that far more people die or suffer serious harm in regular healthcare, as compared to people receiving alternative treatments. But is this a fault of regular medicine? The important question to ask here is: *what kind of medical problems do regular doctors deal with versus alternative practitioners?* It turns out that the overwhelming majority of serious health problems ends up with regular doctors, including care for the frail and elderly. The reason for this is simple: alternative medicine is completely ineffective for treating serious conditions. What's more: alternative practitioners themselves also prefer patients with relatively benign health problems, simply because those patients have a far better chance of treatment being (or seeming) successful.

Hospital admissions are another thing to look at. People end up in hospital for a very good reason: there is something seriously wrong with them, something that they or their family doctor can't deal with, and requires special care. On average, those hospitalized patients have a much higher chance of suffering serious health problems and dying than the average person who consults e.g. a naturopath for lower back pain—but that obviously does not mean that someone with a heart attack should shun the hospital and turn to a naturopath instead.

Oops …

Now all this is not to say that medical errors are not a real problem. Dutch estimates are that each year, some 1,400 people die as a result of mistakes in regular medicine in the Netherlands alone. A far greater number of people suffer harm from mistakes.

In comparison, alternative medicine seems much safer, with only a fraction of the number of deadly incidents mentioned above. And yes, most alternative treatments are inherently quite safe. There are, however, good reasons to believe that alternative medicine is less safe than the above suggests, and the biggest elephant in the alternative room is the very high percentage of bad diagnoses:

* Misdiagnoses can cause severe harm and even death if a patient has a serious condition without knowing it. Many people have died because alternative practitioners failed to recognize heart disease, cancer, and other life-threatening conditions that any regular doctor would have spotted right away.
* Conversely, alternative practitioners often diagnose conditions that patients do not have at all. Many people consulting alternative practitioners are told that they suffer from deficiencies, allergies, toxicities, parasites or failing organs, and need treatment for these completely absent conditions. At the very least diagnoses like these cause stress and anxiety. And of course these people will receive treatments that are complete unnecessary—treatments that may also upset a patient's daily life, e.g. through radical changes in diet.

* Particularly egregious are practitioners falsely diagnosing 'vaccine injury' in children. Not only do these children then receive completely unnecessary (and often costly) treatments for this 'vaccine injury', but their parents will no longer have their kids vaccinated, which exposes these kids to the risk of contracting potentially deadly diseases.
* False and fake diagnoses (and any treatments that are based on those diagnoses) also cause financial harm. People pay for something that they are promised but do not receive: effective healthcare.

Then there are also real errors and incidents, just like in regular medicine. The following are some common risks of various alternative treatments:

* Numerous alternative practitioners actively advise their patients to stay away from regular healthcare, even in the case of very serious conditions such as cancer.[5]
* Orthomolecular treatments can cause vitamin poisoning; many mineral supplements can cause diarrhoea and intestinal complaints if taken in excess, and weight loss and muscle building supplements can even cause heart damage.
* Herbal preparations can cause poisoning, or interfere with other medicines.
* Traditional Chinese herbs and Ayurvedic herbs often contain heavy metals and toxic plants, again causing poisoning.
* There is mounting evidence of patients dying from strokes and neck fractures as a result of chiropractic treatment, especially manipulation of the neck.[6]
* Acupuncture can cause a collapsed lung (pneumothorax) if needles are inserted too deep, and infections if needles are not sterile.

All these things have happened to people, and no doubt are still happening. For instance chiropractic treatments are believed to cause at least half a dozen strokes every year in the Netherlands alone, often resulting in very serious permanent injury (e.g. paralysis from the neck down).

Regular medicine is required by law to report every serious incident so that any incidents can be investigated and hopefully prevented in the future.

---

[5] One particularly egregious example is 'German New Medicine', where cancer patients are told that their disease is the body's response to emotional shock—and that the emotional burden of regular cancer treatment is the 'true cause' of cancer metastasizing and killing people. These practitioners often advise their patients to ignore their cancer and 'simply be happy', after which they will be alright. Which is the most deadly 'advice' thinkable.

[6] Prompting alternative medicine professor Edzard Ernst to come up with the emphatic warning *'Don't let the buggers touch your neck!'*

No such laws or guidelines exist for alternative medicine. This means that a lot of incidents may remain unreported, and usually no action is taken if they occur. Only very rarely are alternative practitioners held accountable if things go wrong and people get hurt. Alternative practitioners also do not learn from their mistakes, nor will they abandon treatments that have been shown to have a negative benefit/risk balance. For instance most chiropractors will continue to perform neck manipulation, even though there is mounting evidence that this manipulation has a small but non-negligible risk of very serious harm, with no evidence of lasting beneficial effects beyond placebo.

What the Science Says

Medical education as well as conventional medical practice nowadays is strongly science-based, meaning that science underpins most of the knowledge and expertise that medical students gather. What's more, if new scientific insights cause old knowledge to become obsolete, then medical practice is adjusted to reflect this. Medical doctors are also required by law to keep up with new developments in their profession, so that they always work in accordance with what is called *the standard of care*.

Simply said: regular medicine is set up in such a way that medical knowledge is not only science-based, but also continuously improves itself, offering patients the benefits of the latest scientific developments. If it turns out that a particular treatment does not work, or if a better treatment is found, then the old treatment is abandoned, and the new treatment becomes part of the standard of care. For instance the recommended treatment for most cases of severe lower back pain used to be lots of bed rest and painkillers. Several decades ago, it was found that a far better treatment regimen was 'pain-guided activity', meaning that people were encouraged to keep going about their daily activities as much as possible, only taking rest and painkillers when the pain became really bad. With this new treatment advice, episodes of serious back pain have more than halved in duration—quite an improvement.

Then there is of course the sheer amount of work that medical students have to put in before they are allowed to call themselves doctors and start treating patients. A full medical education involves on average some 15,000 hours of study and internships, equating to at least eight years of very hard work.

Alternative practitioners are not nearly as well-educated as regular doctors—to put it mildly. Exact figures are hard to find, but simply visiting the Web sites of alternative practitioners already shows that many of these people have no science-based medical training whatsoever.

Admittedly, many practitioners have received some form of medical education, but even the most extensive educational programs such as those for chiropractic or naturopathy suffer from two major problems:

* Even multi-year education programs span 4 or 5 years at most, offering maybe 3,000 hours of science-based medicine altogether. Internships and/or supervised patient contact hours are even worse in comparison to regular medicine.
* A significant part of the curriculum is dedicated to teaching the specific form of alternative medicine, not science-based medicine.

There are of course also alternative practitioners who started out as regular doctors and consequently went through medical school. However, the problem is that their adoption of alternative medicine still means that they deliver healthcare with unproven efficacy.

What this means is that most alternative practitioners at the very best have only basic medical knowledge. At worst, they have no medical education or knowledge at all—and this applies to a large number of practitioners, possibly as much as half of all of them.

Why Does Alternative Medicine Still Exist?

The picture seems pretty clear by now. Conventional medicine is far from perfect, and regular doctors regularly miss diagnoses and make mistakes, sometimes even fatal mistakes. However, alternative medicine is far inferior. A large percentage of alternative practitioners has no relevant training at all; most others have received only a fraction of the medical training that regular doctors have to put in before they're allowed to diagnose and treat patients.

As a result, most diagnoses of alternative practitioners are wrong, and consequently, most treatments based on those diagnoses are useless because they do not address the actual problem. To add insult to injury, many alternative treatments are mostly or completely ineffective, and at best produce a placebo effect.

So why do we still have alternative medicine, if it is mostly useless? Why do practitioners keep offering it? And maybe even more puzzling: why does alternative medicine have so many satisfied customers? Most people would feel tricked or deceived if they found out that they paid significant sums of money for something that doesn't really work. But not in alternative medicine: surveys consistently show that about 8 out of every 10 patients visiting alternative practitioners are quite satisfied with the treatment they received, and would recommend alternative medicine to others. How can we reconcile the reality of alternative medicine, i.e. that it is basically no good, with the far more positive view that both its customers and its practitioners have?

To answer this question, let's look at how health problems typically progress over the course of several weeks to a couple of months, and see where alternative treatments come in.

It often starts with vague and/or not particularly serious problems that regular doctors can't do much about, or for which they advise the wait-and-see approach. The problem is of course that even benign medical issues may still be unpleasant, and people want to do something about them. Those lower back problems at the beginning of this chapter are a point in case.

When it turns out that a regular doctor can't help, then this is often the moment when people start wondering if alternative treatments may offer a solution. At first, people will still wait a while longer and see if the problem goes away by itself. When this does not happen in a reasonable time frame (usually a couple of weeks), they start exploring alternatives. Then, when enough time has passed and/or symptoms appear to get even worse, they opt for an alternative treatment.

Shortly after this treatment, things often get better—depending on the type of treatment, progress may even seem pretty miraculous. From that moment on, and perhaps after another couple of treatments, complaints subside further, sometimes slowly, sometimes fast. And after maybe a few more months at most, the patient is almost or completely healthy again. Viva alternativa!

So given the progression and the timing of events, the treatment surely must have worked, right? Well, not necessarily.

There are several important mechanisms that can create a very strong *illusion* of an effective treatment. Here are some of the most important ones:

- The well-known *placebo effect*, which is the phenomenon that patients often feel better after a treatment—any treatment, regardless whether it had any clinical (measurable) effects or not. This means that even a completely fake treatment can have an effect, but mostly on more or less subjective symptoms such as pain, stress and well-being. Placebo effects can't improve the clinical situation of a condition. Simply said: the placebo effect can make patients *feel* better, but it can't make them *better*.

- Extensive and friendly *personal attention* from a practitioner further enhances the placebo effect. In most forms of alternative medicine, the attention that patients receive from practitioners *is* in fact the treatment.
- Furthermore, the decision to finally *do* something instead of just passively waiting it out also makes people feel better already.
- Then there is what is called the *natural history* of a condition, describing how it develops over time. Many conditions are known to improve spontaneously. When this happens during or shortly after the treatment, this gives a very strong illusion that it was the treatment that helped.
- Another mechanism is *regression to the mean*, meaning many chronic or longer-lasting conditions have ups and downs, and that a particularly bad episode is usually followed by improvement. When do people typically seek treatment? Indeed: when things are really bad. Shortly after treatment, things very often get better—but not necessarily as a result of that treatment.
- There is also what is called *expectation bias*: both the practitioner and the patient expect to see improvement. As a result, their perception of the patient's condition will be more positive after treatment, even if nothing has changed. A human trait called *social reciprocity* can further enhance this expectation bias: the practitioner is optimistic and expects the problem to resolve, at which point the patient more or less unconsciously mirrors this optimistic mindset, and feels better as a result. This again is picked up by the practitioner, who will become even more optimistic, as well as self-assured that they're doing the right thing.
- Yet another effect of seeking help for a medical problem is that patients can become more health-conscious. They may start taking a more critical look at the food they eat, take more exercise, avoid stress, and minimize or quit bad habits. This will also help improving their health, especially in the longer run.

One very important thing to note here is that all these mechanisms and phenomena are not just limited to alternative medicine; they occur in exactly the same way in regular medicine.[7] What this tells us is that it is often impossible to tell if a treatment actually works or not by just experiencing (or administering, or observing) that treatment. Only careful scientific research can tell effective and ineffective treatments apart.

---

[7] Which is why medical science still find ineffective regular treatments almost on a daily basis, up to and including surgical procedures. The big difference with alternative medicine is that regular medicine abandons those ineffective treatments, while alternative medicine does not even test if treatments are effective or not, let alone abandons the ineffective ones.

The problem here is that our brain is hard-wired as well as trained to recognize the pattern of illness → treatment → recovery as a causal chain of events, making the illusion of efficacy and thus the Post Hoc fallacy really powerful—so powerful in fact, that trained scientists and doctors are not immune to it either. Even these people have to remind themselves all the time that a pattern that they see may not be real. Ironically, the success of regular medicine contributes in no small way to this illusion: when we develop a health problem, we consult a doctor in the *expectation* to get better. Already as a child, we were told time and again that if we get really sick, we would go to a doctor, who would then make us better. (This expectation is in fact justified, as modern medicine is capable of treating lots of conditions that were untreatable even a few decades ago.)

Alternative medicine is also attractive because it is invariably characterized as 'mild' and 'natural', with lots of attention from the practitioner for 'the whole patient' (read: people get all the time they want to talk about everything and anything they may have on their mind). All this often takes place in a relaxing, soothing atmosphere, completely different from conventional medicine, where consultation time is limited for reasons of efficiency, and diagnostic procedures and treatments can be pretty unpleasant.

Another common characteristic of alternative medicine is that there is always hope, even if it is false hope. Regular doctors will often have to tell their patients that they can't think of any effective treatment any more, for instance in the case of health problems defying diagnosis, chronic conditions, and terminal conditions. Alternative practitioners will often welcome such patients, especially the first two categories (unexplained and chronic conditions), to start diagnostic and treatment programs that may last for prolonged periods of time. They will rarely admit that they can't do anything any more, and can always think of something else to try. Chances are that in the course of this long time, the condition will eventually improve or even resolve on its own, at which point success is claimed.

Lastly, one not-so-nice reason why people turn to treatments with questionable or even plain out disproven efficacy is their state of mind. Severe stress, grief, mental trauma and other overwhelmingly negative states of mind have a serious impact on people's judgement and decision-making capabilities. Incurable or intractable ailments almost by definition cause a lot of stress and uncertainty, causing patients to try out (alternative) treatments that they would normally have rejected out of hand. This is also why desperate cancer patients sometimes spend fortunes on completely ineffective treatments 'just in case'—treatments offered by unscrupulous practitioners who prey on these extremely vulnerable people.

The Practitioner's Perspective

Just to get this out of the way: it is not my intention to insult or denigrate alternative practitioners, even though a lot of what they do is based on erroneous beliefs and the rejection of science, either implicitly or explicitly, and therefore wrong. The majority of these people genuinely believe that they're helping patients; only a minority of practitioners knows very well that they're selling useless treatments, but keep doing it anyway for a variety of reasons. Then again, even those alternative practitioners with all good intentions are fully aware of what science has to say about their work. Then why don't they accept this science, and go and find another job? There are several reasons for this.

First, the illusory mechanisms described earlier on not only cause patients to believe in erroneous diagnoses and ineffective treatments, but affect practitioners too—maybe the latter even more so, as they see these 'successes' happen every day, while their patients only experience them very occasionally. When practitioners are told that their treatments don't work, by far the most often heard response is 'But we *see* that it works all the time!' This is quite understandable, and very human: we are far more inclined to believe the things we see with our own eyes than what we are told by anonymous scientists.[8]

Many alternative practitioners start out in their profession as a result of a revelation-type experience, often as a patient. Many proponents of alternative medicine also have a rather different notion about what constitutes evidence: they consider the experiences of themselves and their patients to be sufficient evidence that their treatments work. And, of course, because many of their patients get better, they see happy, thankful people all the time, which strongly contributes to the belief that they are doing the Right Thing. Why stop treating people if it makes them happy? As a result, science and any scientific evidence (or rather, the lack thereof) is relegated to the background or simply ignored, as is the very real notion that selling ineffective treatments can be harmful.

---

[8] Recalling one of my personal experiences: I have seen a lady being sawn in half, without any ill effects, and made whole again a couple of minutes later, *with my own eyes*! And I wasn't the only one either—there were hundreds of other witnesses, so it was absolutely real! Now why aren't trauma rooms and surgeons interested in this 'alternative surgery'?

Alternative Training and Education

Another reason why alternative medicine is a popular career choice is that it doesn't involve years of hard study like conventional medicine—in fact, anyone can call themselves for instance 'orthomolecular therapist' and start treating patients with vitamin pills first thing tomorrow morning.

Yes, there are courses and even 'universities' offering multi-year programs in naturopathy, homeopathy, chiropractic and the likes, but even there, students receive only a fraction of the medical science that regular medicine students receive. Also, a lot of those curriculums teach 'Tooth Fairy Science', as the late Harriet Hall called it, i.e. elaborate but ultimately unscientific systems of medicine that simply don't work. Many other institutes are little more than diploma mills, with a curriculum that spans a couple of weeks or months at best, issuing certificates that aren't worth the paper they're printed on. At the very bottom is a veritable thicket of short independent 'training programs', offering training in pseudoscientific tricks of the trade such as live blood analysis and other techniques that are completely useless. Most of these institutes and programs have no truck with conventional medicine or science, and only exist to extract money from gullible people, in this case alternative practitioners and those aspiring to become one. One major problem here is that many of these institutes pretend to offer a science-based education, more or less on par with regular medicine. Together with the 'natural' fallacy, this attracts students who feel that regular medicine pays too little attention to human and natural aspects of medicine. The far less taxing curriculum is also quite appealing.

Then there is what I call the 'investment trap', also known as the *sunk cost fallacy*: when people invest heavily in something, emotionally and/or in terms of money and time, it becomes very hard to abandon again. This also applies to alternative medicine: many practitioners have spent so much time and effort on their alternative medicine of choice that it has become an integral part of their life. This makes it hard to abandon an alternative career, or even to acknowledge its shortcomings. One notable exception is Britt Hermes, who was educated as a naturopath, but realized that in spite of all good intentions, she and her colleagues were often harming patients instead of treating them in an effective way. On one occasion, she suspected acute leukaemia in a child—a medical emergency—and was appalled when a fellow naturopath suggested to just 'look at the gallbladder' instead of referring the child to the emergency room ASAP.

Another example is Natalie Grams from Germany, who studied regular medicine as well as Traditional Chinese Medicine and homeopathy. When working as a homeopath, she did scientific research into homeopathy, and found that there was no good evidence at all that it worked. She stopped practising as a homeopath, and now spends much of her time educating people about the ineffectiveness of homeopathy, while still praising the one good aspect of it: the attention and time that homeopaths spend on their patients.

The subject of investment brings us to another, rather more mundane reason why people choose a career as an alternative practitioner: it is easy money. Most practitioners charge anything between 50 and 200 dollars per hour, which is significantly more than the average hourly wage of 25 dollars in many developed countries, even after taxes and overhead costs. Also, the job is clean and easy, without stringent requirements or responsibilities; good communication skills and a sociable nature are the most important assets for a successful career in alternative medicine. Training and knowledge are optional—quite a few practitioners had completely unrelated jobs before deciding one day that they would henceforth be an alternative medicine practitioner.

The most successful alternative practitioners are the ones who not only are good listeners, but are also great storytellers themselves. As we already explained in the first chapter, humans simply love stories. They tend to trust practitioners who explain in detail what they're doing, how their treatments are supposed to work, and come up with examples of successes in the form of other patient cases. It doesn't matter if those stories are true or not, or if they exaggerate the successes while leaving out the failures. Virtually nobody will check those stories and explanations, especially if the practitioner sounds convincing and self-confident. The most successful, charismatic alternative practitioners have gathered an almost cult-like following of believers (also see Chapter 12) who actively help promote these stories—even if those stories have nothing to do with reality or truth in any way.

Health Freedom

One often-heard argument for supporting or at least tolerating alternative medicine is that it is an important part of 'health freedom', as in: people should be free to choose the type of healthcare they prefer. So why try to abolish it, especially given its popularity?

The fallacy here should be clear: for the most part, alternative medicine is inferior to regular healthcare; most alternative treatments do not have any effect beyond placebo. This means that people are offered a choice between (mostly) effective regular healthcare and (mostly) ineffective alternative healthcare—yet with the strong suggestion that both types are more or less equivalent. In other words: yes, people are offered a choice, but not a very well-informed choice. Alternative practitioners usually do not tell their patients that there is no good scientific evidence for what they do. So the real 'freedom' at stake here is the freedom of alternative practitioners to offer ineffective treatments while claiming or at least suggesting that they are effective.

Conclusion

Diagnosing patients is a science and an art, and requires a lot of training as well as a fair amount of intuition. Even well-trained doctors get it wrong on a regular basis.

Most alternative practitioners do not have a medical education even close to that in regular medicine, and many have no relevant education at all. Their diagnoses are wrong more often than not, and as a result most of their treatments are way off the mark, with success mostly relying on the placebo effect. Many alternative practitioners reject established medical science, and instead claim that they can diagnose and heal people by means of esoteric knowledge and special manipulations that they have mastered.

Nevertheless, alternative practitioners can be quite successful in that they have lots of satisfied patients, and this is in large part due to good personal skills: they spend significantly more time and attention on patients than most regular doctors. It also helps that their treatments are portrayed as safe and gentle—and even though those treatments only have placebo effects, there can be a strong illusion of efficacy.

The next chapter explores the world of medicines in more detail, both the 'natural' ones and those from pharmaceutical companies. We will look at the origins of medicines, both in history and modern times. We will pay special attention to the way that medicines are tested, and what can go wrong in the process. We will of course also look into what is and isn't true about Big 'Bad' Pharma, and how medicines are created and sold in the alternative world.

6

Big Bad Pharma and the Healing Herbs

Good Intentions, Bad Medicine

Breast cancer, lung cancer, chronic leukaemia, rheumatic disorders … And these were just the most serious health problems afflicting Mrs C. at her old age. No wonder she was feeling absolutely horrible, and nobody was surprised when she was admitted to hospital for near-fatal weight loss combined with fatigue. Except that it wasn't the cancer or any of the other ailments that landed her in hospital and nearly killed her.

Over the course of the past half-decade, Mrs C. had seen numerous specialists for increasingly serious health problems, and each one of these specialists really wanted to treat her according to the best standard of care. As her conditions were inoperable for several reasons, it was decided to manage them the best they could with medicines. And medicines is what Mrs C. got. Lots of them. Hydroxycarbamide 500 mg 3 times a week for polycythaemia vera, combined with warfarin 15 mg per day and Bisoprolol 2.5 mg per day. Then there was exemestane 25 mg per day for breast nipple cancer. Osteoporosis was yet another problem, so she got alendronic acid for that, plus omeprazole 20 mg per day to control acid reflux and nausea, which were side effects of alendronic acid (and several other medicines). The rheumatologist prescribed allopurinol 100 mg per day to curb the gout and methotrexate for her rheumatic complaints; the severe back pain was managed with morphine patches, 5 mg per week. And because Mrs C. had developed serious deficiencies, she was also prescribed a host of supplements: folic acid, thiamine (vitamin B1), vitamin B compound, multivitamins, and protein drinks to get at least some nutrition in there.

© The Author(s), under exclusive license to Springer Nature Switzerland AG 2023
R. Rasker, *Mind, Make-Believe and Medicine*,
https://doi.org/10.1007/978-3-031-29444-0_6

When she arrived in the hospital more dead than alive, doctors were astounded – it appeared that Mrs C. not only suffered from three different types of cancer and several other conditions, but had managed to stay alive on almost nothing but this veritable pharmacy of medications and supplements. And in fact, it was this concoction of pills, potions and patches that had almost killed her, as combined side effects made it virtually impossible to keep food down, and also made her feel awful in other ways. She was immediately hooked up to intravenous nutrition, and while she was recovering, both her condition and her medication were closely scrutinized. As it turned out, individual prescriptions were made without paying sufficient attention to all those other prescriptions. The cumulative side effect of all medicines together seriously upset the digestive tract, causing debilitating nausea and general malaise. This in turn set off a downward spiral where lack of nutrition caused Mrs C. to become even weaker, further increasing the impact of these side effects.

After a thorough review of her condition, it was decided that dosages of the most harmful medicines could be substantially reduced, while others were replaced by different medicines with less side effects. One medicine could be discontinued completely, as this substance is normally only used for long-term (as in: many years) suppression of cancer growth. It simply does not make sense to give this treatment to people with a limited remaining life expectancy.

The changes in treatment regimen worked wonders: despite her dire condition, Mrs C. regained her appetite and started putting on weight again – and as of the time of this writing, she is still alive and even enjoying her improved quality of life, though prospects are not good at all. Modern medicine was absolutely to blame for this ordeal caused by overmedication – but then again, she almost certainly would not be alive any more without this very same modern medicine …

The previous two chapters presented a bird's eye view of all of medicine, looking at only a few main categories of treatments in both regular and alternative medicine.

In this chapter, we will concentrate on the one aspect of medicine that most people think of as 'medicine': the medicines themselves. We will take a close look at the history of medicinal treatments and the origins of pharmaceutical products—the basis of what today is often called 'Big Pharma'. For this, we will first look at traditional medicines such as herbs, animal products and other natural substances, and how they were used to treat illness.

Then it is time to address one of the pet peeves of alternative advocates: Big Pharma. Is this industry really as corrupted and evil as it is often portrayed? If so, why are their products still used by billions of people?

Of course it is only fair to also take a critical look at alternative medicines and their manufacturers. Do they work? Are they safe?

Funny Food

Throughout history, people must have stumbled upon 'funny food': plants that had certain special effects when eaten—by humans as well as animals. A lot of those special plants must have been found because animals started behaving strangely after eating these plants. Of course these 'special effects' quite often consisted of getting violently ill or even dying, which, in fact, could be considered intentional—intentional from the evolutionary point of view of the plant, that is. Many plants have evolved toxic substances to discourage animals from eating them. This strategy works quite well, especially because many toxic substances have one thing in common: they have a bitter or otherwise very unpleasant taste,[1] which makes for a universal warning signal right from the first bite. But even less deadly substances were not exactly good for animal survival. Many herbivores living in the wild need to be alert for predators at all times, and getting high on weed or drunk on e.g. fermented fruit is usually a pleasure that is as short-lived as the animal itself.

Humans, however, were not so easily deterred. In fact, quite the contrary: they often considered the intoxicated state to be a religious experience, bringing them closer to their gods (which, in a way, was not always that far off the mark …). Now this of course didn't mean that whole tribes would just stagger around in a chronic drug stupor, because this would still not be very good for survival. In many tribal societies, the use of those special herbs and substances was strictly regulated, and only allowed in special rituals, by special people such as shamans. Rituals like this exist to this very day.

Now those special herbs with their special effects are not quite medicine yet—but that only takes one more step of human reasoning: if eating those herbs makes a healthy person feel sick or otherwise intoxicated, then the opposite could very well apply too: giving special herbs to a sick person might make them better. And it was quite obvious already that some herbs could make people *feel* better, if only for a while.

As a result, virtually all cultures around the world have developed their own medicinal tradition, sometimes featuring a huge collection of herbs and other substances (minerals, animal parts) that are traditionally used to treat all sorts of ailments and problems. The numbers are staggering: in a 2002 paper, German researcher Uwe Schippman estimated that of some 400,000 known plant species, no less than 52,000 were documented as being used as medicines at one time or another—and note that these are just plants.

---

[1] Which, when you think about it, is also the result of evolution—in those animals eating them, this time.

One very important question arises: do all those herbs actually *work*? It seems that the people using them thought so, otherwise those herbs would not have ended up in traditional medicine. However, we have the same problem here that we have with treatments in general, as discussed in Chapter 4: even if someone gets better *after* using a particular medicine, it is often impossible to tell if that medicine *caused* them to get better. We will address this question in more detail further on.

First, we will take a broader look at medicines, and in particular how they work, and what they can and can't do.

Medicines: Cure, Comfort or Curse?

First we have to look at the differences between drugs and medicines, because they are not exactly the same. *Drugs* are best described as chemical substances that have particular effects on people, regardless whether these effects are beneficial or not.

Medicines are a subset of drugs, meant to influence the body's chemistry in ways that make sick people better—as in: they improve a patient's condition. Most of the time, I will use the term 'medicine', to emphasize that we're talking about making people (feel) better.

One of the first and very important things to note about medicines, regardless whether alternative or regular, is that only relatively few of them actually *cure* conditions. Even when medicines work, they usually only treat certain aspects of a condition. Quite often, as many adherents of alternative medicine also say, those medicines 'just suppress symptoms'—as if this were a bad thing. Relieving symptoms or supporting bodily functions can already improve a patient's quality of life tremendously; just ask anyone with e.g. rheumatoid arthritis or asthma what their medication does for them.

Having said this, there are still lots of medicines that *can* cure conditions. Some examples are antibiotics and related substances such as antimalarial drugs. These medicines cure infections by killing off the pathogens that cause these infections. Another example is chemotherapy, used to kill cancer cells. Most medicines, however, have more of a supporting effect, and the actual healing is usually done by the body itself, as described at the beginning of Chapter 4.

Another universal fact about medicines is this: any medicine that works can also have side effects—something that is also the core message of this chapter's opening story. This again goes for both alternative (or 'natural') medicines and regular medicines. If a medicine is promoted as '100% without side effects', then it is very likely also 100% ineffective.[2]

Over the past decades, the public view of medicines, and especially the pharmaceutical industry and its products, has changed quite a bit. In the 1950s, science and technology were universally hailed as the greatest blessings of mankind. Science was making enormous progress, also in the field of medicine, and there was great optimism about the eradication of all diseases—with the pharmaceutical industry at the forefront, producing vaccines to prevent disease and medicines to cure those that couldn't be prevented. But even though this optimism was justified to a degree, there were also several serious incidents and scandals. In 1955, the first mass polio vaccination campaign in the US ground to a halt when it turned out that a serious production fault led to vaccines *causing* polio instead of preventing it. Several years later, an insufficiently tested new medicine by the name of thalidomide caused thousands of children to be born with serious deformities. Pharmaceutical companies were increasingly accused of letting profits prevail over efficacy or even safety of their products—a view that many people have up to this day, and not completely unjustified, when we look at the numerous scandals that Big Pharma got itself into. It also didn't help that the huge sums of money involved in the development and sales of pharmaceutical products attracted people who only cared about getting obscenely rich, no matter if they let their greed prevail over delivering desperately needed medicines for an acceptable price.

Still, Big Pharma is not just the cesspool of evil and greed it is often portrayed to be. Most of their products actually work and are relatively safe,[3] and the most commonly used medicines are in fact very cheap—often even cheaper than their alternative counterparts, i.e. herbal medicines and supplements. Millions of people around the world would not be alive any more if it weren't for the products of Big Pharma, and millions more would have a far lower quality of life with more pain, discomfort, anxiety and lots of other things that can make people pretty miserable. And then just think about this: surgery would be almost impossible without Big Pharma's anaesthetics and other products that are used in almost each and every surgical procedure. So nuance is the keyword here.

---

[2] Apart from the placebo effect, of course. There is *always* placebo.

[3] As in: they have a positive benefit/risk balance. No medicine is safe in an absolute way.

'One Helping of Medicine Please, Hold the Side Effects'

As mentioned already, side effects are a major problem with medicines, and in fact all of medicine: everything that has some kind of desired effect in the human body can almost always have unwanted and often even harmful side effects as well. The humble aspirin may be quite effective as a painkiller, it can also cause bleeding by interfering with blood clotting. Then again, this particular side effect is used in a beneficial manner in people with thrombosis and atherosclerosis—there is good scientific evidence that half an aspirin a day helps prevent dangerous blood clots forming, and thus helps prevent heart attacks, strokes and embolisms [18].

One important drawback of medicines is that they often end up everywhere in the body, even though the problem they're meant to address is just in one organ or location. This is compounded by the fact that the body often uses the same chemical for completely different purposes, depending on the location. One example is serotonin, which acts as a 'feel-good' neurotransmitter in certain parts of the brain, but is also produced by cells in the gut, regulating bowel activity. Too much serotonin here results in diarrhoea—which most people do not exactly associate with 'feel-good'. This is why antidepressants (so-called SSRIs) regularly cause intestinal problems as side effects.

Another problem with side effects of newly developed medicines in particular is that they are not always noticed in trials. If, for instance, a particular side effect only manifests itself after several years of use, then a 6-month trial will not pick this up. And if a side effect only occurs in 1 out of every 200,000 patients, even a trial with 50,000 volunteers will not find it. This is why pharmaceutical companies are obliged to conduct what is called *post-market surveillance*, where they actively monitor what happens with patients who use the new medicine, for an extended period of time. This surveillance has led to numerous medicines to be withdrawn from the market again after initial approval [19].

Also note that it does not matter if a medicine is 'natural' or not; herbs and other natural products can also have side effects. A well-known example is a plant by the name of St. John's wort, which is proven effective as an antidepressant, but also interferes with the way other medicines work.

Traditional Medicine

Every culture in history had their own range of medicines, mostly based on plants, but also on animal and mineral ingredients. So how did the shamans or healers or physicians in those cultures diagnose their patients and choose medicines?

Imagine that you are a tribe's shaman (or shawoman, if you will), and your people succeeded in bringing down a huge buffalo a couple of days ago. Because no-one has invented the freezer yet, the meat is stored in the only place where it can be safely stored: in the tribe's bellies. But after several days of this highly unusual feasting on nothing but red meat, trouble comes calling—people begin to complain about constipation. And now they're looking at *you* to help them.

What to do? The virtues of a plant-rich high-fibre diet are not yet known; one of the main reasons why plants usually are the main diet ingredient is because a lot of the time, there isn't much else to eat. Besides, once the whole number 2 business has already ground to a halt, just taking in some extra fibres isn't going to help much anyway.

What you need is a potent medicine, something to really get things going again. All of a sudden, you remember about a herb that did just that (and explosively so), after one unlucky gatherer ate them. So you go out, and try to find that same plant. Now let's see … yes, on the edge of that grove, those shrubs with the small yellow flowers and the pairs of bright green leaves look the business … And as by a miracle, you got it right in one go! The plant has a spicy, somewhat bitter-fresh taste, and only a handful of mushed-up leaves taken with plenty of water are enough to set off ominous rumbling after just a little while, followed by cramps, with the patient running for the nearest bushes *fast*.

Later that day, you are basking in that warm fuzzy feeling of gratitude from your fellow human beings. The very same fellow human beings, who, in all their good intentions, decide to honour you by throwing yet another feast … at which point going vegetarian seems like a very attractive life choice.

Now this story is of course completely made up, but it is plausible nonetheless: people suffer from a simple, obvious problem, and there are plants out there that do exactly what is needed to remedy that problem. Long live natural remedies!

Unfortunately, things in life are almost never this simple, and this certainly goes for matters of health and sickness. Even as recent as 150 years ago, when people fell ill, doctors usually had no clue what was wrong with them, and at best had only very limited knowledge about what might help them.

Western Traditional Medicine

European and Middle-Eastern cultures diagnosed and treated conditions by means of two principles. The oldest principle, dating back to the ancient Greeks was the *humoral theory*, based on a balance of four types of bodily fluid: blood, yellow bile, black bile, and phlegm. These fluids later became closely associated with four types of temperament named sanguine, choleric, melancholic and phlegmatic. This model was usually the leading principle for doctors to decide on a particular treatment (even if those bodily fluids should not be taken literally all of the time). If a patient was feverish and restless, then this was interpreted as an excess of blood—so bloodletting was the treatment of choice in those cases, together with matching herbs (e.g. mint) to cool down the feverish state. Humoral theory was closely related to the four element model of the physical world, whereby every substance was composed of the four basic elements earth, water, air and fire in particular proportions.

Miasma Theory

Humoral theory tried to explain what disease did in the body and how it could be treated, but not what actually *caused* the diseased state of the body. This latter was explained by the so-called *miasma theory*, according to which disease was caused and spread by 'bad air' or miasmas, usually thought to originate from stagnant water and rotting organic matter. This is also where the name 'malaria' comes from, which literally means 'bad air'—which turns out to be almost spot on: malaria is indeed closely associated with stagnant water, and yes, it spreads through the air—but, as we now know, not as an invisible cloud, but through mosquitoes that breed in this water and spread malaria parasites from person to person by biting them.

Especially during plague outbreaks, doctors tried to protect themselves from these miasmas by wearing their equivalent of our modern-day hazmat suits: long, sealed-off garments, with a breathing mask in the shape of a bird beak, filled with air-purifying fragrant herbs; no doubt, you have seen these depicted [20]. Yes, the general idea of isolating yourself from an infectious environment was pretty good. The idea of filtering breathing air was also quite good. Just too bad that they got it wrong about the *real* disease vector: infected rat fleas, which had little trouble finding their way inside any item of clothing of the time. And no, those 'air-purifying herbs' weren't much good either; at best, they provided the clueless doctors of the time with a pleasant smell while dealing with disease, death and decay. Still, those spooky-looking outfits no doubt contributed to the now all too familiar concept of social distancing, reducing the doctors' chances of getting infected.

Samuel Hahnemann, the inventor of homeopathy, came up with his own, rather peculiar version of the miasma theory. He believed that all chronic diseases were in fact manifestations of three miasmas, two of which were associated with sexually transmitted diseases. He also believed that suppressing acute disease symptoms (instead of fully curing the patient) caused much more serious disease in later life. Which is a bit strange, because homeopathy completely revolves around symptoms—but more about this in the next chapter.

The Doctrine of Signatures

Yet another system of herbal medicine popular in late medieval Europe was the *doctrine of signatures*: by divine design, a plant signalled its medicinal usefulness to us humans by looking like the organ it was supposed to treat. For instance liverwort has leaves resembling the liver's shape, so it was used to treat liver conditions, and lungwort with its spotted leaves apparently resembled diseased lungs. A very obvious example is the resemblance between a walnut and the human skull and brain, leading physicians to proclaim walnut as a good medicine for afflictions of the brain. In most cases though, it took a real stretch of the imagination to recognize a particular organ in a plant, and many doctors also noticed that those organ lookalikes usually didn't appear to do much.

All these disease theories may look silly to us now, but once again demonstrate our human desire to find patterns in things that seem haphazard and random on the surface. And those old doctors were right in a way: medicine *is* based on systematic patterns—it's just that these patterns are more complex than they could have ever imagined.

Traditional Chinese Medicine

Perhaps the best known form of traditional medicine is Traditional Chinese Medicine, or TCM for short. TCM features quite a lot of different types of treatment (so-called *modalities*), including herbal medicine, acupuncture, massage, cupping and much more. Acupuncture is addressed in the chapter on energy medicine; here, we will mostly look at TCM's herbal component, which also is the most used treatment form in TCM.

TCM works with two main principles: the life energy *qi*, which is said to flow along so-called *meridians* in the body, and the balance of yin and yang, which, if disturbed, can cause problems with the flow of qi. Yin and yang again are associated with numerous opposing properties, with hot and cold being the most prominent ones. Other properties are wet and dry, male and female, light and dark, up and down, and so on.

Yin and yang are further connected to organs and bodily phenomena following a system of the 'five phases' wood, fire, earth, metal and water, which themselves are again linked to a natural order of astronomical, seasonal and physical cycles.

TCM also takes into account the actual physical state of the body, including bodily fluids, bodily odours, colour, the way organs feel and much more. However, diagnoses in TCM do not attempt to identify particular diseases, but rather locate the sources of imbalance or disharmony in a patient, by checking the described properties and phenomena. Apart from assessing distinct disease symptoms themselves, diagnoses mostly take place by taking the patient's pulse and observing their tongue in great detail; this is combined with other symptoms and signs, and interpreted in terms of yin and yang patterns, hot or cold, wet or dry etcetera.

Treatments are then chosen based on the imbalances that are perceived. For instance stomach pain is often diagnosed as an excess of heat in the abdomen, so the medicine to treat this must be classified as 'cold'. As this heat is believed to burn off bodily fluids and thus cause dryness, the medicine must also have a 'damp' or 'moistening' property. In addition, this dryness in turn blocks the downward (as opposed to upward) flow of qi, causing 'stomach stagnation', constipation and nausea—necessitating a treatment that restores the downward flow of chi and works as a laxative. All this can be accompanied by three possible types of pulse: rapid, slippery, or full, and a tongue that is red in the middle, with a yellow coating.

There is much more to TCM than can be explained in these few paragraphs; extensive books have been written on the subject. The main idea here is that herbal medicines in TCM are primarily based on a complex of properties rather than efficacy for a particular disease, so that they can counteract the diagnosed state of yin and yang in organs, and restore the proper flow of qi in a patient.

Ayurveda

Ayurveda is an oriental system of medicine from the Indian subcontinent with even more ancient roots than TCM. It is similar to TCM in that it relies heavily on herbal medicine and the use of mineral components. Also, its basic tenets involve five elements that are partly analogous to TCM's five phases.

In many other aspects, however, it differs considerably from TCM. For instance health and sickness are determined by a balance of three 'impurities' or *doshas* called *vāta, pitta* and *kapha* (translated as wind, bile and phlegm), instead of the Chinese dualistic model of yin and yang. Also, Ayurveda does not use animal ingredients as extensively as TCM, although products from cows (such as milk, urine and dung) still play an important role.

Ayurveda is mentioned here because together with TCM, it is one of the more popular oriental systems of medicine found in western countries, and because it is mainly based on herbal and mineral ingredients.

Big Books of Medicine

Both in Europe and Asia, lists of medicines called *pharmacopoeias* were compiled, naming and describing each medicine, what its properties were, and what it was used for. This of course made it much easier for physicians to find a medicine for patients with a particular ailment, but it also enabled a rudimentary form of pharmaceutical research as well as quality control: medicines that were found useless or even harmful could be mentioned as such, so that these were no longer used. Especially in seventeenth century Europe, pharmacopoeia committees slowly began to use a more scientific approach, trying to cut down on the ever growing number of medicines in pharmacopoeias, and weeding out unnecessary ingredients. Yet even in the early eighteenth century, some pretty icky substances such as dog poo and moss grown on the skull of a corpse were still listed as legitimate medicinal ingredients. That's traditional medicine for you!

So far, we saw how medicines were identified and selected, carefully avoiding the elephant in the room: their actual efficacy. How well did those traditional herbal medicines work? Did they work at all?

The answer is: sometimes.

All those doctors in history ran into much the same problem we already discussed in Chapter 4: when patients get better, it is often difficult to tell if it was the medicine (or other treatment) that did the trick, or that the problems went away by themselves. Even with the sophisticated scientific tools we have these days, it can still be difficult to judge if a medicine has an effect or not, especially when the effect is small, or only emerges after prolonged use.

In some situations, the causality is pretty clear, such as in our story about constipation: the problem is obvious even for laypeople, and so is the remedy, in the form of a plant that can, erm, get things going again on very short notice.

But cases like this are the exception, not the rule. Until relatively recently, people had no clue as to what caused diseases, and treatments were based on a mixture of traditional knowledge (which was often wrong), a doctor's personal experience (which was also not much good) and sometimes new (but usually wrong) insights. Before the advent of the scientific method, testing of medicines usually was limited to one doctor giving a new concoction to at most a couple of patients, and see what happened:

* Patients did not get better. This, even while disappointing, was at least a clear indication that the medicine didn't work.

* Patients got better after treatment. But was it the medicine that did it? Most of the time it was not, because a lot of the time, the body just heals itself. But how could these people know what really happened? The best course of action was to keep prescribing the medicine to patients with the same condition, just in case it did actually do something useful.

'Used for' Is Not the Same as 'Effective For'

This practice to keep using medicines that *might* make patients better was quite sensible at the time, especially if there were no serious side effects. Even today, this principle is expressed by the rather curious[4] saying *If it doesn't help, then it doesn't hurt.*

This tendency to consider herbal remedies effective 'just in case' resulted in pharmacopoeias growing ever larger—with TCM as the absolute champion, with historical records listing a staggering 100,000 different medicinal recipes altogether, based on 13,000 ingredients. And however sensible it might have seemed to keep adding medicines 'just in case' simply because patients recovered after receiving those herbal concoctions, the truth of the matter is that the overwhelming majority does not work. Sure, many of these herbs probably provide some valuable nutrients such as vitamins, minerals, antioxidants and more, but those don't count as medicines.

This problem is also affecting herbal medicine in this day and age. Almost all practitioners and books touting the virtues of herbal treatments make the same mistake: when a plant is traditionally *used* for certain problems, it is automatically assumed that it also *works* for those problems. This is not by definition the case.

Let's take a look at a very popular herbal medicine by the name of *echinacea purpurea*, a species of coneflower. On the Internet, you will find claims that it is quite effective against the common cold and other airway infections, and can reduce symptoms of these diseases by as much as 75%. Many commercial products based on echinacea make similar claims (albeit often disguised as 'strengthening the immune system', for reasons that will be explained shortly). As a clincher, it is often mentioned that it has been used by the indigenous North Americans for well over 400 years. So echinacea is a time-tested remedy that must work for sure, right?

Alas, when we look at the actual scientific evidence, the results are far less compelling. Some research finds that taking echinacea extract at the onset of colds might somewhat reduce the duration of symptoms, while other research

---

[4] Because things that don't help can absolutely hurt.

finds no benefits. Yes, echinacea extracts show clear antiviral activity in vitro (in test tubes), but as any pharmacology student can tell you, this only very rarely translates to useful medicinal effects in living humans (in vivo). So far, the scientific verdict on echinacea is that at best, it has only very limited antiviral effects [21]. Despite this, echinacea products are used by millions of people worldwide, making it pretty Big Business.

The same goes for most other herbal products: they may have been used in traditional medicine for centuries or even millennia, but that is no guarantee that they actually work. In many (if not most) cases, they don't.

Herbal Successes

The news on herbal and traditional medicines is not all bad, and there have been some striking successes. Arguably the biggest success was a traditional medicine that turned out to be effective against malaria.

In 1967, China started a secret military research program to see if their vast pharmacopoeia of traditional medicines contained any effective remedies against malaria. At the time, China's ally North Vietnam was at war with South Vietnam, and malaria was taking a heavy toll on their armed forces. After whittling down the list to the 2,000 most likely compounds, a group of scientists started the painstaking work of testing each of these medicines for antimalarial activity. In 1972, a group led by researcher Tu Youyou found that the extract of a plant named artemisia was indeed effective—more so, in fact, than any existing antimalarial medicine at the time.[5] In 1980, the active substance named artemisinin was also found to be effective against schistosomiasis, the most widespread parasitic infection after malaria. In 2015, Tu Youyou was awarded the Nobel Prize in Medicine, shared with two researchers who discovered avermectin, another very effective medicine for parasitic diseases.

There are several dozen other herbal medicines with scientifically proven efficacy. One example mentioned earlier is St. John's wort, which turns out to be just as effective for mild or moderate depression as commonly prescribed pharmaceutical products.

One advantage of herbal medicine is of course its simplicity: you can just go out there and gather the plants that you need. You don't have to rely on pharmaceutical companies that sometimes charge extortionate prices for their products. Also, most medicinal plants also contain important micronutrients

---

[5] It should be noted, however, that in Traditional Chinese Medicine, artemisin was never used for malaria; this particular indication was first discovered by Tu Youyou and her team.

such as vitamins and minerals, which, if not directly medicinal, at least may contribute to overall health.

Looking Things up at the NCCIH and RationalWiki

If you want to see what a particular herbal medicine can and can't do, the best source of information is often the National Center for Complementary and Integrative Health (NCCIH) [22]. This American institute was founded in 1991 as an initiative to give the world of alternative medicine a more robust, scientific foundation. Unfortunately, even their well-funded research (costing a total of almost 4 billion dollars to date) failed to identify any really effective forms of alternative medicine; almost all of their trials came up negative. However, their information on herbal medicine is quite good, and far more trustworthy than the overly positive information on the Web where herbal treatments are promoted and sold. Another good source of information is RationalWiki [23].

What the Science Says

In the late 1700s, science began to make inroads in medicine, including pharmacology. Doctors and scientists began to realize that many traditional medicines weren't much good, and also found out that medicines were in fact a kind of chemistry. Plants did not have magical healing powers, but contained chemical compounds that interacted with human physiology in (hopefully) beneficial ways. This was further supported by earlier findings in alchemy, where for instance mercury compounds were found effective for treating bacterial infections. Unfortunately, many mercury compounds are highly toxic, and in the long run, these treatments often caused far more serious problems than they solved.

Drawbacks of Herbal and Traditional Medicines

The main drawback of herbal/traditional medicines has already been mentioned: it appears that the majority is not effective, or only has very little effect when properly tested. Of the tens of thousands of known TCM medicines, only a couple of hundred have been found effective so far. This is to be expected, given how these herbal treatments ended up in pharmacopoeias in the first place. The people who tried out and approved these herbal treatments were not stupid, they just lacked the scientific means and knowledge to verify if something really worked—so they used the 'just in case' strategy.

Environmental Damage

We just mentioned that gathering medicinal ingredients in nature can be easier and cheaper than having to pay through the nose for Big Pharma products. Unfortunately, this has serious environmental consequences: many plants and animals used in traditional medicine and especially in TCM are now threatened with extinction. This is compounded by the unfortunate human tendency to consider exotic, rare species to be more effective and desirable than very common species. We all know about the madness of the illegal but still ongoing trade in rhino horn and tigers bones—both of which are of no therapeutic value whatsoever, but are nevertheless very popular in TCM. However, numerous less-known plants are also becoming rare as a result of excessive, non-sustainable exploitation [24].

On the upside, most herbal products sold in Western countries today are no longer gathered from nature, but grown commercially.

Dosage Problems

One important aspect of using medicines is of course the dosage: how much do you need to get the desired effect? Too little, and nothing much will happen; too much, and you run the risk of serious side effects and sometimes even death. The problem with medicinal herbs is that it is often hard to tell how much of the active substance is present. One individual plant may contain barely enough to treat even one patient, while the plant right next to it may have enough for five or even ten patients. This is further compounded by the fact that not all parts of the plant may contain the active substance. With some, it is only present in the leaves, with others in the flowers or the root, and others again have the desired substance in every part (but even then in varying amounts).

With many medicines, herbal or otherwise, it is not too much of a problem if you get several times the minimum effective dose. But with other medicines, the correct dose is vitally important. For instance in 1785, it was found that foxglove could be quite effective for treating certain heart conditions. Unfortunately, the active substance (digitoxin) is very easy to overdose, with a toxic dose being on average just twice the effective dose (the ending 'toxin' in the name is also a bit of a hint here …). This means that the so-called *therapeutic index* (the average toxic dose divided by the average effective dose) of digitoxin is only 2. For comparison, morphine, which is considered a pretty risky drug (and rightly so) has a therapeutic index of 70. This means that herbal medicines should always be used with caution, especially the ones with strong effects.

Interactions, Side Effects, and What Happens in Your Body

Then there is what I like to call the new household pet problem. Suppose you already have a dog or a cat, and you want to introduce another pet. Then the inevitable question arises: will they be friends? Or will they start chasing each other, maybe try to rip each other apart, causing complete mayhem in the process? (Yes, I may have watched one too many Tom & Jerry cartoons …) Something similar can happen when you are already on one medicine, and then start taking another one: they don't get along very well, and your interior will end up in shambles. This problem of course is not unique for herbal medicine—as our opening story also clearly shows.

The point here is that herbal medicine is usually regarded as 'natural' and thus mild and harmless. Because of this, people who get prescribed medicines may forget to mention that they're also using herbal products. In some cases, this can cause unexpected trouble. For instance St. John's wort is proven effective in treating moderate depression, but it also influences the liver's functioning in ways that may reduce the effects of other medicines [25]. This can have serious consequences if someone's life depends on those prescription medicines. So here's a bit of important medical advice:

If your doctor prescribes you a medicine, always mention any herbal medicines or supplements that you may be taking. If you plan to use over-the-counter medicines, at least research potential interactions yourself.

Any doctor worth their salt should of course ask you about this, but hey, they're only human too, and sometimes make mistakes or forget things.

Then there are side effects of the medicine itself. Herbal medicines can have side effects too, just like pharmaceutical products. But unlike pharmaceutical products, which contain one or perhaps two active substances at most, herbal products often contain lots of different compounds (as in: hundreds or even thousands), many of which unidentified, with largely unknown effects, and in unknown quantities. As mentioned before, a lot of these substances are harmless and may even be healthy, but there may also be some that do have unexpected effects—for better or for worse, and there's no way to tell.

Lastly, there are the complementary and closely related principles of pharmacokinetics and pharmacodynamics. *Pharmacokinetics* (PK) basically describes how a medicine gets into the body, how it is transported inside the body, and how it is excreted. *Pharmacodynamics* (PD) tells us what it is that a medicine actually *does* inside the body, so what effects it has (if any), how it is processed and by which organ(s), and what products it is metabolized into. In more detail, PK and PD tell us.

* how a medicine is administered (pills, injections, IV's etcetera),
* what happens after it is introduced to the body (lots of medicines don't survive the digestive tract, so these have to be administered by injection or another more direct route),
* how and where they can and can't spread through the body (most medicines can't pass the so-called blood–brain barrier, but some can),
* how our body responds to the medicine (which should be the desired effect and little else, but also includes any side effects),
* how the medicines are broken down, and what they are broken down into, and/or
* how they are excreted from the body.

All these things are important, not just for pharmaceutical products, but also for herbal products. E.g. people with kidney problems should not take medicines that are exclusively excreted through the kidneys (and this should also be listed in the label).

When medicines are taken orally, a lot of the administered dose may deactivated by enzymes in the intestines and the liver before it even becomes available to the rest of the body. This mostly depends on the medicine in question; sometimes as little as a few percent of a medicine actually reaches its destination inside the body. Well, no real problem there: just increase the dose sufficiently to overcome this loss, right? Yes—but there's a snag: some *other* substances can really mess up this deactivation process, and one of these (a so-called *furanocoumarin*) is present in grapefruit. You know, those healthy, vitamin-packed breakfast bombs full of sunshine. When you eat grapefruit and then take a normal dose of medicine—a dose based on the expectation that 90% doesn't make it past the liver—then what you *get* can turn out to be a tenfold dose. In other words: a serious overdose. This is why several medicines come with big warnings that they should not be taken together with grapefruit or grapefruit juice.

Now this whole PK and PD stuff may be hugely interesting to pharmacology geeks, but what does it have to do with herbal medicines in particular you ask? After all, it affects herbal medicines and pharmaceutical products alike. The difference is that pharmaceutical manufacturers are obliged by law to carefully study the pharmacodynamics and pharmacokinetics of their products, and mention any relevant results in the label. This way, doctors and pharmacists can see when two or more medicines won't be friends, so the combination should be avoided. They are also alerted to so-called contraindications, so conditions which preclude the use of a particular medicine (most often liver and kidney problems).

None of this is required for herbal medicines, and this means that manufacturers and sellers of herbal medicines often can't tell you what it is that their products actually do in people. After all, doing this kind of research is expensive …

The following says it all, really:

Herbal medicine: taking an unknown dose of an unknown combination of largely unknown substances with unknown effects.

Quality and Regulatory Problems

Yet another problem with herbal medicines is that in most countries, they are not regulated as strictly as pharmaceutical products. Manufacturers of herbal products do not have to provide evidence of efficacy or even safety before their products are allowed onto the market. The only concession those manufacturers have to make is that they can't advertise their products as medicines, which means that they are also not allowed to make claims of efficacy for any specific condition. They are however allowed to use more general claims such as 'supports the immune system', or 'helps in case of colds and flu'.

In many countries, herbal products only have to comply with food and general consumer regulations, meaning that they should be generally safe for use, and that the ingredients should match what the label says.

Most herbal products that are manufactured by larger, well-known companies and sold by major western retail chains are usually OK, even though dosage of the active substance can still vary considerably. But herbal products directly ordered from abroad over the Internet are best avoided, and this especially goes for traditional Chinese and Ayurvedic herbs, for reasons discussed next.

Toxic Ingredients, Contamination and Adulteration

Traditional Chinese Medicine and Ayurveda may be the oldest systems of medicine we know, they are unfortunately fraught with problems and risks. Sometimes, the true toxic nature of a traditional medicine was not recognized until recently. Or perhaps TCM ingredients were not properly documented, or simply not available. In those cases, practitioners tend to resort to using other plants with more or less similar names. For instance birthwort (aristolochia, literally 'excellent birth' in Greek) was given to pregnant women from the days of ancient Greece well into the twentieth century. Little did anyone suspect that this plant was actually very toxic, and came with serious risks of permanent kidney damage and even cancer—something that was only discovered in the 1990s in Belgium, when over fifty health spa visitors developed chronic kidney failure after taking Chinese herbal supplements containing aristolochia. One major reason for this serious incident is that Chinese medicinal herbs are deemed interchangeable if their names sound more or less the same. Here, the relatively harmless plant by the Chinese name of *han fang ji* (stephania tetrandra) was substituted with a highly toxic aristolochia variety named *guang fang ji*. The use of aristolochia in TCM is also implicated in the relatively high number of cases of kidney cancer in Taiwan [26].

How Would You Like Your Arsenic Sir, Boiled or Roasted?

One of the biggest problems with Ayurveda but also TCM is the traditional use of heavy metals such as mercury, lead and arsenic in these medicines— a tradition that is still alive and well today (something that can't be said of quite a few patients). Ayurvedic and TCM practitioners claim that the special way in which those highly toxic metals are processed makes them not only completely safe, but even beneficial for people's health.

They are wrong.

While toxicity of mercury compounds can vary considerably, and some mercury compounds have indeed a low toxicity, the problem is that the preparation of those safer forms requires strict quality control during and after production, and this quality control and testing almost never takes place. Lead and arsenic compounds are almost never safe, in any chemical form.

Even as recently as 2017, testing 252 random samples of Ayurvedic medicines found lead in 65% of samples, mercury in 38% of samples, and arsenic in 32% of samples [27]. In almost one third of these, the amounts found exceeded safe limits by thousands of times, turning those 'medicines' into a very serious health hazard.

Especially children are susceptible to the toxic effects of lead and other heavy metals, so they should *never* be given oriental herbal medicines. But adults too are regularly poisoned and even killed by these products, even though many cases go unnoticed—heavy metal poisoning is often a slow process that can go unrecognized for a long time, and can look a lot like natural degenerative or neurological diseases. Also, most doctors in western countries don't expect to see these kinds of poisonings, which may delay a correct diagnosis considerably. This is yet another reason to always tell your doctor if you are using herbal products or supplements.

Traditional Medicine with Modern Effectiveness

Research into TCM herbs brought yet another problem to light: not only did quite a few 'traditional herbs' contain heavy metal or toxic plant ingredients, many were also laced with unlisted real medicines, most likely to make certain that they worked as claimed [28]. One cause of this type of dangerous fraud is the fact that for the Chinese, TCM is a very important source of national pride, as a result of Mao Zedong's propaganda in the 1960s. TCM has an official status as a system of medicine, on par with western medicine, even though it is arguably far less effective. As a result, Chinese studies into TCM are often falsified and TCM products are adulterated with pharmaceutical products, just to keep up appearances.

All this is why it usually advisable to stay away from traditional Chinese and Ayurvedic herbal products: there is a far bigger chance that they will harm and poison you than that they will benefit your health.

Pharma Time!

We have seen that traditional and herbal medicines have lots of shortcomings and drawbacks, the most important of which is that generally, they aren't very effective. This is not strange, given that they were identified and used when people had virtually no knowledge about health and disease, and especially about what caused patients to get better. The upside is that herbal medicines, having less of an effect, also have less risk of (serious) side effects than their pharmaceutical counterparts[6]—at least when they don' t contain toxic ingredients or secret pharmaceutical ingredients.

The big question now is if things are any better with Big Pharma's products. Let's find out!

Our modern-day pharmaceutical companies of course didn't just pop up out of nowhere, selling their chemical pills 'n potions as a more modern alternative to time-trusted herbal remedies. Modern pharmacology is very firmly rooted in historic herbal medicine, and still makes extensive use of numerous plant and even animal and mineral ingredients.

What really changed things was introducing science throughout the process of identifying, testing and producing medicines, instead of just administering medicines to patients based on traditional knowledge, and hope for the best. This progress of science also enabled another major change: the extraction, processing, manufacturing and marketing of active substances on an industrial scale.

These new developments started when chemists began to study herbal medicines that clearly worked, and tried to figure out what it was that made them effective. One of the earlier successes was the isolation of salicin from willow bark in 1828. Willow bark extract had been known as a pain and fever remedy for thousands of years, and it turned out that this salicin was the active ingredient (derived from *Salix*, Latin for 'willow'). Now as a chemist, of course you don't stop when you've found your active ingredient. You start experimenting with it, such as cooking it up with other substances to see if you can improve or change it—and it wasn't too long that some test tube tinkerers created salicylic acid and, some time later, acetylsalicylic acid. This last compound turned out to be effective against pain and fever just like its predecessors, but with far less side effects. Around 1900, it became a huge sales success for Bayer under the brand name Aspirin. Together with Merck, another German company selling chemical products, Bayer can be considered as one of the first incarnations of what we now call Big Pharma.

When you sell products that claim to improve people's health, great success comes with great responsibilities. Unfortunately, public health was not always the first priority, to put it mildly. The same Bayer that blessed the world with its cheap, effective and relatively safe Aspirin painkiller started selling heroin (yes, the drug) as an over-the-counter medicine in 1895. And not just that, they marketed it as a 'non-addictive substitute for morphine'. Nothing could be further from the truth. The fact that it took almost 20 years before US governmental regulation first restricted its sale in 1914 tells us that Bayer

---

[6] On a side note: many supplements and herbal products that are popular in the alternative world (known for its aversion to Big Pharma) are produced by—you guessed it—pharmaceutical companies.

either hadn't bothered to actually research the addictive nature of its product, or that they just cared more about the money. And even far worse: history repeated itself a century later, with America's opioid crisis destroying countless lives. And again the blame squarely lay with pharmaceutical companies who aggressively marketed their highly addictive products, ignoring or playing down the very real risk of addiction.

So yes, Big Pharma absolutely deserves a lot of the flak that they get. Then again, they have also done some absolutely great things for humanity. Without Big Pharma's efforts, Alexander Fleming's discovery of penicillin in 1928 would not have led to the mass production of the world's first antibiotic, and thousands upon thousands of allied World War II soldiers would not have survived the war. Vaccines are another example: widespread smallpox vaccination has saved hundreds of millions of lives in the twentieth century alone, and even completely wiped this horrible disease from the face of the earth. None of this would have been achieved without the pharmaceutical industry.

Generally speaking, the majority of Big Pharma's products is safe and effective, although this did not exactly happen all by itself: many necessary improvements were only carried through after ever more stringent laws were enacted, and/or when serious incidents brought equally serious failings to light.

How Pharmaceutical Products Are Made

The following sections present a clearer picture of how medicines are actually developed, and what obstacles scientists and pharmaceutical companies have to overcome before they are allowed to sell a new product. In this instance, the US situation is described with the FDA (Food and Drug Administration) as the official authority supervising the quality of (indeed) food and medicines, but the general procedure is largely the same in other countries.

'A Promising New Substance'

It all starts out with a candidate for a new medicine, for example a particular chemical substance or a plant that has caught the attention of scientists. In the past, finding such candidates was a matter of endless trial-and-error, aided by checking out the effects of substances similar to already proven compounds, old pharmacopoeias and other sources that hinted at possible efficacy.

Nowadays, a more targeted approach is often used, where scientists for instance look for certain receptors in our body that may be tied to a particular condition, and try to find or create substances that might interact with those receptors. Also, existing medicines may have unexpected effects that hint at usefulness for other conditions than just the ones it is currently registered for.

These scientists usually carry out this basic research in academical institutions, who in turn license any promising substances to pharmaceutical companies. These companies then take over further research and development based on the scientific findings.

When potential candidates are identified (and this can run into the hundreds or even thousands of initial candidates), selection and early testing begins. In FDA jargon, this is called *discovery and development*, where lots of tests are done to weed out the ones that are clearly no good [29].

After this first crude selection, a few of the most promising candidates are chosen for the next step, called *preclinical research*. This is where testing intensifies, first in test tubes (in vitro, literally 'in glass'), then also in living animals (in vivo). This early testing stage is also the point where regulatory bodies such as the FDA start getting in on the act. They check if research is done by qualified people, in suitable laboratories, with the right equipment, under proper conditions … the list of requirements goes on an on.

Clinical Trials

When preclinical research is successfully concluded, a plan must be submitted to the FDA describing not only the proposed clinical trials with humans, but also the outcomes of all trials carried out so far. When FDA approval has been secured, trials with human volunteers can begin. These clinical trials are typically carried out in three phases:

- Phase 1: testing safety, dosage and the way the medicine is metabolized in less than one hundred volunteers. This phase usually takes several months, with 30% of prospective medicines failing at this stage.
- Phase 2: testing safety and efficacy in several hundred volunteers; this is where the first tests against placebo take place. This phase can take anything from several months to several years, with one in three medicines making it to the next phase.
- Phase 3: testing safety and efficacy in thousands of volunteers; this is where statistical information on common side effects is gathered, as well as all sorts of other information, such as the potential influence of age, gender, combination with other medicines, etcetera. This phase usually takes between 1 and 4 years, with 25% of candidates getting through this stage.

Phase 1 and phase 2 trials may take place with healthy volunteers, but also with people suffering from the condition that the medicine is meant to address. Phase 3 trials always include large numbers of people with the condition, and are preferably carried out as so-called double-blinded randomized controlled trials (RCTs), which is the best way to assess the efficacy of a potential medicine (and also named 'gold standard' for this reason).

After phase 3 clinical trials have shown the new medicine to be both safe and effective, the manufacturer of the medicine can file a New Drug Application (NDA) with the FDA, which then again reviews all studies and data gathered so far—which may take up to 10 months. If the FDA finds everything in order, then the new medicine is approved, and it can be registered for sale.

However, even after phase 3, the pharmaceutical company can't just lay back and watch the money rolling in. They still have to do what is called *post-market surveillance*, where they actively monitor what happens when ordinary patients out there use their new medicine over longer periods of time. This way, even very rare or long-term side effects can be recognized.

Summarized: the whole journey from 'promising new substance' to just one new medicine on the market can take up to 12 years and cost several billion dollars. Only a tiny fraction of promising candidates makes it all the way through, maybe one in a thousand. All the others fall by the wayside because they don't work as hoped for, or have too many or too serious side effects, or have other major drawbacks. Any money invested in an ultimately unsuccessful candidate is considered lost, so pharmaceutical companies are very keen on weeding out any failures as soon as possible. Having to ditch a product in sight of the finish is extremely costly—not only in terms of money, time and effort, but also reputation: late failures are considered a sign of incompetence.

However, the products that make it should be safe and effective, right? Well, yes, generally speaking. But then again, even this is not always the case.

Problems with Pharmaceutical Products

Even investments of billions of dollars and strict governmental regulations can't guarantee that every pill or potion made by pharmaceutical companies does what it is supposed to do. Here, I will touch upon some of the most important problems.

The Money Problem

The main issue with Big Pharma is money: the whole business model is based on investing huge sums of money in projects that have a high risk of failing—money that must be recouped through the few ones that succeed. Which means that projects *must* succeed on a more or less regular basis. And this is where a whole lot of trouble comes in, often in the form of conflicting interests. There's the public interest, which is best served by medicines that are safe, effective and cheap. On the other side there are pharmaceutical companies whose prime interest is getting a return on investments. In fact, it is even stronger: they *must* recoup those investments, otherwise they will go bankrupt—which also means that they will no longer make medicines that can serve the public interest.

Making the situation even more problematic is that a pharmaceutical company only has a limited amount of time to earn back their investment, due to the way that patents work. A patent is valid only for 20 years, the first 10 years of which are usually lost in research and development. This gives a pharmaceutical company just 10 more years for earning back investments. After that, the patent expires and anyone can copy and sell the medicine if they like, usually at a far lower price, since those competitors don't have billion-dollar investments to earn back. There are several tricks to extend patent protection, but those don't always work.

The Mechanistic Fallacy

A completely different problem with medicines in general is what I like to call the *mechanistic fallacy*: yes, the medicine does what it was designed to do—but without actually benefiting patients in terms of lower mortality or improved quality of life. If for instance a patient has a somewhat irregular heartbeat, then this can often be corrected with medicines (a 'mechanical' solution). However, this treatment, although technically effective, is useless when patients in general don't live longer or feel better as a result. When such a medicine has noticeable side effects, it can even be worse than useless, because it lowers instead of raises the quality of life. (Please note that this does not mean that all heart medicines are useless—several types of cardiac arrhythmia are in fact very dangerous, and taking the right medicine is then a matter of life and death.)

This mechanistic fallacy also applies to for instance orthomolecular treatments: if a patient's blood test[7] shows one or more deficiencies, then those deficiencies are treated by prescribing supplements—but in many cases, getting vitamin and mineral levels back to 'normal' are not what makes the patient's health complaints go away.

Hail the New Pill, just Like the Old Pill

A lot of pharmaceutical R&D is aimed at improving existing, effective medicines. If you come up with a new medicine that is essentially no better than an old and (by now) cheap one, then you are in trouble—because it simply won't sell. The way this is often tackled is by marketing: convince your buyers that the new product is somehow better still, and that they should no longer use the old 'obsolete' one, even though there is no real difference. Yes, this sounds an awful lot like consumer advertising for e.g. dishwashing liquid: if you add up all the countless 'improvements' touted over the years, you could by now do a year's washing up with just one drop of SuperBrand X, and a bottle would last you a lifetime. Which it clearly doesn't.

New cancer medicines regularly suffer from this problem: at best, they only add weeks or a few months to the life of cancer patients, while at the same time being extremely expensive—money that could have helped far more people in far better ways.

It can also be very tempting to just fudge the numbers to ensure that a new medicine can be sold, and recoup the money already spent. After all, who will know? Luckily, this type of fraud is rare, if only because it will come to light sooner or later.

More common is promoting so-called *off-label use* of already approved medicines, meaning that they are used to treat other conditions than what they were approved for. This is not normally allowed, because no studies were done to assess the benefits and risks for this new application; pharmaceutical companies have been fined billions of dollars for committing this type of fraud [30].

Not exactly fraudulent but still ethically undesirable are (some times lifesaving) medicines that are so expensive that many people can't afford them. This happens a lot with medicines developed for rare diseases.

But still, the current system mostly works: in general, products from Big Pharma can be trusted to work as claimed, and especially the older, so-called generic medicines are usually quite cheap as well. For instance one 500-mg

---

[7] As in: a legitimate blood test, not live blood analysis.

dose of paracetamol (or acetaminophen, for our American readers) costs just 2 cents.

Big Pharma and the Alternative World

From what was discussed in this chapter, it almost seems that there could be no bigger contrast: on the one hand there are herbal medicines that are selected and used based on tradition and practitioners' own experiences. On the other hand there are Big Pharma's products, which may take many years and billions of dollars to develop and test in high-tech laboratory's, and must comply with countless rules and regulations.

Then again, a lot of Big Pharma's products have their origins in herbal medicines, and some are still made from plants. For instance the chemotherapy medicine taxol is still (partly) made from yew trees.

Then there is the fact that many (if not most) 'alternative' products including supplements and herbal extracts are in fact made by Big Pharma—simply because they have the equipment and the experience to produce these things in a hygienic way on an industrial scale (those jars were certainly not filled by old ladies who hand-picked the herbs themselves …). It may be a bit ironic, but Big Pharma producing and selling products for the alternative market simply shows that they won't turn their back on an opportunity to make an easy buck—all the easier because those herbs and supplements don't have to comply with the same strict regulations that most of their other medicines do.

Conclusion

Herbal medicine is still quite appealing to proponents of alternative medicine, as it is 'natural', and of course has a tradition as long as our own human history. But when we take a more rational look, there are several problems with herbal medicine. The biggest problem is that, with a few exceptions, herbal medicine is generally far less effective than Big Pharma's products; most herbal products don't work as claimed. Also, oriental herbal products often contain highly toxic substances such as lead and mercury.

All this does not automatically mean that there's nothing wrong with the pharmaceutical industry. Research and development of even one medicine involves a highly risky investment of huge sums of money, which can make it very tempting to exaggerate the benefits and downplay the drawbacks of a medicine. Sometimes, pharmaceutical companies even fudge the numbers or break the law in other ways. All this means that Big Pharma's bad name is not completely undeserved, even though most of their products can be trusted.

The simple fact that most pharmaceutical products actually do something also means that they tend to come with a bigger chance of side effects. If you are using several medicines and supplements(!), it is always a good idea to plan at least one annual 'pharma check' with your doctor, to discuss your medication and what it does for you. If you think you suffer from side effects, then maybe one or more medicines can be stopped, or maybe a different medicine may have fewer side effects in your case.

But whatever you do, always check with your doctor.

The next chapter is dedicated to one very special type of alternative medicine: homeopathy. The special thing about homeopathy is that it involves no active substances whatsoever. So read on to find out what *is* in it!

7

Shaken, Not Stirred

A Most Wonderful Remedy

Jason was not a happy boy, and Colleen was beginning to worry. It had been over two weeks now, and her little eight-month-old still wasn't his old self. A visit to the family doctor hadn't been much help either. If anything, it had made her feel worse, what with the GP only taking a couple of minutes to explain that things like this are quite normal for children that age, that he couldn't see any alarming symptoms, and that Jason would probably be fine in another week or so. If not, call again. And that with Jason clearly feeling uncomfortable and even crying. So no help there. She'd done everything right, hadn't she? As advised, she'd started Jason on a more varied diet with solids a few months ago, even taking care to avoid the really sugary stuff such as fruit juice. So what could be wrong with her little boy? Maybe she could ask that natural practitioner guy Eileen mentioned, what was it, that homeopath, Mr Aldern? Eileen said he'd been a great help when her kid had some minor health issues. And homeopathy is after all a natural and completely harmless treatment, wasn't it? So what's there to lose?

'Yes, he's been like this for almost three weeks now, fussy with eating and drinking, listless, crying a lot... I try comforting him as much as I can, and that seems to help, but he often starts crying again the minute I put him in his cot or leave him with his toys. He also wakes up a lot at night, crying. He calms down when we cuddle him and take him into our bed, but that's no real solution of course.'

Mr Aldern nodded understandingly. 'Well, we see a lot of this, of course, and quite often we can help out. But I'll need more information in order to find the most appropriate remedy for your little boy. So tell me, how would you describe Jason's character and health up until now? Were there any particular episodes of interest? Did he have any illnesses? Did he get the scheduled vaccinations? And how did he respond to those? I see he's quite shy, but that's only to be expected; this must be just as intimidating as a visit to the GP.'

Colleen felt more reassured by the minute. This man was really asking questions, and obviously knew what he was doing. Yes, there had been the regular series of jabs during the first four months, and yes Jason did have a bit of a reaction every time. Nothing to worry about, according to the GP, so she thought nothing of it at the time. Besides, the side effects always wore off in a few days. 'Could the vaccines have anything to do with this? The last ones were well over four months ago now.'

Mr Aldern explained 'Well, we do see quite a bit of negative reactions to vaccines, and especially what we call latent effects can take many guises, such as what little Jason is going through right now. So I can't really rule that out. But let's just see what his symptoms are.'

Every now and then after asking a few questions, Mr Aldern turned to his computer. Colleen's curiosity was roused. 'Ah, you're filing everything, just like our doctor?'

'Well, yes, and then again no. This program does a lot more than that. It also sorts through and weighs all the symptoms I just entered, and helps me find the most suitable remedy for your Jason. Let's see what we found, shall we?'

Mr Aldern entered a last few things and studied the screen for a moment. 'Ah, yes, just as I expected, Pulsatilla is the first remedy of choice here. A higher potency of 30C would be in order, because the symptoms have been going on for a while. I have it here in my apothecary, and if you're OK with it, we can give the first dose right now.'

Colleen wasn't quite certain. 'Well, if you say so … And what is it with this potency? Is really harmless? And is it expensive, by the way? I had these special antibiotics once, and they cost well over two hundred pounds for only a week's course…'

'Nothing to worry about.' Mr Aldern said. 'All homeopathic remedies are completely harmless by their very nature, they're nothing like regular allopathic medicine at all; a homeopathic remedy doesn't do anything by itself, but works by activating the body's own healing mechanisms. It's as natural as you can get. If you're interested, I can explain a bit more, since you're the last visitor for today anyway. The remedy is only ten pounds, plus another thirty for the consultation. And since you seem really interested in my work, I'll just waive the normal intake fee of eighty pounds.'

With that, he stepped out the room for a few moments, and returned with a little bottle containing round white pellets. 'These little pills called globules are the remedy. They're basically sugar pills, but with a homeopathic imprint of the active ingredient; simply give Jason five globules at a time, three times a day.'

Jason at first shied away and started crying again, but after Mr Aldern handed Colleen the bottle, she managed to pop a pellet in her son's mouth. Only moments *later, Jason stopped crying, and took the other four without trouble. Within minutes, he clearly perked up, taking in his surroundings with new interest. Colleen was speechless. 'This is amazing! Does it always work this fast? How can this be? And how can people say that homeopathy doesn't really do anything?'*

Mr Aldern smiled, and explained 'Well, not always, but yes, we see this quite a lot, especially in children. Please note that since this is a higher potency remedy, relief may take a short while to set in. But you should see general improvement in a week or so. If not, please contact me again, so that we can see how to build on the improvement. And yes, now you see with your own eyes that homeopathy absolutely works. Of course, we homeopaths have known this all along, and see this every day; and what's more: it has also been scientifically proven.'

Colleen was astounded, and happily paid Mr Aldern's fee. She was also determined to find out more about homeopathy, especially since Mr Aldern had said that it isn't really all that difficult to understand. And yes, Jason did great; within a week he was his own happy self again, his smile returned, even revealing his first teeth for his parents to admire.

This story is played out countless times every day in lots of different places. And yes, it would seem an open-and-shut case for homeopathy: a child with vague complaints that the family doctor is unable to resolve is carefully examined by a homeopath, who then administers the best matching remedy, resulting in instant improvement, and a completely healed child after just a week. This is a far cry from the harsh scientific view that homeopathy is just a placebo treatment without any real effectiveness. After all, toddlers can't be fooled into believing that they are receiving an effective treatment, now can they? A child that age can't possibly fathom what the meaning is of 'sickness' and 'healing'; he just knows that he isn't feeling well, and that's what he is showing by fussing, crying, and seeking comfort with his mother. So, homeopathy works, at the very least in this case, right? And how can science be so very wrong about homeopathy? Or is there something more going on than this?

Well, yes, as a matter of fact, there is. There is quite a bit more going on, even though things may be difficult to spot at a first glance. But this story isn't quite finished yet…

A month later, Colleen gets a phone call.

'Hello, who is this? Oh, hi Mr Aldern, it's you! No, no problems at all, your remedy worked wonders every time, just as you said. And within days, our little man was quite OK again! He even had his first teeth! … Yes, thank you for following up on this, that is most thoughtful of you! … So no, there isn't anything right at the moment … oh, wait, there is one little thing we'd like your opinion on. In two months' time, when our Jason turns one, it's time for his jabs again. Now I

remember that you mentioned vaccines, and I've also been doing some more reading on the Internet ... yes, that's right ... well, we'd like to ask you for your advice on this before we go to the doctor with Jason. ... We wondered if you could do something about the side effects ... yes, especially those that you mentioned. What exactly was that again? ... 'Latent vaccine injury'? ... And that can last a really long time? But why doesn't our GP or the NHS tell us about that? ... OK, you don't know that either ... yes, on the Internet, and on Facebook too ... yes ... Oh, that is interesting, you have a homeopathic treatment for this 'vaccine injury'? And even a homeopathic alternative? Now that may be something for us! Oh yes please ... yes, next Monday afternoon will be fine. A full consultation, yes. How much is that? Oh, sixty pounds, plus remedies, well ... No, no problem. When it's about our son's health, we only want the best. And after I've seen what you can do ... Ha ha, you're welcome! Until then, bye bye!'

So what is going on here? Does Mr Aldern really know what's best for baby Jason? Is Colleen right to trust her gut feeling in this matter? And what's with those vaccinations? It also would appear that the poor family doctor has been largely sidetracked, even though he is the only one here with a medical education. How could this have happened? One could of course argue that the most important thing is that Jason is well again, and leave it at that. But that is not very satisfying, simply because it leaves too many questions unanswered. It is time to take a closer look at homeopathy.

Exactly What Is Homeopathy?

It is a common misconception that homeopathy is herbalism of a kind. Herbalism is based on the medicinal effects of plant material such as willow bark, which contains a natural painkiller, or St. John's wort, which is a natural antidepressant. Herbalism is the ancestor of our modern-day pharmaceutical industry. Even today, lots of medicines are still made from plants, as also explained in the previous chapter.

The essential difference between herbalism and homeopathy is that most homeopathic products do not contain an active ingredient at all. Also, many homeopathic remedies are not based on plants, but on other substances. More about that later, first a bit of history.

Homeopathy was invented in 1796 by a German physician by the name of Samuel Hahnemann. Hahnemann was trained as a doctor, but he wasn't very happy about his profession, and with good reason: medical treatments were not only largely ineffective, they were often far more harmful than the ailments they were supposed to cure. Instead of starting a regular medical practice, Hahnemann set out in search for better medicines, mostly by testing all sorts of medicines on himself. One day, he experimented with cinchona bark, which in those days was already known as an effective malaria medicine. After taking a dose of cinchona, Hahnemann was surprised to notice symptoms resembling malaria itself, such as shivers and fever-like sensations. He thought he had stumbled upon something very important. He did several further tests, and eventually posited that every substance had a special signature or imprint, and that this imprint would stimulate the body's self-healing mechanism in such a way, that it would cure the symptoms that it evoked in a healthy person. He called this the *Law of Similars*: 'That which causes symptoms of a disease in a healthy person, can cure those symptoms in a sick person.' This is often shortened to 'Like cures like'.

Problems Right Away

Already from the beginning, all sorts of problems cropped up. The first problem is that the *Law of Similars* doesn't appear to work for most substances, at least not in their undiluted form: if something causes certain effects, it usually does so in healthy and sick persons alike. In fact, there is not a single example of a substance that consistently produces opposite effects, depending on the state of health of a person.

Hahnemann 'solved' this by claiming that the beneficial effect (the imprint that supposedly stimulates the self-healing mechanisms of the body) could only dominate if the substance was highly diluted and also shaken (not stirred[1]) between dilution steps. He even claimed that these beneficial effects would *increase* by diluting and shaking (something Hahnemann called *potentization*).

However, this contradicts the very observation on which Hahnemann based his *Law of Similars*: cinchona bark was only effective against malaria when taken in significant amounts, not in a highly diluted form. And Hahnemann himself experienced malaria-like symptoms from cinchona bark, but again only when taking a significant dose, not a diluted dose. So was his crucial first observation a fluke? Does the *Law of Similars* normally only apply to highly diluted substances? It would appear that way. But even when that would be the case, there were more problems:

- From the very beginning, many people failed to duplicate Hahnemann's findings. Already then, many doctors noticed that it didn't seem to make

---

[1] So now you know the *real* origins of James Bond's favourite drink.

much of a difference if people were given plain water or a homeopathic dilution. Sick people didn't recover faster or better, and healthy persons did not develop any particular symptoms. This was also the outcome of the *Nuremberg salt test of 1835* (see the Science section at the end of this chapter).

- More generally, people had been diluting and shaking things for thousands of years, both accidentally and on purpose. The observation had invariably been that any effects, regardless whether beneficial or harmful, decreased with higher dilutions, never increased. Not even homeopaths could demonstrate a consistent increase in effect at higher dilutions.
- The beneficial effects were supposed to come about because the imprint of a diluted substance stimulated self-healing of the body in a very specific way, depending on the substance. Even if this were somehow true, it doesn't explain how a diluted substance would *cause* symptoms in a healthy person. And indeed, these symptoms were rarely, if ever, observed by others than homeopaths.

Despite these problems, Hahnemann claimed that he consistently saw his laws confirmed with lots of substances, and insisted that the other doctors and scientists must have been doing thing wrong.

But It Works so Much Better!

One of Hahnemann's major arguments for the efficacy of homeopathy was that patients treated with his new method often fared much better than patients who received traditional medical treatments; and yes, this was certainly true. But we now know that this was not because homeopathy is so effective, but because regular medicine was so bad. Many regular treatments did far more harm than good. Homeopathy simply boils down to doing nothing, which in many cases is the best way to deal with medical problems, even though nobody realized it in those days. Also, homeopathy can have a strong placebo effect, which further contributed to the illusion of effectiveness. For these reasons, it wasn't all that strange that homeopathy quickly became quite popular, even though its underlying principles seemed rather shaky (pun intended) already then.

Hahnemann's Miasma Theory

In the previous chapter, we talked about several ways that people historically explained the effects and spread of diseases. One of these old theories was the *miasma theory*, whereby disease spread in the form of 'bad air', emanating of rotting organic matter.

Samuel Hahnemann adapted the miasma theory into a homeopathic disease model by defining three fundamental miasmas: psora, syphilis and sycosis, each manifesting itself initially as a skin rash or lesion. In his view, psora was the primary miasma that lay at the root of most diseases. The syphilitic and sycotic miasmas were associated with syphilis and gonorrhoea respectively. He believed that it was essential to treat these miasmas themselves, and not the superficial symptoms, because 'suppressing symptoms' would only lead to far more serious problems later on.

His idea of suppressed symptoms causing problems in the future possibly stems from the natural progression of untreated syphilis, which at first shows relatively minor symptoms, which eventually disappear by themselves. The infection can then remain dormant for many years, after which it flares up again in a far more devastating manner. When this happens, it can affect almost any part of the body, causing a bewildering array of symptoms—which is why this disease is also known as 'the great pretender', as these late-stage symptoms often resemble those of completely different diseases.

Humoral theory and later also the miasma theory became obsolete in the course of the nineteenth century, after it became clear that bacteria and other pathogens were the main cause of infectious disease. Only homeopaths still believe in miasmas to this day, and especially in the claim that 'suppressing' disease symptoms (read: treating it in a science-based way) will cause far more serious problems later on. There is no evidence that this is the case—in fact, this is where homeopathy shows its self-contradictory nature once again, as the very foundation of homeopathy consists of treating (read: suppressing) symptoms instead of diagnosing and treating the underlying conditions.

Dilution or Oblivion

Then there is the dilution process itself. How diluted are homeopathic preparations? To give you an idea, we'll do a bit of practical diluting ourselves. Travel to the coast, find a seaside pub, and order a pint of beer. Now (and this is the difficult bit) *don't drink the beer*, but instead walk down the beach or seaside cliff, and tip the beer into the ocean.[2] You can watch the waves sloshing it about if you like. Diluting and shaking: homeopathy in action! Then wait a while, to make sure that the beer is mixed up well and good with the world's oceans. Finally, take a plane to the other side of the world, wade into the ocean, and scoop up a pint of water. Do you now have a typical homeopathic dilution of your beer? As a matter of

---

[2] You may want to explain your actions and motivations to the publican beforehand.

fact, no. *It is still far too concentrated.* Assuming for the sake of the argument that the beer is fully mixed with the world's oceans, even that pint of seawater still contains hundreds of molecules of the original pint of beer. Most homeopathic preparations are diluted more than that. Way more, in fact.

What we now know, but wasn't known in Hahnemann's day, is that substances can't be infinitely diluted. After a few dozen dilution steps at most, a homeopathic remedy contains not a single molecule or atom of the original substance any more (this is further explained in the Science section at the end of this chapter). So how can a substance have any effect if it completely absent?

Homeopaths these days admit that most of their remedies have no active ingredient left. They even go one step further, and claim that this is the very reason why their preparations are absolutely safe, with no harmful side effects. However, they also claim that each remedy contains a special beneficial imprint as postulated by Hahnemann, and that this imprint is what stimulates the healing process in a subtle yet very precise manner. This again may superficially sound like a plausible principle, but here too, problems arise—many problems, and big ones, at that.

The first problem is again the simple fact that even if this 'imprint' mechanism works as claimed, it offers no explanation at all how such an imprint could *cause* symptoms in healthy persons. After all, it is supposed to stimulate *healing*, not sickness.

However, the second and perhaps biggest problem is that nobody ever succeeded in finding even a smidgen of a trace of this purported 'imprint'. And these elusive imprints must have some remarkable properties indeed: they must not just be present in the homeopathic dilution, but somehow either their number or their effect must *increase* at every dilution step—after all, one of homeopathy's base principles is that remedies get more potent at higher dilutions. This is nothing short of bizarre, and flies in the face of not just common sense, but simple everyday experience.

Also, each individual imprint is associated with very specific symptoms, so each imprint must have a quite unique and intricate structure. This means that a highly diluted homeopathic preparation must contain this very specific imprint, derived from what was once dissolved in it, but is no longer present any more. Or to put it in simpler terms: water must have a memory. And for a short while in the late 1980s, a respected scientist by the name of Jacques Benveniste thought that he found evidence for this water memory.

But no. In the end, Benveniste's results could not be reliably replicated, and even the most sensitive and advanced scientific equipment can't find anything even remotely resembling an intricate imprint or memory in any form, right down to the molecular and even quantum-physical level. No special structure or 'energy' was ever found. Also, nobody can distinguish a homeopathic preparation from plain water. Even homeopaths can't tell the difference. There is, for all intents and purposes, no difference at all.

Another strange property of these imprints is that they can ostensibly be transferred from water to sugar pills without any problem. Most modern-day homeopathic remedies are not sold as liquid, but in the form of sugar pellets (so-called *globules*, just like the ones given to baby Jason), made by moistening the pellets with the final homeopathic dilution, and subsequently letting the water evaporate. This means that sugar too must have this very special memory.

Pure and Simple

And there is no end of problems still, another one being the water used to dilute the homeopathic preparation. Water is never just water, as in 100% pure H_2O; it inevitably contains other substances, such as minerals. Just read the label on a bottle of 'pure' mineral water: there's quite a lot of other stuff there, mostly minerals such as salts of sodium, potassium, calcium and magnesium. But even if homeopaths use distilled or even so-called ultra-pure water as a diluent, there will still be contaminants in that water. And if that wasn't enough, all kinds of substances will leach from any glass or metal containers used—not only minerals such as those already mentioned, but also trace amounts of lead, arsenic, and other substances. Then there is the air. Every cubic metre of air contains thousands of microbes, such as bacterial and fungal spores, and viruses. From the very first dilution step, all these things inevitably end up in the preparation. Yes, we're talking about very small amounts from a chemical point of view—parts per million or even parts per billion—but in homeopathic terms, those are *huge* amounts.

So what happens with these impurities and contaminants? Is the effect of their 'imprint' not also increased ('*potentized*') in the process? And oh, at every dilution step, a fresh batch of contaminants is added, together with the water. What effect does that have? And what to think of preparations based on the very same substance as one of the contaminants? *Arsenicum Album*, for instance, is a commonly used homeopathic remedy, based on (yes, you guessed it) arsenic. When preparing this, should the homeopath take into account the minute traces of arsenic that may leach from the glassware or the metalware used?

Or, in simpler words: if water has a memory, *how does the water know which substances to remember and potentize*? Why, it would appear that water not only has a memory, but also intelligence and even telepathic abilities—it seems to know *exactly* which substance the homeopath wishes to potentize, completely ignoring the host of other substances that are inevitably present too!

Still, homeopaths stick to their claims, and insist that this imprint is really there. After all, they *see* the effects of their homeopathic remedies, so they must be right and the imprint *must* exist—a wonderful example of circular reasoning, in other words. As it is, there are other, quite mundane explanations why homeopaths think they see effects, which we will discuss in a moment.

Homeopathic Proving

After inventing his laws of homeopathy, Hahnemann set out to test as many new remedies as possible. Since it was quite infeasible to test all those homeopathic substances on himself, he came up with a new, systematic procedure to test substances for their usefulness as a homeopathic remedy.

In a so-called *proving*, a dozen or so healthy volunteers take daily doses of a new homeopathic preparation for days, weeks or sometimes even months on end. During this time, they keep a journal, documenting any 'symptoms', which means anything out of the ordinary that they experience. Symptoms reported by multiple participants are attributed to the homeopathic preparation, and these are by definition also the symptoms in sick people that could be cured by this preparation. One notable thing here is that these 'symptoms' can be almost anything, not merely physical phenomena. For instance, 'a dream about robbers' can be a symptom, as well as 'coughing when playing the piano'.

Provings of hundreds of substances were carried out this way by Hahnemann and his assistants, and new provings still take place today. Homeopathic remedies thus identified are entered into two large books: the *Repertory*, which is a systematic list of all possible symptoms and their associated remedies, and the *Materia Medica*, which works the other way round, listing all remedies in alphabetical order, naming all symptoms that are associated with each one of those remedies.

Finding a remedy is then simply a matter of obtaining as many symptoms as possible from a patient, and then looking up the best matching remedy in the *Repertory*.

This is how homeopathy was practised in Hahnemann's day, and it is how (classic) homeopaths still work today. The only concession to modern times may be a computerized system for the *Repertory* and the *Materia Medica*, which makes finding the best matching remedy easier and faster.

Homeopathic Proving as a Medicine Trial

Maybe you already noticed the glaring problem here: a homeopathic proving does *not* involve sick people or even diseases *at all*. A new remedy is identified by having a dozen or so healthy volunteers take a new homeopathic preparation, and see what symptoms they report back. It is then simply assumed that the new remedy will cure anyone suffering from those symptoms, without actually testing it on patients.

Also, participants in such a proving are of course expecting symptoms. This means that they will experience 'symptoms' that they normally would not notice at all, and many symptoms are likely imaginary. As if this wasn't already reason enough not to trust provings, participants in provings usually *know* what kind of substance they are testing—in scientific terms: there is no *blinding*. If the proving involves for example chilli peppers, reported symptoms almost inevitably are along the lines of 'burning', 'stinging', 'hot', 'face flush' etcetera, even though the homeopathic preparation is diluted down to nothing but water. And indeed, this adequately describes the basic symptoms associated with a remedy called *Capsicum Annuum* [31]. For homeopaths, this is compelling evidence for the validity of homeopathy. Scientists, on the other hand, are not impressed at all; to them, this is proof that proper blinding is absolutely essential to rule out *expectation bias*, and that homeopathic proving is a useless ritual.

If any regular pharmaceutical company were to 'test' their products in this manner, they would be seriously punished or even forced to shut down completely. By law, regular medicines must be extensively tested for both efficacy and safety, before they are allowed on the market. Homeopaths have the curious privilege that they are allowed to sell homeopathic medicines that have not been properly tested in any meaningful way, least of all for efficacy.

Some interesting and sometimes plain nutty examples of provings are discussed in the Science section of this chapter.

The Verdict on Homeopathy

In all, there are many, many problems with homeopathy. It has all kinds of inconsistencies and contradictions, and makes wildly implausible claims that are not confirmed by science or even casual observation. It would appear that homeopathy cannot possibly work as claimed, and this is further confirmed when we look at it from a scientific point of view. If homeopathy would actually work, this would mean that a lot of our scientific knowledge in the field of chemistry, physics, and medicine must be wrong.

To put it like this: the first one to produce sound scientific proof that homeopathy actually works, would likely be awarded Nobel prizes for at least chemistry and medicine. So far, this kind of proof has never been delivered.

In fact, there is *not a single repeatable experiment* supporting any of homeopathy's 'laws' and principles. There is also not a single homeopathic product that shows any effects in a consistent, repeatable manner. All that we have are claims of homeopaths that they 'see it work'.

But if homeopathy doesn't really work, then why is it still one of the most popular forms of alternative medicine? Patient satisfaction is quite high; a recent Dutch survey showed that some 75% of people who consulted a homeopath were quite positive about the treatment and its results. Or, as homeopaths themselves often say, 'So many satisfied patients can't be wrong.' And why are most homeopaths too still convinced that it *does* work? Then there's still baby Jason: one would say that homeopathy achieved some pretty amazing results there, even if this is just one anecdote.

Alas, we're sorry to say that homeopathy indeed is nothing more than a bogus treatment, relying mostly on several simple principles that we already discussed in Chapter 4: the placebo effect, and the fact that most ailments resolve naturally, given sufficient time. There are some more mechanisms at work here, mostly of a psychological nature; those are explained in the Science section.

Yes, it would be absolutely wonderful if homeopathy would work as claimed: a perfectly harmless yet effective treatment, at a very low cost indeed, because the huge dilution factor means that you need only a minute amount of base substance; for all the rest, just add water and give it a good shaking at every dilution step. It all sounds too simple and above all too good to be true, and yes, it *is* too good to be true.

So let's dive further into what is *really* going on.

What About Baby Jason?

The story of baby Jason from the beginning of this chapter is based on two true anecdotes of mothers who consulted a homeopath with their baby.

One of the unsatisfying things about this story is that we never really found out what was wrong with Jason. The family doctor merely said that there didn't appear to be anything seriously wrong, and that Jason would probable be fine within another week or so. The homeopath also didn't come up with a real diagnosis, apart from a vague hint about 'vaccine injury'. Then again, homeopathy doesn't really deal with diagnoses or disease mechanisms, only with symptoms. The idea is to determine as many symptoms as possible as precisely as possible, and that should lead to the most appropriate remedy; disease mechanisms play no role in this.

In fact, the family doctor was right. Jason's condition is quite common for a baby his age. At eight months of age, a lot happens: the maternal antibodies which protected Jason from infectious disease for the first six months of his life are running out, and his immune system is now on its own to deal with all the microbes that it comes into contact with. This often results in several minor infections one after another,[3] until the immune system has learned how to handle the most common ones. Also, Jason was teething, and that too is a very common cause for fussiness and crying. But whatever caused Jason's problems, the vaccinations four months prior had nothing to with it. The reason why the homeopath mentioned this is that many homeopaths have jumped on the anti-vaccine bandwagon, and are often even openly hostile towards vaccination—more about that in a moment.

The mistake that our poor family doctor made was that he was probably in a hurry, and neglected to explain the situation to Colleen in more detail. This gave her the feeling of being given the brush-off instead of being taken seriously.

But what about the miraculous cure of Jason? Wasn't that brought on by the homeopathic remedy? Well, yes, and then again, no. Yes, it *was* the remedy that caused the sudden improvement. But is wasn't the elusive active ingredient, the shaken dilution of *pulsatilla* (a small, poisonous plant) that did it. Ironically, it was the other ingredient, the one that is considered 'inactive' by homeopaths—it was the sugar that homeopathic pellets are made of. In plain English: Jason was given candy. There's a lot of research confirming that a bit of sugar is very effective to make babies stop crying and fussing almost instantly [32]. Dipping baby's pacifier in a bit of sugar water is also a tried and tested home remedy in case of sleeping problems.

As the family doctor had predicted already, Jason was fine after another week or so, especially after his first teeth had broken through. The candy, erm, 'homeopathic remedy' may have made him more comfortable, but hasn't really contributed to his getting better. Jason would have been just as fine

---

[3] And this can happen again when Jason goes to daycare for the first time, when he not only makes acquaintance with new playmates, but also with new microbes; ditto at his first school day.

without it. So no, even in this case, homeopathy didn't work; it was merely an effective placebo.

Older children and adults of course are not so easily soothed with just a few grains of sugar. In these cases, the placebo effect consists of the time and attention that a homeopath spends on a client, together with several other mechanisms. See the Science section for a more in-depth discussion of these mechanisms. The most important reason for homeopathy's success, however, is that most ailments resolve naturally. If this happens while taking a homeopathic remedy or shortly thereafter, the illusion can be very convincing that it was the remedy that did it.

Ethical Considerations

Even if homeopathy does not actually work and only has a placebo effect, there are many proponents who argue that at least it makes a lot of people happy, and that it should therefore be left to people's own discretion whether to use it or not. Also, homeopathic remedies contain no active ingredients, so what is the harm in offering and using it?

The foremost problem is that placebo treatments involve an element of deception: people believe that they pay for an effective treatment, whereas all they get is a placebo, a bogus treatment, so to speak. The fact that homeopaths also believe that homeopathy really works can be considered a mitigating factor, but it does not change the fact that they charge money for something that they do not actually deliver, i.e. an effective medicine.

Also, there are real risks involved: if someone has a serious medical condition without knowing it, resorting to a homeopathic treatment as a first choice can delay proper medical care, sometimes with dire consequences. Also, most homeopaths have no medical training to speak of, so they often do not recognize serious conditions for what they are. An important bit of advice is in order here:

If you suspect that you have a medical problem, always consult a regular doctor first, not a homeopath or other alternative practitioner.

When a regular doctor is reasonably certain that there is nothing seriously wrong with you, consulting a homeopath is usually safe, provided that you keep an eye open for any signs that your condition isn't harmless after all. And always realize that the best that homeopathy or any other alternative treatment can do, is make you *feel* better. It does *not* actively cure any medical problems, regardless what homeopaths claim.

With this said, there is a much darker side to homeopathy, where trusting a homeopath can be very harmful indeed. This is the case with homeopaths who actively oppose regular medical treatment, or offer homeopathic treatment as an alternative for essential regular treatments.

Homeopathy and Vaccination

The second part of our opening story, the phone conversation about Jason's vaccinations, was explicitly added to highlight a more serious problem: the fact that in recent years, increasing numbers of homeopaths and other alternative practitioners are taking a stance against vaccination (more on vaccination in the next chapter).

The principle of vaccination was discovered by Edward Jenner in 1796, the same year that Hahnemann came up with homeopathy. Simply said, vaccination prevents people getting sick from harmful diseases by infecting them with a small bit of a disease, or with a similar but harmless disease; Jenner discovered that smallpox, a very deadly and contagious disease, could be prevented by infecting people with cowpox, a mostly harmless variety of pox. Vaccination has arguably been one of the greatest achievements in medical history, saving hundreds of millions of lives over the past two centuries, at a low cost and a very low risk.

Vaccination received praise from Hahnemann himself, not just because it helped preventing one of the most feared diseases on the planet, but because he saw it as a confirmation of his homeopathic principles. Modern-day homeopaths also often explain the *Law of Similars* by comparing homeopathy with vaccination: a tiny bit of what makes you sick is also what cures you. This is, however, not a valid comparison, even if homeopathy would actually work as claimed: vaccination *prevents* disease; homeopathy, on the other hand, is supposed to only *cure* (not prevent) disease. Furthermore, we know that vaccination works, and we also know how it works: a small amount of a pathogen is presented to the immune system, which recognizes it as 'bad', and in response starts creating antibodies to eradicate this pathogen from the body. Homeopathy does not work by any known mechanism, and a homeopathic preparation usually does not contain any active ingredient at all. And according to its own principles, giving a healthy person a homeopathic preparation should *cause* symptoms, most certainly not prevent them.

This, however, has not stopped a homeopath by the name of Isaac Golden from claiming that he actually created a homeopathic alternative to vaccination, called *homeopathic prophylaxis*, or *homeoprophylaxis* for short. According to Golden, his homeopathic prophylaxis is just as effective in preventing serious diseases as regular childhood and travellers' vaccines, and many homeopaths worldwide offer it as an alternative for regular vaccination.

This alone is a very worrisome development, because Golden's homeopathic prophylaxis cannot possibly work. Anyone who relies on this as an alternative to real vaccination is sold a false sense of security, and is just as susceptible to disease as a completely unvaccinated person. Golden claims that research proves that it does work, but that research is of a very poor scientific quality.

As if this wasn't bad enough already, many homeopaths also claim that regular vaccination causes lots of health problems they call 'vaccine injury' or 'post-vaccination syndrome', ranging from being a bit under the weather to more serious problems such as brain damage. *This is absolutely untrue.* Continuous scientific research into the effects and safety of vaccination shows no link between vaccination and any significant negative health effects whatsoever. None. Once again, homeopaths make the same old Post hoc mistake of false causality: according to them, any health problems that crop up *after* vaccination are in their view *caused by* this vaccination. And sure enough, when they treat these 'vaccine-injured' children with homeopathic remedies, the problems eventually go away, leading to yet another case of false causality—because those children would also have gotten better without the remedy.

These are very problematic developments, because parents are told that regular vaccination can be harmful for their children and should not be trusted; and they are sold useless sugar crumbs in lieu of proven effective vaccination, leaving their children fully exposed to potentially deadly and crippling diseases. This is bad for public health, not just because it contributes to outbreaks of serious diseases, but also because it undermines the public's trust in regular medicine.

If you want to consult a homeopath, verify their opinion on regular medicine beforehand. It is best to steer clear of those who endanger public health in general and children's health in particular by rejecting regular vaccination and offering homeopathic alternatives.

The same goes for homeopaths who advise against other regular treatments such as chemotherapy for cancer or psychotropic pharmaceuticals for mental problems. Their advice actually endangers the lives of sick and often desperate people.

What the Science Says

Science and homeopathy have never really been on friendly terms, and with good reason. Homeopathy is considered a pseudoscience, by claiming to adhere to scientific principles, but in actuality violating many of those principles.

One of the main problems is that homeopaths use a rather tenuous definition of 'truth'. They tell the general public that homeopathy has a 'scientifically proven' effectiveness, whereas the actual scientists unanimously agree that this is not the case.

Homeopaths also insist on adhering to methods and principles that were proven wrong already long ago; the whole concept of proving as a means to test remedies is an example. If you want to test the medicinal effects of a substance, the only proper way is to give this substance to people suffering from a particular condition, and see if they recover faster or better than without that substance. Homeopaths 'test' a substance by administering it to healthy people, to see what symptoms they develop. The only thing that this may tell you is whether a substance is harmful or not. It tells you nothing whatsoever about its use as a medicine. This was already demonstrated in Hahnemann's time, in the Nuremberg salt test of 1835.

Proving Disproved

The *Nuremberg salt test of 1835* was a major scientific milestone, as it was probably the first so-called double-blind randomized placebo-controlled trial in history [33]. In this type of experiment, a medicine is tested by comparing its effects with the effects of a fake medicine (a *placebo*), but without anyone knowing who receives the real medicine (the *verum*) and who receives a placebo. Potions or pills are all given a random code, and only at the end of the trial this code is looked up, revealing which ones were placebos and which ones were the real thing. This is the best way to determine if a medicine has significantly more effect than a placebo.

The Nuremberg salt test was such a test, and it was amazingly well set-up, even by modern-day standards. In this test, a total of 50 volunteers were given a small vial containing either a homeopathic preparation of *Natrium Muriaticum 30C* or pure water, without anyone knowing who received what. Apart from this blinding, the trial was carried out as a normal homeopathic proving. Participants were asked to take a few drops of the preparation every day over the course of several weeks, and write down any unusual symptoms in a journal.

Homeopaths supporting this trial were convinced that people receiving the homeopathic remedy would quickly notice particular symptoms, thereby proving that homeopathy's principles were sound. It turned out that they were wrong. Out of 50 participants, only 8 had noticed any unusual 'symptoms', 5 of whom had received the homeopathic remedy, while the other 3 had received plain water. This difference was far too small to be significant. Also, the very nature of this 'remedy' is another reason for doubt: *Natrium Muriaticum 30C* is nothing more than sodium chloride, or plain table salt, diluted into oblivion. Average adults have some 200 g of table salt in their body, and it is *extremely* unlikely that the homeopathic ghost of a single grain of salt can make any difference at all.

Nevertheless, until this very day, *Natrium Muriaticum* is associated with well over a hundred distinct symptoms in the *Materia Medica*, and it is still commonly prescribed by homeopaths as a remedy for all sorts of ailments [34].

But, notwithstanding the Nuremberg salt test, how is it possible that homeopathic provings consistently produce outspoken symptoms, both in Hahnemann's time and today? The answer is simple: the volunteers doing the proving usually *know* what kind of substance they are testing, and thus what symptoms to expect. And sure enough, the symptoms almost always closely match the substance's known or perceived properties. A recent proving of a homeopathic preparation based on jellyfish evoked *exactly* the symptoms one would expect:

Burning, stinging. Pins and needles, electric currents, tingling, throbbing, pulsing.

- *Feels like jelly, weakness, collapse of structure, numbness, empty.*
- *Itching, crawling ... (etcetera)*

In fact, the following quote from the supervisor of another homeopathic proving says it all:

I experienced strong symptoms from the remedy even though I did not take it [35]

Yes, you read it right: this person, himself a homeopath, literally says that the effects he experienced were *not* caused by taking the homeopathic remedy itself, but by just being involved in the proving. There is a scientific, down-to-earth explanation for this: *expectation bias*. All these people are keenly expecting certain symptoms, so their mind and body obligingly produce the appropriate symptoms—which is in fact just another manifestation of the placebo effect.

The previous paragraphs merely demonstrate that the whole concept of proving is fatally flawed, even though the materials tested, such as minerals and plants, are still within the realm of common sense. Things become truly bizarre when we take a look at what other things were subjected to proving.

* In 2002, a British homeopath by the name of Mary English did a proving of an old shipwreck, lodged in a sandy beach in Wales. The participants in this proving had detailed knowledge of the background of this shipwreck, and sure enough, the 'symptoms' they described exactly matched the ship's log of its final hours
* In 2009, a homeopath named Patricia Maher performed a proving of the light of Saturn [36]. This once again shows that many homeopaths are quite disconnected from any scientific world view, and are rather prone to magical thinking. These are not people who you want to trust with your health.
* Homeopaths have even come up with a 'remedy' based on debris from the Berlin Wall [37].

There are many more examples of bizarre provings and other homeopathic practices, sometimes involving 'energy' of a kind, and/or fancy equipment, and one proving even involves antimatter (which begs the question where this was obtained, as it is currently only produced as single atoms in huge machines called particle accelerators). Other homeopaths claim that simply writing down something on a scrap of paper and then placing a glass of water on top of that paper will somehow imbue that water with whatever the text says. Even Hahnemann himself would turn in his grave, could he see what is done in the name of homeopathy.

Crunching the Numbers on Homeopathic Dilutions

Hahnemann's *Law of Infinitesimals* posits that diluting (and shaking) a substance will reduce harmful effects, but *increase* its beneficial effects. This claim once again goes against all human experience, both in the everyday sense and in a scientific context: diluting something will *always* reduce whatever effect it has. Add more water to lemonade, and all you get is increasingly watery lemonade, nothing else (and you can shake it all you want, but that doesn't change a thing). Dilute a medicine, and it will have less effect—and from a certain point onwards, it will have no effect at all any more, period. There is not a single example in science where diluting a substance consistently leads to a stronger effect, regardless whether that effect is beneficial or not. Yet homeopaths claim that they see this happen all the time with their remedies. Clearly, someone is wrong here.

Homeopathic Dilution Scales

Stepwise dilution in homeopathy takes place in steps of 1:10 (the D or X scale), or 1:100 (the C or K scale). The most common homeopathic dilution is 30C, which means diluting of 1 part of the previous dilution with 99 parts water, repeated 30 times in a row.

This doesn't sound like a big deal, but it actually means that there is not a single atom or molecule left in the final dilution. To demonstrate this, we'll make our own homeopathic sleep medicine—and yes, feel free to try this at home.

Making Your Own Homeopathic Remedy

Let's say that you suffer from sleeplessness. According to homeopathic principles, this means that you first need to find a substance that is known to *cause* sleeplessness. Yes, you guessed it: coffee is the potion of choice here, with caffeine being the active ingredient on which we will base our homeopathic remedy.

We begin with one small cup of black coffee, 100 millilitres (ml) in total. Then we simply follow homeopathy's methodology: dilute it with water by one part in a hundred, thirty times in a row, shaking it in between dilutions, and we're there: we have created a homeopathic remedy by the name of *Coffea Cruda 30C* in our own kitchen!

However, as we're taking the scientific approach, we want to keep track of what happens to the caffeine (the active ingredient) while we do this. So first, let's look up how much caffeine we start with. It turns out that 100 ml of coffee contains roughly 40 mg of caffeine. With a bit of high school chemistry we can then calculate the actual number of caffeine molecules in those 40 mg. For this, we simply divide the weight of the caffeine in grams (0.04) by the so-called molar mass of caffeine (194), and then multiply the result with the *Avogadro constant* (6×10^{23}). This gives us roughly 1.2×10^{20} caffeine molecules.

As a first step, we take 1 millilitre (ml) of coffee (approximately 10 drops), which contains 1% of those 1.2×10^{20} caffeine molecules, so 1.2×10^{18} or 12,000,000,000,000,000 molecules. This is a huge number, so a bit of diluting shouldn't be a problem, right? Well, let's see ....

We dissolve this 1 millilitre of coffee in 99 ml fresh water (one teacup). Cover the top, shake it properly, and presto, we have our first 1:100 dilution, or 1C in homeopathic jargon. The new number of caffeine molecules has of course decreased by a factor of 100, which is simply a matter of removing two zeros from our big number:

1C: 12,000,000,000,000,000 caffeine molecules

Now we repeat the procedure over and over again, so that we get 2C, then 3C, etcetera:

2C: 120,000,000,000,000
3C: 1,200,000,000,000
4C: 12,000,000,000

...

7C: 12,000
8C: 120
9C: 1.2?
10C: 0.012??

Hang on, what's going on here? We're still only at 9C, and we're already down to the last molecule! And what happens if we go one step further? We can't have less than one molecule of caffeine, because it wouldn't be caffeine any more—just like 0.012 of a car is not a car any more. From 10C upwards, *not a single molecule of caffeine remains in the dilution.* Yet homeopaths merrily keep on diluting, in effect diluting water with water, for another 20 steps.

This is one of the big problems with homeopathy: after the tenth or eleventh dilution step, there is no active ingredient left, regardless of the original substance. What is left is water, nothing else. So how can this still have any effect? The answer is simple: it can't. Homeopaths claim that the caffeine has left an 'imprint' in the water, and that this imprint is not only preserved but even increased at every dilution step, but neither this imprint nor its effects (let alone increasing effects at higher dilutions) have ever been observed, neither by scientists nor by homeopaths.

What About Our Oceanic Beer?

In a previous paragraph, we tipped a pint of beer in the ocean, and explained that the resulting dilution was still more concentrated than most homeo-pathic remedies. Now that we know a bit more about the actual numbers, you may wonder what dilution we actually have, homeopathically speaking.

As it turns out, that calculation too is fairly simple: we simply diluted one pint, say half a litre, in all the world's oceans. So we turn to the Internet and look up the amount of water in the oceans, which apparently is 1.3 billion cubic kilometres, so 1.3×10^9 cubic kilometres. As one cubic kilo-metre contains $1000 \times 1000 \times 1000 = 10^9$ cubic metres, and one cubic metre contains $1000 = 10^3$ L, all the world's oceans contain a total of $1.3 \times 10^{(9+9+3)} = 1.3 \times 10^{21}$ L of water. Half a litre divided by this amount gives us a dilution of 1 on 2.6×10^{21}, so about eleven 1:100 dilution steps, or 11C. This is indeed way less than the often used 30C dilution.

However, our beer experiment still has a major flaw: it would take centuries before that one pint of brew is evenly distributed throughout the world's oceans. So it is probably best to just drink your seaside beer after all and do the whole homeopathic dilution thing as a thought experiment.

The Case of *Oscillococcinum*

Another bizarre example is the story of a rather well-known homeopathic product called *Oscillococcinum*, which supposedly prevents or shortens a flu infection.

In 1918, a French army doctor by the name of Joseph Roy was one of the many doctors searching for the cause of the catastrophic influenza pandemic then ravaging the world, causing between 50 and 100 million deaths. When he examined a flu patient's blood under a microscope, he observed vibrating round objects, and he thought that he had found the bacterium responsible not only for the 1918 flu pandemic, but for many other diseases as well. He called them *oscillococci*, which simply means 'vibrating ball-shaped bacteria'.

He decided to create a homeopathic remedy based on these oscillococci, and set out to find a reliable source of this bacterium, which he thought he found in duck liver. Up until this day, *Oscillococcinum* is produced by fermenting mashed-up duck liver and heart, then creating a 200C dilution of this putrid liquid, the end result of which is sprayed on sugar pellets which are dried. Once again, this may sound somewhat plausible at a glance, but in reality, every single step in producing this remedy is completely wrong or absurd:

- Oscillococci do not exist, as they have never been observed by anyone else. Joseph Roy probably wasn't very good at using a microscope, and most likely mistook small air bubbles in his slides for bacteria. The vibrations he noticed were almost certainly caused by so-called Brownian motion.
- The cause of influenza is not a bacterium, but a far smaller pathogen called a virus—something that Roy could not have observed in 1918.
- Even though ducks are indeed known to carry influenza viruses that may infect humans, these avian flu viruses are not normally present in the liver or the heart, but in the intestinal tract.
- The final dilution is 200C. This means that the original substance is diluted by a factor of 1 to 10^{400}. This is spectacularly absurd, as our known universe only contains approximately 10^{80} atoms.

Scientific research also confirms that Oscillococcinum has no effect on any disease whatsoever. Yet in spite of this, this 'remedy' achieves gross sales of over 300 million dollars annually.

Why Homeopaths and Patients Think Homeopathy Works

The effects of homeopathy are usually attributed to the placebo effect, but there are more mechanisms that play a role here. The following are the most significant mechanisms that contribute to homeopathy's perceived effects and popularity. Most of these mechanisms were already explained in Chapter 4, but if can't hurt to bring them back to mind:

- **Most health problems resolve spontaneously**. When people don't feel well, they will usually try to do something about it. And when things subsequently improve, the illusion can be very strong indeed that this was due to whatever was done, be it hot tea with honey, 'sweating it out', or homeopathic sugar crumbs. This is the single biggest mental trap for both homeopaths and their customers: any improvement *after* taking a remedy is automatically attributed *to* that remedy. This is the fallacy of false causation, or *post hoc ergo propter hoc*.
- **People usually seek treatment when complaints are quite severe**. In other words: when people don't feel well, they usually wait a little while to see if the problems resolve on their own. When instead things get worse and they really become uncomfortable, they will start looking for help. But as the majority of ailments eventually clear up by themselves, there is a very

good chance that this happens *after* consultation of a doctor or a homeopath. This principle is called *regression to the mean*, and is a well-know cause for falsely attributing healing to the effects of a treatment. When the ailment goes away *before* seeking help, this of course is not linked to any treatment, so those cases are not counted.

- **The placebo effect.** The placebo effect can make people feel better almost instantly, simply because they *expect* to feel better. A scientist by the name Ted Kaptchuk has done a lot of research in this field, and he discovered that the placebo effect sometimes even works when people *know* that they take a placebo. There is also the opposite effect called the *nocebo* effect. Both effects are almost always observed in regular placebo-controlled medicine trials: participants who receive a placebo without knowing it often report both beneficial effects and side effects.

  In homeopathy, the placebo effect is mostly due to the amount of time and attention that someone receives from a homeopath. In a very real sense, this attention *is* the remedy.

  The placebo effect can, however, be dangerous, because it can mask the symptoms of a really serious condition. In one experiment, asthma patients who received a placebo reported feeling almost as well as patients who received real medication. However, the lung capacity of the placebo group was still far worse than the medicated group, putting them at risk of a potentially deadly asthma attack.

- **"But we see that it works with our own eyes!"** This is the single most common defence of homeopaths when confronted with scientific arguments that homeopathy cannot possibly work. And yes, they are right, they 'see it work with their own eyes'. But we all know that looks can be deceiving; our own eyes fool us on an almost daily basis. This is what happens with homeopathy too.

- **Social reciprocity and positive attitude.** As already mentioned, homeopaths spend a lot of time and attention on their customers, and positive attention at that. A good homeopath lends their customers a listening ear with a very patient and understanding attitude. Anyone who receives this kind of attention will unconsciously tend to return this in a positive manner, often reporting more progress than there actually is.

  This is stimulated further by the homeopath urging to 'look out for any sign of improvement', as that is supposed to mean that the remedy is working. And if the chosen remedy doesn't appear to help after several weeks, well, there are many more remedies that can be tried, so there is always hope! It is not unusual for a homeopath and a customer to keep 'trying' for several months, until either the problems have disappeared (which is then of course chalked up as another success for homeopathy), or the customer finally gives up. Many homeopaths also keep a warm customer relationship by actively following up on a treatment at a later date: they call people to ask if everything is still all right, and if there is anything else that they can do. This is also what happened in the case of baby Jason.

• **The nature of the health problems**. Homeopaths preferably deal with rather vague and/or chronic complaints, rather than acute clinical problems such as obvious infections. Again, the story of baby Jason is a case in point. Health problems of this category are the most likely to elicit the placebo effect, or at least show some improvement over time (even if that improvement is temporary), strengthening the illusion that homeopathy is working.

• **The nature of the treatment**. Homeopathy involves no unpleasant examinations or invasive procedures; even its remedies cannot possibly have side effects. And if homeopaths and/or customers insist that the treatment really works, it is of course very tempting to give it a try. Who would not want to be cured of his or her ailment, without any risk or even uncomfortable things happening? Alas, a treatment that is guaranteed without side effects is also guaranteed ineffective.

Conclusion

Homeopathy is form of medicine that violates not just everyday experience, but many scientific principles. Homeopathic preparations usually contain no active substances, and the effects that homeopaths claim they see are based on imaginary 'information patterns' in water and even sugar—patterns that no-one has ever observed in any form or way.

In the end, there is one simple fact that disproves all of homeopathy: even after well over two hundred years, homeopaths have not succeeded in coming up with even one 'remedy' showing significant and independently repeatable effects in experiments or trials.

Many other forms of traditional and alternative medicine have led to at least a few successful treatments that have since become part of real medicine, but not homeopathy.

So far, we discussed several different ways to treat people suffering from illness. The next chapter goes one step further, and deals with one particular, sometimes hotly disputed way to *prevent* disease: vaccination.

8

An Ounce of Prevention …

Not Anti-vaccine

'*Today we will discuss vaccines in general and childhood vaccines in particular with our special guest Mr K. He is an expert on this sometimes controversial subject, with no less than three books to his name. So welcome Mr K!*'

'*Hello Dylan, thank you for having me here! I really hope that I can bring some sense and clarity into this whole debate that's been going on, and that your listeners can finally make up their own mind in a well-informed way.*'

'*So, Kyle, just to kick off with a blunt question: would you describe yourself as anti-vaccine?*'

'*No, I would certainly not describe myself as anti-vaccine! I am in fact very much pro-vaccine, and think that it is always best to prevent disease whenever possible. But any vaccines out there should be 100% tested and safe – so I'm basically pro-SAFE-vaccine.*'

'*But aren't the vaccines out there safe? I'm sure I read that they were extensively tested, and this is also what doctors and scientists claim, and of course the pharmaceutical companies that make those vaccines.*'

'*Yes, I heard those claims too, but I don't think those vaccines are properly tested at all. Did they do a proper double-blind test of fully vaccinated children versus fully unvaccinated children? No, they didn't. Did they test for long-term side effects? No, they didn't. Did they test the vaccines on children at all? No, they didn't – testing was done on healthy adults, not on children with immune systems that were still developing. They just tested the vaccines on maybe thirty thousand people for half*'

R. Rasker, *Mind, Make-Believe and Medicine*, https://doi.org/10.1007/978-3-031-29444-0_8

a year or so, but now they give them to billions of innocent kids. So you see? No real testing at all!

And just think about it: who is doing the testing? Is it the government? No. Is it an independent lab? No, it is the vaccine makers themselves who test their own products. Can you trust them to get it right? Of course not!'

'Well, you may have a point there, but haven't those childhood vaccines proven themselves in practice by now? After all, some have been used for thirty or forty years now, without any problems as far as we know.'

'There, you just said it: as far as we know. Because all those vaccines have not really been tested, we don't really know if they're safe or not. In fact, there are a lot of health problems these days that we didn't use to have, such as allergies, auto-immune problems, obesity and autism, to name just a few.'

'Are you saying that these conditions are all caused by childhood vaccinations?'

'Well, what else can it be? If you look at the graphs, you can clearly see it: number of shots going up since the eighties, and at exactly the same time, autism diagnoses suddenly went through the roof. Also, those vaccines have all sorts of toxins in them that are very harmful to the development of young children, such as mercury, formaldehyde and aluminium. All these things are known to cause brain damage and other problems.'

'But don't those vaccines at least protect children from all sorts of very dangerous diseases?'

'That's another thing they want you to believe. No, vaccines have done almost nothing to protect our children. Here, let me show you another graph, with measles deaths over the past century and a half. You see? Almost no children died of measles any more before they started those vaccination campaigns. And why do children still get whooping cough, if those vaccines work so well?'

'Well, Kyle, we've got a commercial break coming up, so we'll have to make it short for now. You're saying that vaccines should be tested far better, is that right?'

'Yes, they really should do a double-blind fully vaccinated versus fully unvacci- nated test, with at least a couple of million children. Half should get the vaccine, the other half placebos.'

'OK, clear. And earlier, you mentioned something about long-term effects?'

'Yes, that is also a major issue. Vaccines are put out there after maybe one or two years of study. That's way too short for any serious long-term side effects to show.'

'Then how long do you propose testing should take?'

'As long as need be, so that we can be sure that our children are safe.'

'So what you're basically saying is that vaccines should be tested on several million children volunteers, for up to ten or twenty years, and double-blind at that, with another group of millions of children left fully unvaccinated. And only after this long-term study is concluded should the results become available. And oh, this study should not be done by pharmaceutical companies. Am I right?'

'Yes, that about sums it up pretty neatly. As I said, I am very much pro-SAFE- vaccine, so this testing should be done properly, with results you can trust.'

'OK, well, there you have it folks, we need to do much better in those vaccine studies. After all, the safety of our children is at stake here! Kyle, thank you very much for being here!'

'All my pleasure, bye!'

There is probably no health intervention that has sparked so much emotionally laden debate and controversy as vaccination, even before the Covid-19 pandemic with its vaccine mandates in several countries around the world.

Anti-vaccine people sometimes go out of their way to portray vaccines as something inherently evil, causing almost all and any health problems that can't be easily explained otherwise. Some of these problems were already mentioned in the preceding (fictional) interview[1]; there are however many more health conditions attributed to vaccines: infertility, cerebral palsy, chronic fatigue syndrome, paralysis, pancreatitis, cardiac arrest, intestinal problems, brain inflammation, vertigo—you name it, and vaccines have been named as a culprit at one time or other. Some people even go as far as to use hyperboles such as 'vaccine holocaust'. Some others claim that vaccination programs are really a conspiracy to give some sort of 'shadow elite' full control over us mortals, with 5th generation wireless networks (5G) used for controlling us via microchips in vaccines, as puppets on strings as it were.

In this chapter, we will try to explain why some people have such an aversion towards something that arguably saved hundreds of millions of lives. We will look at what vaccines actually *do* (and, importantly, do *not* do). To explain this, we also need to look at what happens when we catch a bug, so to speak, and how our immune system responds to this invasion of our body.

No Trespassing

The British have this saying *My Home is my Castle*, to express the sentiment that their home should be inviolate, and with good reason. You don't want just anyone to enter your home and do whatever they like, because that would seriously upset your personal life. Rather quickly, you would not have a personal life any more, or even a place to call home.

The same goes for your body: you really don't want just anything to be able to take up residence inside your body, plunder the fridge and make itself at home—let alone use your body as a nursery. Simply said, you don't want to catch an infection—which is a bit of a problem, as microbes are literally

---

[1] Made up by yours truly, but based on real talking points from real anti-vaccine activists.

everywhere. So like almost all higher organisms, we evolved a tough outer layer (read: skin) to keep out unwelcome guests.

Unfortunately, we necessarily need to have at least some holes in this skin in order to breathe, eat, and drink, among other things, and those holes are sort of an open invitation to lots of pathogenic microbes to come on in and party. Also, it is possible to poke new holes in skin.

This means that plan A—skin alone—even though quite helpful already, isn't enough, and evolution came up with plan B: a system that is capable of fighting off any microbes that may make it into our body. This system to ward off disease-causing infectious microbes (so-called *pathogens*) is of course the immune system, and it is pretty clever: it can distinguish between cells and proteins that belong in our body, and things from outside. When the immune system recognizes something as 'non-self', two things happen:

1. The intruder is immediately attacked and destroyed by immune cells.
2. A 'fingerprint' of the intruder is made, meaning that a sort of copy of its characterizing proteins is made. This copy is then used to create so-called *antibodies* that can latch on to exactly these proteins, effectively inactivating any new specimens of this particular pathogen. This fingerprint is also memorized in (yes, you guessed it) memory cells, so that a future infection with the same bug can be fought off much faster.

The first action is done by what is called the *innate immune system*. The second, more elaborate procedure is carried out by the *adaptive immune system*. The adaptive immune system is far better and more efficient at eliminating intruders, except at the very first encounter: then it needs time to start up the production of antibodies for that new pathogen, which usually takes a week or so.

This time delay between the actual infection and the production of large numbers of antibodies is a bit of a problem, because a virus or bacterium can multiply relatively unhindered during that time. This means that getting infected is the start of a race—a race between the pathogen on one hand, and the immune system on the other hand. If the pathogen multiplies slowly and doesn't cause serious damage, then the immune system wins the race easily, and you may not even notice the infection before it is eradicated. However, if the pathogen multiplies fast and causes significant damage, you may get pretty sick before the immune system gets on top of it and you get better again. And if you're really unlucky, you suffer critical damage or even die before the immune system manages to produce enough antibodies.

Once the infection has been successfully fought off, things look a lot better: you are protected against renewed infection, often for a long time, and in some cases for the rest of your life. Because as soon as the pathogen returns, any antibodies still circulating in your blood immediately attack it. Also, the immune system's memory cells holding this bug's mug shot kick into action again, and start the production of fresh antibodies right away. This usually happens so fast that the intruder has no time to multiply and make you miserable before being eradicated; in most cases, a renewed infection goes completely unnoticed.

Enter the Vaccine

The concept of vaccination is extremely simple: take a dangerous pathogen, break it into pieces or render it harmless in another way, and then inject it into people. Or even simpler: trick cells in the body into making some of the parts of a dangerous pathogen.

Either way, the immune system then recognizes those weakened bugs or their parts as harmful intruders, and responds in exactly the same way as if the real disease had infected the body: by making antibodies and storing a fingerprint of the offending material in memory cells.

I will explain how vaccines are made in more detail in the Science section. First, we will look at two natural ways that provide us with immunity against infectious diseases: natural immunity and maternal immunity.

Natural Immunity

Natural immunity is the immunity that you get by living through an infectious disease. Many anti-vaccine people and proponents of alternative medicine claim that this immunity is superior to vaccine-induced immunity, and there is indeed some truth to this: being sick for a week or so means that your body is overrun by pathogens, causing a very strong and extended immune response (and you feeling pretty awful). This is quite different from receiving a vaccine with only a very limited dose of antigens.

Getting through an infection often elicits better and longer lasting immunity than getting vaccinated for the same disease. So is it better to rely on natural immunity than on vaccines, as anti-vaccine activists often claim?

The thinking error here should be obvious: in order to get natural immunity against a deadly disease, someone must first *survive* this disease—and getting sick with a disease is what vaccines are supposed to prevent.

Contracting a potentially deadly disease first in order to become immune to this dangerous disease is putting the horse behind the cart. Another snag is that some diseases (for instance tetanus) don't produce any immunity, even if you survive them.

Maternal Immunity

Maternal immunity is a type of so-called *passive immunity* that babies are born with, and is conveyed by the antibodies that passed from the mother's blood via the placenta into the baby's blood. These antibodies typically last for about six months after birth, at which point the baby's immune system has to learn to recognize and fend off the countless microbes it encounters all by itself. This also explains why many babies start having one minor infection after another at six or seven months of age.

Also note that this maternal immunity only includes the diseases that the mother has developed antibodies against. If she was never infected with a particular disease, then her baby is also susceptible to that disease from the day it is born.

Some vaccination critics argue that this maternal immunity makes it unnecessary to vaccinate children. Even though this argument is generally incorrect, there is an extra twist to it that can explain some peculiarities with some childhood diseases, as explained in the sidebar.

The Polio Mystery

For most of human history, paralytic polio was so rare that people didn't even know that the sparse cases of childhood paralysis that occasionally occurred were in fact caused by one specific disease. Things changed in the 1800s, when clusters of paralysis cases began to appear in Europe and the United States. From 1900 onwards, outbreaks grew into epidemics, with ever increasing numbers of victims, and by 1916, it was clear that some sort of mysterious infectious disease was the cause. Doctors and scientists were caught off-guard: lots of other infectious diseases such as cholera and typhoid fever became less of a problem with improving living standards and better hygiene. So why this totally unexpected and dramatic increase in polio cases?

It turned out that hygiene indeed had something to do with it, together with maternal immunity and the characteristics of the disease itself. Polio is a highly infectious intestinal disease that mostly spreads via the so-called faecal-oral route. This means that in unhygienic conditions, virtually everyone is exposed to the virus almost on a daily basis. Because small infants still have maternal immunity, this exposure has no consequences for the first six months of their life. By the time this immunity starts to wane, the immune system has had ample opportunity to get to know the virus, and start producing its own antibodies and memory cells against it. In a way, this can be seen as 'natural vaccination'.

This pre-emptive exposure to the polio virus decreased as hygienic living circumstances improved with better sanitation. This became problematic when infants did not have contact with the virus until after their maternal immunity had disappeared: the virus had free rein to wreak havoc in the body, until the immune system caught up with events and got its antibody production up and running—taking at least a week.

What made things worse was that a polio infection goes completely unnoticed in two thirds of cases, and only produces mild to moderate cold-like symptoms in most other cases. Only about one percent of infections leads to paralysis. This means that polio could circulate in the greater population without being noticed, making it impossible to recognize (and avoid) infected persons, as only a few unlucky ones developed clear polio symptoms. From about 1920 until the advent of mass polio vaccination in 1957, every cough and runny nose was cause for alarm. These cold-like symptoms were especially dreaded during the summer season, when polio spread more easily via uncooked food, contaminated swimming water and even insects such as house flies, which could carry viruses from sewage to fresh food.

The Anti-vaccine World

So far, vaccination seems like a good way to prevent people (and especially children) from getting sick and sometimes even dying. Just trick the immune system into making antibodies by presenting it with a weakened version or even just a few parts of a pathogen, and they're protected! No big deal, technically speaking—and indeed, modern medical science can make vaccines that are extremely safe and still very effective. So why do quite a few people still have a deep-felt aversion against vaccination?

First off, anti-vaccine sentiments are nothing new; they started out basically from the moment that Edward Jenner came up with the first smallpox vaccine in 1796. This vaccine was based on cowpox, a close relative of smallpox, but far less dangerous—close enough, in fact, that the antibodies made by the immune system against the cowpox virus were just as effective against smallpox virus. Now of course in those days, nobody knew about viruses or antibodies or even the immune system. All that people saw, was that pus from cowpox blisters was used to deliberately infect healthy people, after which they were supposedly protected from smallpox. This prompted an 1802 cartoon artist to draw the first anti-vaccine meme ever: *The Cow Pock— or—the Wonderful Effects of the New Inoculation*, where vaccinated people developed all sorts of horrible cow-related growths, including horns, udders and even partial miniature cows [38].

Over the course of the years, people have come up with lots of reasons to distrust or even shun vaccination. Some of these reasons are more or less valid (or at least understandable), while other reasons are simply wrong. The following paragraphs will discuss the most common ones.

Integrity of the Human Body

One reason to be wary of vaccination has to do with the instinctive aversion of almost all living creatures to anything intruding into the body. Getting stung by something or having the skin pierced in another way is usually not good news. Best case, it is merely a painful warning to stay away from a plant or an animal, but getting bitten by disease-carrying insects can have really serious consequences. Then there is of course the always present risk of infection. So having someone poke needles in you is not something that we would naturally welcome.

Anti-vaccine activists often invoke the right to bodily integrity to reject vaccination, especially for children, as they're too young to give informed consent. This argument is however largely fallacious, as getting infected with a potentially deadly disease constitutes a far bigger violation of someone's bodily integrity than an injection with virtually no risk at all.

Vaccine Mandates

Related to the previous point is the question of mandatory vaccination. This too is a legitimate concern: is it ethically justified to make vaccination compulsory for everyone, even adults? If so, under which circumstances? Two things should be noted:

* In many countries, vaccination is already mandatory in certain situations, such as for medical students and healthcare personnel, and for children's access to daycare and public schools. Also, lots of countries require visitors to be vaccinated against certain tropical diseases.
* Governments already have legal power over their citizens, including the right to intrude upon someone's bodily integrity, e.g. when someone is a crime suspect. To this end, most constitutions that guarantee a person's right to bodily integrity also stipulate exceptions to this right in certain well-defined situations.

Still, it is desirable to keep vaccination voluntary as much as possible, if only because history shows that mandatory vaccination is often counter-productive. This means that mandates should only be used in emergency situations, where not vaccinating would endanger the lives of a significant part of the population. (And of course the bone of contention then becomes what qualifies as an emergency.)

'Vaccinating = Medically Treating Healthy People'

Vaccination by definition means that *healthy* people are subjected to a medical intervention, and this is another thing that feels instinctively wrong. You treat people when they're sick, not when they are healthy. When taken together with the next point, you get the additional problem that there is risk involved as well, making it even more unattractive to get yourself or your children vaccinated. We also have several sayings along the lines of *If it isn't broken, don't fix it* to express the notion that you shouldn't interfere with something that is working just fine—in this case a human body.

But even though this too is quite an understandable argument, it is still fallacious. We do preventive things all the time, such as buying home insurance, or wearing seatbelts or a motorcycle helmet. All these things cost money or limit our freedom in some way, even though no-one expects to be the victim of a burglary, a fire or a traffic accident. Yet we accept that these things can happen nonetheless, and that preventive measures indisputably prevent far worse things such as financial ruin, severe injuries or death.

'Vaccines Can Have Serious Side Effects'

It is a fact that vaccines can have side effects, sometimes even serious side effects, up to and including death. However, vaccine side effects are almost always harmless. Serious side effects are very rare, usually in the range of one per tens of thousands or even hundreds of thousands of vaccinations. Those serious side effects almost always involve a severe allergic reaction, so an overreaction of the immune system to the vaccine. Vaccine-related deaths are much rarer still—so rare, in fact, that it is hard to put a number to. Most estimates peg the incidence at something of maybe one death per every 10 million vaccinations, mostly among people with pre-existing health problems.

Still, even these extremely small chances are reason for some people to decline vaccination. The fallacy here is twofold:

- The disease in question usually comes with a far, far higher risk of serious side effects (read: physical damage) and death.
- Everyone takes far greater risks on a daily basis. For instance here in the Netherlands, simply leaving the house comes with a risk of 1 in about 10 million of getting killed in traffic—*every single day.* Yet nobody stays indoors for this reason.

A reason why vaccines have less serious side effects than regular medicines is that vaccines are distinctly different from medicines. Vaccines don't work by changing chemical processes inside the body, but by merely 'showing' the immune system the distinctive features of a pathogen. In fact, all vaccines basically do the exact same thing, and this thing already happens naturally in our body every day: our immune system is continuously faced with potentially harmful microbes, which it then eliminates and remembers for future infections. Vaccines only differ in the details how this is done. More about this in the Science section.

'What About Long-Term Side Effects?'

Another often-heard concern about newer vaccines in particular is the potential risk of long-term side effects. Again, this is a reasonable question. After all, there have been medicines as well as herbal products that caused serious health problems in the long run [39]. So what about vaccines?

There are several reasons why it is extremely unlikely that vaccines would cause any long-term health problems. The first reason is that there are in fact very few substances that can cause long-term damage after just incidental exposure; most long-term harmful effects arise from continuous exposure to something harmful—smoking is a point in case. Vaccines are administered only occasionally. And indeed, in the 226 years that vaccines have been used, not a single one has had long-term effects. (Well, except for one intentional long-term effect: immunity against a particular disease.)

The second reason is the way vaccines work: they just present the immune system with (parts of) a pathogen, and the immune system responds by destroying this vaccine material, as well as programming memory cells to respond to any new encounters. Vaccines don't alter the body's chemistry, they don't influence hormonal systems or anything like that. Basically, they do exactly the same that pathogens do every day—but without causing serious disease in the process. And, as already mentioned, the vaccine material is cleared from the body in just a couple of days or weeks at most.

'Vaccines Have Not Been Properly Tested'

The argument that vaccines have not been properly tested, also featuring prominently in our opening story, is another major reason for to be wary of vaccines. This is in a way a weakened variant of the previous arguments about potentially serious and/or long-term side effects: even if we don't see any serious side effects, we should not just assume that vaccines are safe. They should be thoroughly tested and proven safe, especially as they are intended to be given to healthy children—*all* healthy children. Until such testing has been done, we should not use them. This is an application of the *precautionary principle*, which argues that anything new should be considered dangerous until proven otherwise.

So are vaccines properly tested or not? The contentious word here is *properly*. Even vaccination critics admit that vaccines are tested, but argue that this testing is not done thorough and long enough. These are the two main arguments:

'We Need Real Vaccinated Versus Unvaccinated Trials'

Anti-vaccine activists claim that there is only one way to find any detrimental effects of mass childhood vaccinations: through a huge double-blind randomized 'vaccinated vs unvaccinated' trial. This is, however, a bad argument in several respects. There have been many studies comparing the health of vaccinated and unvaccinated children. The simplest and at the same time biggest studies simply looked at children's health before and after introduction of mass measles vaccination in several countries. The outcome was that measles vaccination had one very clear effect: vaccinated children were healthier, simply because they no longer got measles or one of its serious complications (deafness, brain inflammation, death). For al the rest, vaccinated children were just as healthy as the unvaccinated ones. One example is the so-called Finnish study, where a total of 1.8 million people were followed before and after MMR vaccination (Measles, Mumps, Rubella), for a total of 14 years [40]. No problems were found.

This was also the outcome from later studies comparing unvaccinated children (usually from anti-vaccine parents) with vaccinated children: there was no difference in health. And when the HPV vaccine was introduced in the Netherlands, only half of all eligible girls got the vaccine, with the other half rejecting it for fear of possible negative health effects. While undesirable from a public health point of view, this presented the perfect opportunity to compare the health of two very large groups of vaccinated and unvaccinated girls. The outcome once again was that there was no difference at all. All sorts of health problems that anti-vaccine people attributed to HPV vaccination (such as chronic fatigue syndrome and infertility) occurred in exactly the same numbers in both groups.

Then there is the ethical point: with their 'vaccinated vs unvaccinated' trial, anti-vaccine activists in fact demand that a very large group of children is left completely unvaccinated, exposing them to harmful and even deadly diseases, without knowing. There is no medical ethics committee in the world that would ever approve of such a trial, especially since the efficacy of these vaccines in protecting children has been established beyond a shadow of a doubt. In other words: even for an individual child, the risk of harm posed by disease when left unvaccinated is still greater than any risk of harm from the vaccine itself.

'Vaccines Aren't Tested for Long-Term Effects'

Earlier on, it was already discussed why it is extremely unlikely that vaccines have any long-term side effects. Still, an often-heard claim is that vaccines have not been actually *tested* for any long-term effects, and thus should still not be trusted. Well, this is true to an extent; most phase 3 clinical trials (see the previous chapter) test a vaccine for something between 1 and 2 years. The argument, however, is disingenuous: the only way to test something for effects that may perhaps surface after 20 years is *to test that something for 20 years*.

So should vaccine manufacturers really spend 20 years testing each of their products on millions of people before concluding that it is safe? The answer is of course that this is utterly impossible, if only for the astronomical cost that this would entail. And what if something bad happens after 25 or 30 years? Also think of those millions or even billions of people who will suffer and sometimes even die from the disease in question while waiting for long-term tests to be completed—tests that with almost 100% certainty will not find any problems.

The bottom line is that these arguments and demands simply aren't realistic. Vaccines are deemed safe enough for general use after several years of testing without serious problems. This demand that a pharmaceutical product should be both 100% safe and 100% effective is called the *nirvana fallacy*—nothing is 100% safe and effective.

Many anti-vaccine activists also know this, but still use these arguments to make themselves look less radical than they are, while still completely rejecting vaccination: 'Hey, we are not anti-vaccine, we are pro-SAFE-vaccine!'.

'Vaccines Don't Prevent Infections'

One important argument for vaccines is that they prevent infections, yet anti-vaccine groups claim that vaccines *don't* prevent infections. As it turns out, both claims are right: vaccines indeed don't prevent *individuals* from getting infected, but they do prevent infections at the population level.

This is how it works: if someone is vaccinated, this doesn't mean that viruses or bacteria no longer enter this person's body. So these vaccinated people absolutely get infected. However, those infections are far less severe (and often even go unnoticed), because the body gets on top of the infection very quickly. This means that a vaccinated person who is infected will be less infectious to other people, and for a shorter time span, than an unvaccinated person who is infected. Quite logical, when you think about it.

'Those Diseases Are Very Rare, so We Don't Need Vaccines Any More'

Another argument for declining vaccination (and especially childhood vaccinations) is that the risks of contracting dangerous childhood diseases these days is vanishingly small, so that even the tiny risks of vaccination quickly outweigh the risk of the disease.[2] And yes, the first premise is true: most childhood diseases that we vaccinate against are in fact very rare in our western world. So why vaccinate against something that has all but disappeared?

As soon as you encounter this argument, you should ask yourself a question: *why* are those diseases so rare in our western world? Could that be because vaccination *made* them rare? As an example, let's look at measles. Before the introduction of the MMR (Measles, Mumps and Rubella) vaccine in the 1970s, every child would contract measles, usually before the age of five. This would kill 1 out of every 1,000 children and cause permanent hearing loss in 1 out of every 300 children.

After the MMR vaccine became available, the annual number of measles cases dropped from hundreds of thousands to just a few hundred in 1995 and later. Unfortunately, anti-vaccine propaganda has prompted several larger

---

[2] This concept that the disappearance of childhood diseases automatically causes people to focus more on the risks of vaccination is also prompted by a human trait know as *loss aversion*. This human trait, first described by Daniel Kahneman and Amos Tversky in 1979, says that people award a disproportionate amount of weight to a particular loss (potential or real) compared to a gain of equal size [41]. In the context of vaccination, this means that people will tend to emphasize the extremely small chance of serious side effects of vaccination over the much bigger gains of vaccination. This is especially the case when they are no longer confronted by the losses caused by the infectious diseases themselves.

communities to shun childhood vaccinations, causing measles outbreaks that landed one in every four infected children in hospital—outbreaks that could easily have been prevented.

What this tells us is that it is vitally important to keep vaccinating our children, otherwise those diseases will return within just a couple of years.

'But All Those Toxic Chemicals in Vaccines Can't Be Good!'

Apart from the viral or bacterial ingredient, vaccines contain several other ingredients, some of which can be considered toxic—in larger doses, that is. Suffice to say that no, those chemicals added to vaccines are not harmful. In fact, most of them make vaccines *safer*, if anything. We will look into this in more detail in the Science section.

'You Can't Trust Vaccines'

One of the claims of anti-vaccine activists is that vaccines can't be trusted. After all, they're made and sold by large, pharmaceutical companies that are only interested in making easy money, not in delivering high-quality, trustworthy products. Which means that vaccines are far more harmful and less effective than they tell us.

As already discussed back in Chapter 1, distrusting large, more or less anonymous organizations as opposed to the proverbial friendly neighbour is in fact completely normal. But is the distrust justified in this case? Just ask yourself a question: what would those pharmaceutical companies stand to gain by producing and marketing bad vaccines, and then lying about it in order to keep up sales?

Let's look at the main motivation according to anti-vaccine people: money. What is the best way for big companies to make lots of money for a long time? Is it by making unsafe, unreliable products, and then lie to people in order to sell them? No, not exactly. In fact, the opposite applies: the best way to make lots of money and stay in business as a multi-billion-dollar corporation is to make high-quality products. Any company selling bad or even dangerous products will lose their customers and end up going bankrupt, sooner rather than later.

The same goes for vaccine manufacturers. It is far more profitable as well as easier to make high quality vaccines than to spend a lot of effort and money on making bad products and then keeping this hushed up indefinitely in order to keep up sales. This also touches on another argument: you can't keep things like this secret for long, as also explained in Chapter 12.

Then let's take a look at the actual money involved. Contrary to what many anti-vaccine activists believe, vaccines are not exactly a big cash cow for their makers. For instance the MMR vaccine makes its manufacturer (Merck) about 2 billion dollars in annual sales—and about a quarter of that (some 500 million dollars) is profit. Yes, this is a lot of money for the average Joe, but in the world of multinationals, this is peanuts, and represents only 5% of Merck's total annual sales [42].

No vaccine maker would get it into their head to commit very serious fraud to boost their profits by just a few percent. If the vaccine wouldn't work as claimed, measles cases would be much higher than expected; and if the vaccine would cause significant damage, this too would be noticed almost immediately.

Other Anti-vaccine Propaganda and Myths

At the time of this writing, a slick, professional-looking video production titled *Died Suddenly* was spread over the Internet, claiming that lots of completely healthy and often young people dropped dead as a result of Covid-19 vaccination. By way of 'evidence', the video showed footage of people suddenly collapsing in live TV broadcasts and other situations captured on camera. It also featured two coroners who claimed to see massive blood clots in deceased people, which they attributed to Covid-19 vaccination.

This video is an exceptionally vile piece of anti-vaccine propaganda, because it is One Big Lie: the people shown collapsing did not die at all, but merely fainted—and even this fainting could not be caused by Covid-19 vaccination, because those clips all dated from before the Covid-19 pandemic. By the same token, those blood clots that were found in deceased people were in fact completely normal post-mortem blood clots.

Unfortunately, this video has reached millions of people, resulting in a tidal wave of anti-vaccine propaganda, to the extent that virtually every unexpected death or health problem was immediately linked to vaccination.

Other false claims about vaccines are that they alter the DNA[3] of the recipient, or do other detrimental things. We can be very short about this: all these claims are untrue, and only meant to spread fear, uncertainty and doubt (FUD) about vaccines.

---

[3] Interestingly, some viral infections *can* change our DNA; these viruses (among which HIV) have found a way to integrate their genetic material in our DNA. When this part of our DNA is later expressed, this results in new virus particles.

The fact is that vaccines may well be the safest medical intervention ever—and vaccine deaths are so rare, that they can't even be properly counted.

What the Science Says

So far, many common arguments against vaccination have been presented, complete with reasons why they aren't valid. However to really understand the safety of vaccines, it is important to know more details about how they work and how they're made.

Making Vaccines

As already explained, vaccines do exactly one thing: they show the immune system a pathogen or parts of a pathogen. The immune system then responds in the same way as if a real infection had happened, resulting in immunity to the pathogen several days later. This sounds simple, and in fact it *is* simple—just look at how Edward Jenner worked: he collected a bit of pus from a cowpox blister on the tip of a blade, and then scratched the skin of a person with that blade to transfer the cowpox material into that person. That is how vaccination was done for over a hundred years, and it worked quite well—even though this came with the risk of a secondary infection, so other pathogens hitching a ride with the cowpox material.

Modern vaccines are much safer, and contamination with other pathogens hasn't happened for at least a half-century. Let's take a closer look at how the various vaccines are made, and what ingredients are used.

Attenuated vaccines contain a weakened version of the complete pathogen. This pathogen can still multiply, but no longer causes serious illness. The MMR vaccine (measles, mumps and rubella) and the oral polio vaccine are examples of attenuated vaccines, containing weakened versions of the viruses in question. Because these vaccines basically infect people with live viruses that still multiply inside the body, they produce an excellent immune response, and protect recipients for many decades, often even the rest of their life. The drawback is that the multiplying virus is dangerous for people with a weakened or damaged immune system, so these people should not receive attenuated vaccines.

Another drawback of attenuated vaccines is that they require growing the original pathogen. This can be pretty tricky, especially if the pathogen can only reproduce in human cells (e.g. the measles virus).

Subunit vaccines and **conjugate vaccines** do not contain live pathogens any more, but just parts of the pathogen, usually characteristic proteins or so-called polysaccharides (what we earlier on called 'fingerprint'). The hepatitis B and acellular pertussis vaccines are examples of subunit vaccines. Because the limited amount of pathogenic material that the immune system can respond to, these vaccines do not always elicit a strong immune response; in many cases, so-called *adjuvants* are added to enhance the immune response. More about adjuvants and other additives in a moment.

These vaccines too used to rely on live cultures of the pathogen. Nowadays, those specific pieces of protein or polysaccharide are often produced by genetically modified yeast or bacterial cells, which is a lot easier as well as safer.

Toxoid vaccines such as tetanus and diphtheria vaccines cause an immune response to the toxins produced by pathogens, not the pathogens themselves—because it is ultimately these toxins that can cause sickness and death. These vaccines too usually have adjuvants added to enhance the immune response.

mRNA vaccines are a relatively new type of vaccine, developed over the past 25 years, and first used in mass vaccination for Covid-19. These vaccines do not contain pathogens or parts of pathogens for the immune system to respond to; instead, they contain part of the genetic information (mRNA) of the virus. When this mRNA is introduced into cells of our body, those cells start making viral proteins (the viral spike protein in the case of Covid-19), which then ends up at the outside of the cell. Here, the immune system responds to those proteins in exactly the same way as with subunit vaccines.

The advantage of mRNA vaccines is that you no longer need to grow bacteria or viruses. You just have to assemble a strand of mRNA, and package it in such a way that it can enter cells after injection. This process can speed up the vaccine development process enormously; vaccine production and testing can start almost as soon as the mRNA code of a virus is known.

There are several other, less common techniques to make vaccines, but they all have one thing in common: they present the immune system with the characteristics of the disease that they protect against.

Invasion Tactics

Most people (and certainly doctors) know that antibiotics are useless against viral infections, but not *why* this is the case. This has to do with the completely different ways that bacteria and viruses live and reproduce.

Bacteria are self-contained living creatures, taking in nutrients from their surroundings, and reproducing by dividing, much like most cells in our body.

Bacteria cause disease by either producing toxic compounds, and/or by invading and damaging tissues. Because bacteria need to take in nutrients from their surroundings, they are vulnerable to antibiotics that can interfere with this food uptake or get inside bacteria and destroy them from the inside out. Bacteria can often be grown in a Petri dish, without the need for any host cells.

Viruses, however, are a completely different kettle of fish. Viruses are in fact little more than a little blob of genetic material, coated in a protective shell, the so-called *envelope*. Viruses don't take in nutrients and can't reproduce by themselves; there is even a debate going on whether viruses are alive.

When a virus encounters a suitable host cell (e.g. an epithelial cell in your airways), it first sticks to that cell using special proteins on its outside. In the Covid-19 virus, those special proteins are the spike proteins.

As a second step, the virus merges with the cell, at which point its genetic material (RNA or DNA) ends up inside the cell. This RNA or DNA contains the instructions necessary for making all parts of the virus. The cell responds by reading this RNA or DNA code, and translating it into new virus particles.[4] These new virus particles move to the outside of the infected cell, where they break free and start infecting new cells, repeating the cycle. Some viruses don't move to the outside of the cell, but simply multiply in such large numbers that the cell bursts. These infected and damaged cells are recognized by the immune system, which then starts to clear up the mess—at which point you begin to feel ill.

Simply said, a virus hijacks the cell's molecular machinery to make copies of itself. Normally, the cell's DNA, which is securely stored in the nucleus, is copied into small pieces of so-called *messenger RNA* (mRNA), which are processed by the cell's machinery to keep the cell itself going. Some mRNA has code to make more cellular proteins, other bits of mRNA are the recipe for making mucus etcetera. You can compare the DNA with a cookbook, containing all the recipes of a posh restaurant, kept in a secure place (the cell's nucleus). Every time when customers order a specific meal, the recipe for that meal is copied onto a small scrap of paper (an mRNA copy is made), and sent down to the kitchen (the main interior of the cell). The kitchen then follows the recipe to cook the ordered meals (proteins etcetera), after which the copy is discarded (the mRNA breaks down again).

In this analogy, a virus can be seen as a bad guy (e.g. from the competition) who disrupts the whole business by flooding the kitchen with his own recipes. These fake recipes take up all available food and other ingredients, and some even order the kitchen to send copies of those fake recipes to other restaurants, spreading the infection.

mRNA vaccines also send 'fake recipes' to the kitchen, but these are only designed to attract the attention of the immune system, without spreading or multiplying any further.

---

[4] Note that this is a simplified description, especially in the case of DNA viruses.

Other Vaccine Ingredients (and Why They're Safe)

Apart from the actual antigens (i.e. the 'fingerprints'), vaccines can contain several other ingredients. Generally speaking, all these ingredients are inherently safe, either because they already occur naturally in the body or because their total dose is very low. As the saying goes, the dose makes the poison—also see the next chapter, which deals with toxins.

Adjuvants are substances that cause a stronger immune response, making the vaccine more effective. They are mostly used in vaccines that contain only parts of a pathogen, which by themselves often only cause a weak immune response. The most used adjuvant is a compound of aluminium (or aluminum, as Americans say), about 500 µg per vaccine. This adjuvant disappears from the body within one or two weeks.

Aluminium has been associated with Alzheimer's disease in aluminium factory workers, but these people were exposed to thousands of times a normal vaccine dose, for years on end. There are no indications that normal vaccine doses cause any problem. This is further supported by the notion that babies are also naturally exposed to aluminium through their mother's milk, with doses up to 50 mg per day, without any ill effects.

Preservatives make vaccines much safer by preventing them from spoiling. In the beginning of the twentieth century, there were several incidents where vaccines with bacterial contamination killed dozens of children. One commonly used preservative was thimerosal, a mercury-based substance that anti-vaccine people linked to autism. Even though science as well as common sense could not find any evidence that thimerosal caused neurological problems, this preservative is no longer used in normal vaccines. More about this further on.

Stabilizers and emulsifiers are substances that prevent the vaccine ingredients from degrading or separating out after manufacture, which would render the vaccine useless. One regularly vilified emulsifier is a substance by the name of polysorbate 80. This is in fact a very common food additive; for instance one serving of ice cream can contain up to half a gram of polysorbate 80—which roughly equates to ten thousand times the maximum amount in one vaccine. No problems were ever found with this additive, both in food or in vaccines.

Manufacturing residues are traces of chemical substances that are used in vaccine manufacturing. Examples are formaldehyde, certain antibiotics and egg protein. Especially formaldehyde is often mentioned as a 'vaccine poison'. And yes, formaldehyde is indeed a harmful, toxic substance—in larger doses. In small doses, it is not only harmless, but even essential for our body to function, and even a newborn already has at least 1 mg of formaldehyde in their body. Vaccines contain less than 0.1 mg. Also, lots of fruits and other food contain formaldehyde; just one pear can contain as much as 5 mg of formaldehyde—50 times the amount present in one vaccine. This is no problem at all. The only substance that warrants some caution is egg protein (used in the manufacture of influenza vaccines), which can cause an allergic reaction. However, serious allergic reactions to vaccines are exceedingly rare.

Buffer substances are salt and other simple substances that are added to make the vaccine isotonic to your body—this reduces irritation, pain and swelling.

It is important to note that those vaccine ingredients were deliberately added to make vaccines safer and less painful, not to taint the vaccine and poison its recipients.

Testing Vaccines

New vaccines are tested in three clinical trial phases, just like any other (also see the previous chapter). In all, any new vaccine is tested for something like one to two years on tens of thousands of human volunteers before being approved for sale. One exception to this course of action was Pfizer's novel Covid-19 mRNA vaccine, which had a shortened phase 3 trial of just three months before receiving emergency approval. However, this does not mean that this new vaccine technology itself was only tested for three months; prior to these developments, mRNA vaccines had been tested on human volunteers for at least a decade already, without any serious problems.

Keeping an Eye on Things

Once a vaccine has been approved for sale, something called *post-market surveillance* starts. This is a mandatory process in which vaccine manufacturers have to monitor what happens to vaccine recipients in several different ways. *Active monitoring* means that thousands of vaccinated people are asked about their health at regular intervals. These people are encouraged to report any health problems (or adverse events in jargon) they experienced since receiving the vaccine, even if those problems seem insignificant. This is relatively labour-intensive and has only a limited reach, but produces relatively good data.

Passive monitoring relies on vaccinated people reporting adverse events themselves. One such passive reporting system in the US is called VAERS, short for the Vaccine Adverse Event Reporting System [43]. Other countries have similar passive reporting systems in place. Here, anyone can report a health problem experienced after vaccination, but the data quality is lower than with active monitoring. For instance almost nobody will be bothered to report mild, common side effects such a redness and swelling at the injection site, which automatically skews the reported events towards more serious problems.

One of the problems of both monitoring systems is that it is often difficult or even impossible to tell if a reported adverse event was caused by vaccination, at least without further research. This means that a large percentage of reported adverse events most likely had nothing to do with vaccination—which is also reflected in reported events naming drowning or trauma from accidents as a cause of death. What's more, healthcare providers (doctors etcetera) *must* report certain health problems (including death) following vaccination, even if the vaccination almost certainly played no role.

One issue with VAERS is that the anti-vaccine movement uses it to 'prove' that vaccines cause large-scale harm to people, simply by attributing most reported events to vaccination. In response, VAERS shows prominent warning messages such as the following:

VAERS reports alone cannot be used to determine if a vaccine caused or contributed to an adverse event or illness.

These adverse event reporting systems can only be used to signal potential problems that weren't observed up in earlier research. If such a signal is picked up, further investigation must establish if there is a link between vaccination and the event.

That these systems work very well, was shown in 2009 in the Netherlands: over a time frame of just a couple of months, three infants died within two weeks after receiving a pneumococci vaccine. This was immediately signalled, and vaccination with that particular batch of vaccines was put on hold, pending an investigation. In the end, it was found that two of the deceased infants died from causes not related to vaccination; the exact cause of death of the third child was still unclear, but a connection with vaccination seems very unlikely, as already millions of vaccine doses had been administered without any serious side effects. After a year, the investigation was concluded, and no similar events have happened since.

The Vaccination-Autism Myth

One of the most persistent anti-vaccine claims is that childhood vaccination causes autism. The main argument these days is as simple as it is fallacious: autism diagnoses have risen sharply in the past decades, and the number of childhood vaccines has also risen in that time period. So vaccines must cause autism. This is again our old friend the Post hoc fallacy, also known as *false causality*. One could just as easily claim that organic food causes autism, because organic food sales have also risen dramatically in the past few decades. Or that cell phones cause autism, or social media, or ….

The 1998 Lancet Paper

The alleged link between vaccines and autism was first published in 1998, in a scientific paper by one Andrew Wakefield, published in The Lancet. In this paper, he claimed that he had studied twelve children with autism, and found a link between the measles vaccine, autism, and a new type of intestinal disease. In particular, he claimed that in eight of the twelve children, symptoms of autism suddenly appeared within two weeks of receiving the measles, mumps and rubella vaccine.

This paper immediately led to controversy, mainly because scientists failed to find any supporting evidence for Wakefield's results. Instead of working with other scientists in order to solve the questions and problems, Wakefield actively sought publicity for his paper and his claims in press conferences, urging to stop MMR vaccinations. His critics accused him of 'doing science by press conference', sending a scary message into the world before science had a chance to properly evaluate his findings.

The anti-vaccine community of course immediately seized upon this opportunity to cause even more commotion, scaring parents into no longer vaccinating their children. As could be expected, measles cases began to rise alarmingly within just a few years.

It's Mercury Poisoning!

The dust from Wakefield's controversial paper had barely settled when in 1999, a then-common vaccine ingredient by the name of thimerosal was implicated as causing autism. Superficially, this is somewhat plausible: many mercury compounds are indeed potent neurotoxins, so maybe exposing the developing brain of young children to even minute amounts of mercury could indeed have devastating effects. Again the anti-vaccine movement made head-lines with claims that the use of this poison had damaged millions of children, and should be halted immediately. In 2001, they got what they wanted: the US stopped using thimerosal in all childhood vaccines. Vaccine critics were elated, and predicted that the number of new autism cases would sharply drop in years to come.

However, there were already some major problems with the thimerosal-autism link. The first problem was that most western countries had already abandoned thimerosal decades earlier. Yet there too, increasing numbers of children were diagnosed with autism. The second problem was that the symp-toms and clinical effects of mercury poisoning are completely different from autism symptoms. What's even more: some countries with high autism rates used far less childhood vaccines, and vice versa. Just look up some country's vaccination schedules and autism prevalence: the numbers are all over the place; there is not even a correlation, let alone causation. Unfortunately, most anti-vaccine activists only looked at US data.

Now what happened in the US after 2001 you ask, when thimerosal was banned from childhood vaccines? Well, nothing. There was no trend break in the health of American children whatsoever. The number of autism diagnoses kept rising slowly, and nothing remarkable happened with other conditions such as allergies or auto-immune disorders either. In turned out that thimerosal was completely safe. So what the did anti-vaccine community do? Did they admit that they were wrong? No, of course not. They simply picked the next ingredient on the list to demonize: aluminium adjuvants.

Wakefield's Fraud Exposed

We're now well into the 2000s, and thimerosal wasn't the bogeyman that the anti-vaccine crowd had insisted it was. However, there was still Wake-field's paper, linking the MMR vaccine (which, by the way, contains neither thimerosal nor aluminium) to autism. This piece of anti-vaccine evidence would soon be discredited too. In 2004, journalist Brian Deer discovered that just before publishing his paper and embarking on his anti-MMR campaign, Wakefield had applied for a patent on a 'safe' measles vaccine that he had developed, and expected to make millions in sales from it.

At the same time, more disturbing facts about his research began to emerge: it turned out that Wakefield had lied about a lot of things. Three out of nine children he reported as having regressive autism had no autism at all; claims that all twelve children were 'completely normal' before MMR vacci-nation turned out to be untrue, with five children already showing clear signs of developmental problems beforehand; the claim that the onset of autism symptoms happened within two weeks of MMR vaccination turned out to be false as well: symptoms sometimes started after several months, not weeks; laboratory tests of children's intestine were falsified to show the 'inflammation' that Wakefield claimed to have observed. In addition, Wakefield had received a substantial amount of money from solicitors who planned to earn money by suing vaccine makers for damages. Wakefield also overstepped ethical boundaries by using autistic children in his research without approval from an ethics committee, and subjecting these children to unnecessary invasive and potentially harmful diagnostic procedures such as colonoscopies, lumbar punctures and blood-drawing (the latter at a children's birthday party, of all places …).

In 2010, Wakefield's paper was finally retracted for reasons of fraud, and Wakefield himself was struck off the medical register for multiple counts of serious medical misconduct.

In spite of all the evidence against him, Wakefield, now living in the US, maintains his innocence to this day. He has also joined the anti-vaccine community in the US, where he enjoys a status of martyr and guru, earning money by giving anti-vaccine lectures.

Unfortunately, there is no way to undo the damage that Wakefield has done, as his fraudulent claims have instilled uncertainty and doubt about vaccination in countless people, especially parents of young children. Also, many people still believe the myth that vaccines somehow cause autism—even though study after study failed to find any link between autism and vaccines [44–46].

Explaining Autism Diagnoses

Anti-vaccine activists are right about one thing: the number of autism diagnoses has increased significantly over the past 50 years. But everything suggests that they are wrong about the cause: vaccination is with very high certainty not the cause of this 'autism epidemic'. So where do all these autism diagnoses come from?

One important thing to note is that 'autism' is not a simple, well-defined condition, but covers a broad spectrum of developmental and behavioural disorders. Symptoms can vary from almost imperceptible to very serious. The definition of autism has also been broadened considerably in the past decades, which in fact explains most of the increase in diagnoses of what nowadays is called autism spectrum disorder (ASD). Many people who used to be regarded as 'slow', 'introvert', 'inattentive', 'antisocial' or 'eccentric' are now often diagnosed with ASD. There are some other factors at play here as well. One of these is that there is a lot less of a taboo surrounding mental issues. It is now completely normal for children with learning or behavioural problems to see a psychiatrist and get diagnosed with things such as ASD, ADD, dyslexia, and other disorders. Such a diagnosis often enables these children to take advantage of adapted learning programs, helping them get through school, lowering the threshold for seeking help even further.

The Bad Thing About the Vaccine-Autism Myth

Anti-vaccine activists who keep claiming that vaccines are the cause of the 'autism epidemic' are not exactly doing the world a service—and certainly not the people with autism. In their almost religious fervour, they not only discourage people from having their kids vaccinated, but they also portray autism as an absolute horror that should be averted at all cost. This is very insulting for a lot of people with ASD who live perfectly happy lives, and hate being seen as having an unspeakable mental condition. Certainly, autism can sometimes be very bad, and it would probably be a good thing if those cases could be prevented in the future. But some of the most celebrated scientists and artists in history almost certainly had what we now call ASD, with Newton and Einstein just two of the most prominent examples.

The Immune System Going Rogue

Another category of health problems often linked to vaccination is immune disorders, and especially autoimmune conditions.

Autoimmune conditions happen when the immune system mistakes one or more of the body's own proteins for an intruder, and starts attacking the cells that have these proteins. This can have very serious and often even deadly consequences. Some well-known examples are rheumatoid arthritis (affecting cells in the body's joints and cartilage), type 1 diabetes (where insulin-producing cells in the pancreas are destroyed) and multiple sclerosis (where the immune system attacks the insulating outer layer of nerves).

Autoimmune diseases are still one of the bigger unresolved problems in medicine. In many cases, it is unclear what exactly triggers the immune system to attack its own body; once this happens, there is no way of stopping it—the immune system cannot easily 'unlearn' certain proteins that it has marked and memorized as a target. This means that there is also no cure.

In most cases, treatments can only suppress the immune response and thus the disease symptoms.

Some autoimmune conditions run in families, suggesting a hereditary factor. In some cases such as with type 1 diabetes and rheumatoid arthritis, genetic mutations seem to play an important role, whereas for other conditions, viral infections might be a causative factor. The hypothesis is that a viral protein closely resembles one of the human body's own proteins. When the immune system has learned to recognize and attack the viral protein, it inadvertently also destroys the body's own protein as a sort of 'collateral damage'.

This latter mechanism makes it superficially plausible that vaccines might also cause autoimmune conditions, as it causes the immune system to attack new proteins it has not yet encountered before. However, there are several arguments against this hypothesis:

* Most autoimmune conditions were known well before the introduction of vaccines.
* The diseases that we vaccinate against are not known to cause autoimmune conditions, which makes it unlikely that the vaccine does so after all.
* Clinical trials and post-market surveillance do not show a higher incidence of autoimmune conditions in vaccinated people.

In short, there are no indications that vaccines are somehow linked to autoimmune conditions.

Conclusion

There are some pretty good and very human reasons to be wary of vaccination: we have an instinctive aversion to getting stung or injected with something, and the fact that most vaccinations are given to healthy people also feels a bit uncomfortable.

Yes, vaccines can have side effects, ranging from mild to very serious. However, virtually all common side effects are mild, and serious side effects are very rare. Most things we do in life are far more risky than getting vaccinated.

Vaccines are in fact among the safest and most rigorously tested products in medicine—precisely *because* they are given to healthy people, and especially children. Vaccine makers have to comply with very strict regulations for testing and manufacturing vaccines, even though vaccines are by far not their biggest cash cow—after all, most vaccine are given only a few times during a person's lifetime; it is far more profitable to make pills that patients have to take every day. In short: there's nothing wrong with vaccines.

Despite all this, the anti-vaccine movement is still quite vocal and has a lot of followers—and they still perpetuate the long-debunked myth that vaccines cause autism, allergies, autoimmune diseases and other health conditions. Huge amounts of scientific research as well as common sense says that they're wrong.

In the next chapter, we will investigate substances that *do* cause harm—we shall visit the world of toxins. Which ones are real and should be avoided? And which ones are fake, and only used to sell products? Read on and find out!

9

Toxins Everywhere

Whodunnit?

In the early spring of 1862, a doctor by the name of Thomas Orton was called to the house of one Richard Turner in London's East End, where three-year-old Ann Amelia Turner was very ill. Her desperate parents told Dr Orton that in the past few months, they already lost three of their four children, and feared that their only remaining child would suffer the same fate.

When their first child became ill and died in February, another doctor they consulted believed that their children were dying from diphtheria, a common and often deadly disease in those days. Within weeks, the other Turner children all started showing the same symptoms: a sore throat, difficulty swallowing, severe stomach and intestinal pain, and increasing exhaustion. Even though quite a few of these symptoms matched diphtheria, there were some things that did not make sense. For one thing, no-one else in the cramped living conditions of the local neighbourhood showed any signs of diphtheria, even several months after the first Turner child fell ill. This was strange, given that diphtheria is highly contagious. Also, not all symptoms fit the disease, common diphtheria treatments didn't seem to help the sick children at all, and the Turner family had always been the paragon of health up until Christmas, when the children first contracted measles and then diphtheria.

Dr Orton was puzzled, and started having doubts about the original diagnosis of diphtheria. Determined to do his best to find the cause of the unfolding drama, he decided to meticulously record his findings, including the family's living conditions. He noticed that the house was clean, well-aired, and in excellent condition; also, there seemed to be no problem with the drinking water – a prime cause of cholera

© The Author(s), under exclusive license to Springer Nature Switzerland AG 2023
R. Rasker, *Mind, Make-Believe and Medicine*,
https://doi.org/10.1007/978-3-031-29444-0_9

in those days. Dr Orton suspected that something else than infectious disease was at play here, but could not put his finger on what exactly that could be. He did however notice one detail: the children's bedroom had recently been decorated with wallpaper in vivid green colours.

Unfortunately, he could do nothing more but try and make little Ann Amelia as comfortable as possible. Dr Orton left, and some time later, the last Turner child also tragically died. Following this last death, one doctor Henry Letheby, a public health official, performed a post-mortem on the child's body. The verdict was clear and confirmed Dr Orton's suspicions: little Ann Amelia Turner had not died from diphtheria, but from arsenic poisoning, and it was very likely that the same fate had befallen the other three children. But what had caused it? Where did the poison come from?

Immediately, Dr Orton recalled the bright green wallpaper in the children's bedroom. The green colour was a well-known arsenic compound called Scheele's Green, and doctors had suspected for quite some time that it might pose health risks. Arsenic-based pigments had already been banned in mainland Europe for many years, after French and German doctors associated these green pigments with severe health problems and even deaths.

Orton and Letheby decided to bring the case to court, in an attempt to have these arsenic compounds banned in Britain as well. The problem was, however, that both British wallpaper and arsenic mining were Big Business, with millions of rolls of wallpaper being produced every year, and that arsenic was used in countless applications. Manufacturers of arsenic-laden goods vehemently denied any toxicity of their products, and insisted that arsenic was only dangerous when ingested.

Unfortunately, the judge refused to accept the findings of the good doctors, and reportedly even said that Dr Letheby's conclusions were "objectionable", after which the jury ruled the death of all children due to natural causes. And even though public awareness of the dangers of arsenic compounds steadily grew, no legislation was passed to regulate its use in domestic products for many years to come.

It is not recorded how Richard Turner and his wife reacted to the verdict, but one can imagine that they must have been absolutely devastated. The culprit had been identified with almost 100% certainty, and the death of all four of their children could probably have been prevented, had Britain followed mainland Europe's example. But in spite of all this, both the judge and the jury swept the evidence aside, and decided that there were no unnatural causes involved, let alone culpability on anyone's behalf.

It took many more years and many more deaths before increasing public mistrust of arsenic-containing products led to a subsequent drop in demand, finally forcing manufacturers to switch to using arsenic-free pigments for their products. Only in the early twentieth century, Britain began implementing legislation restricting the use of these highly toxic substances for household purposes.

This historic tragedy sets the backdrop for this chapter, where we will explore all sorts of toxins, real and imaginary. Also, we will see how Big Business and its hunger for profit as well as political indifference and incompetence can poison innocent people, not only in the nineteenth century, but even as recent as only a few years ago. Then again, we will also explore toxins in the alternative world, with several surprises along the way.

In the Science section, we will learn how toxic certain substances are, and why these days, we don't have to worry too much about toxins, especially in our privileged corner of the world.

What Is a Toxin?

It would appear that this question is easily answered: a toxin (or poison, more correctly) is a substance that causes harm to an organism by upsetting the body chemistry of that organism. However, things are not as simple as that: many substances are quite harmless or even essential for life in small amounts, only to become toxic (and sometimes life-threatening) in larger amounts—**the dose makes the poison**, as the old saying goes. Some substances are almost universally toxic, while other substances are harmful only to certain creatures, but not to others.

Some toxins have almost instantaneous effects, while others slowly damage organs such as the liver, the kidneys or the brain, leading to deteriorating health and sometimes death—which can happen so long after the actual exposure that victims have no idea what is harming them. Some toxins also have the nasty property of slowly accumulating in the body.

Many of our food plants are toxic, which means that we must process these plants before eating them. Some plants have edible parts and toxic parts. Then there are substances that are not toxic by themselves, but become toxic when processed in the body.

Other toxins again can be used medicinally, some of which even as potent anti-cancer drugs, albeit usually with serious side-effects. More on this in the Science section.

And oh, there are also quite a few toxins that many of us take voluntarily, not seldom with detrimental effects on our health. (Still fancy that beer?).

One important and scary aspect of toxins is their insidious nature: toxins often can't be easily recognized for what they are—not until it is too late anyway. Toxins can be found in plants, fungi or meat that may appear perfectly edible; some toxins can even do harm by touch alone. We can be exposed to environmental toxins for many years unknowingly.

And if this weren't unsettling and confusing enough already, all sorts of false claims are made about toxins and things purportedly containing toxins, usually out of fear and a lack of knowledge, but often also to scare people into buying 'detox' products.

It is no wonder that many people are afraid of 'toxins', even completely imaginary ones.

How Toxins Work

All living creatures rely on complex chemical reactions to function. A toxin is defined as any substance that interferes with these chemical reactions in a way that is harmful to the organism.

For instance, each and every living cell in our body needs a constant supply of oxygen in order to survive. For this, we breathe air containing oxygen. In our lungs, the oxygen is taken up by the blood, and more specifically by *haemoglobin*, a complex protein in our red blood cells, capable of trapping oxygen directly from the air in the lungs and delivering it anywhere in our body.

Unfortunately, oxygen is not the only thing that can bind to haemoglobin. A substance called carbon monoxide can do this too, and even stronger than oxygen at that. When this happens, the haemoglobin can't carry oxygen any more, killing the unfortunate victim by suffocation from the inside, as it were.

This is just one example of how a toxin can work. There are literally tens of thousands of ways that our body chemistry can be upset by toxic substances. *Toxicology* is the huge scientific area that studies toxins and their effects, and it is closely linked to several other sciences such as medical science, general chemistry, biochemistry, biology, botany (the study of plants), entomology (the study of insects) and even geology.

Toxins, Poisons and Venoms

For those who wondered about the differences between the three distinct terms: a **poison** is a general term for a harmful substance, regardless of its origin. A **venom** is defined as a toxic substance from animal origin that is injected through stinging or biting, whereas the term **toxin** is mostly used for poisons produced by microbes and fungi.

However, I will be less strict in my definitions here, and use 'toxin' and 'poison' more or less interchangeably. So please forgive yours truly for calling e.g. a synthetic chemical substance a toxin on occasion.

Toxins in Evolution and History

Toxins have been a fact of life from the very beginning of life on earth. Even the earliest self-replicating creatures relied on specific chemical substances and reactions for their energy and building materials. Any other chemicals blocking those reactions would be toxic to those creatures. Also see the sidebar 'Poisoning the world' for a dramatic example.

It is believed that most toxins produced by living creatures themselves came about by accident, as a by-product of metabolic processes, and that evolution subsequently favoured organisms who could use these substances to their benefit, for example as a deterrent or to subdue prey.

Poisoning the Planet

One poisoning event known as the *Great Oxidation Event* happened on a truly global scale. This started several billion years ago, at an age when the earth's atmosphere held no free oxygen at all. Most of the existing life-forms at that time were so-called anaerobic bacteria, which got their energy from several types of chemical reactions that did not involve free oxygen.

About 2.5 billion years ago, some bacterial strains evolved special chemistry that was capable of trapping the energy from sunlight, and using this energy to combine carbon dioxide and water into bigger molecules—molecules that were both a source of energy and a building material. These bacteria had stumbled upon a wonderful new source of food and energy, one that was far more abundant than the often scarce supply of special chemicals that their ancestors needed. There was only one problem: this completely new and efficient type of metabolism had a nasty waste product: oxygen gas. This free oxygen interfered with the chemical reactions that other bacteria depended on, depriving them of energy and building materials—the very definition of toxicity. As a consequence, most of these anaerobic bacteria went extinct.[1] The world was taken over by bacteria and (later) other lifeforms that evolved the capability to use oxygen to their advantage. As it is, the Great Oxidation Event kick-started the evolution of multi-cellular lifeforms, turning the single most devastating global poisoning around into a unique success story that continues to this day.

So we humans are definitely not the first creatures to poison our atmosphere with our own waste products.[2]

The Great Oxidation Event was the biggest and also one of the earliest examples of toxins having a huge influence on living creatures. However toxins have been a fact of life during all of the history of life on earth. Some environments are naturally toxic to lots of organisms due to the presence of chemical substances, e.g. areas of high volcanic activity, or places with high natural concentrations of arsenic in the soil and drinking water.

Many toxic substances are produced by organisms as the result of what can be seen as an evolutionary arms race. Snake venom, for example, evolved from saliva, and benefits snakes in several ways: it not only subdues and sometimes even helps pre-digest their prey, but it is also a defensive measure against other predators. This is quite a successful strategy, as only few creatures are known to hunt and eat snakes.

Plant Toxins

Many plants produce toxins. This is makes sense, as plants have rather less options to defend themselves against being eaten than animals. Toxicity is quite an effective strategy if you can't run away or fight when someone starts nibbling on your leaves. By producing toxins, plants make sure that eating them really ruins your day, so that next time, you will avoid them and eat something else instead.

As already mentioned, many of our food plants are toxic in one way or another. We learned to solve this problem by avoiding the most toxic parts (e.g. we can safely eat rhubarb stalks but not rhubarb leaves), or by processing (raw beans are toxic, but cooked beans are quite safe). Other toxic plants have

---

[1] Contrary to what the name 'Great Oxidation Event' suggests, this was a slow process that probably took hundreds of millions of years. Also, many strains of anaerobic bacteria still exist today, living and thriving wherever free oxygen is scarce or absent.

[2] Which is of course *not* an excuse to lean back, do nothing about it, and simply wait until we evolve traits to deal profitably with excessive heat, raised sea levels and other consequences of our wasteful lifestyle.

become safe to eat through cross-breeding, repeatedly selecting the safest, most nutritious plants to breed with.

Avoiding Toxins

The notion that certain things can be quite unhealthy is of course not a uniquely human trait. Even single-celled creatures can be observed moving away from harmful substances, and most animals have evolved mechanisms to avoid poisoning—and they are actually being helped by those toxic organisms themselves: many poisonous and venomous animal species have evolved bright colours as a clear warning signal, and many plant toxins taste unpleasantly bitter, including a large family of so-called *alkaloids*.

Higher animals and particularly social animals have also evolved social behaviour to avoid poisoning. If one member of a group becomes unwell after eating something, the whole group can often be seen to avoid that particular food from that moment on, at least as long as there are alternative food sources.

Still, natural toxins make lots of victims. According to WHO estimates, each year, somewhere between 80,000 and 140,000 people are killed by snakebites alone, and food poisoning (where bacterial and plant toxins play an important role) accounts for even more deaths, some 420,000 annually.

Dealing with Toxins

The picture is clear: toxins are everywhere, and can't always be avoided. What is even more, lots of processes inside the body produce toxic substances that we have to get rid of. This means that all organisms have evolved ways to deal with toxins.

In higher animals, two organs in particular are responsible for handling toxins: the *liver* is perhaps best described as a universal chemical processing plant that (among other things) breaks down many substances into simpler, less noxious[3] waste products, while the *kidneys* remove many of those waste products from the blood and excrete them in urine. Between them, these

---

[3] Unfortunately, this does not always work: the liver sometimes turns substances into *more* harmful products before getting rid of them. Methanol ('wood alcohol') is a point in case: methanol itself is no more toxic than ethanol (normal alcohol)—but the liver turns it into highly toxic formic acid, causing blindness and death in relatively small amounts (10–50 millilitres).

organs can get rid of a huge amount of different substances that would otherwise kill us within days—most of which are, incidentally, produced by the body itself.

But obviously, even these wonderful organs have their limitations, and can't handle everything.

Toxins and Poisons in Human History

Like all life-forms, humans too have always had to deal with toxins. For a long time, the only toxins humans had to be wary about originated from plants, animals and the environment. However, from the moment that we humans discovered the use of fire, our own activities exposed us to an increasing number of new unhealthy substances, often without realizing it. Here is a quick go-through of our own toxic history:

Fire produces lots of poisonous substances such as carbon monoxide and smoke. From prehistoric times right up to this day, open fires for cooking and heating, especially indoors, have been the cause of all sorts of health problems—the same problems that we in the western world associate with smoking tobacco: lung cancer, heart and lung disease, and respiratory problems. It is estimated that a typical cooking fire produces the equivalent amount of toxic smoke of several hundred cigarettes. Per hour, that is.

Metal production from the bronze age onward exposed people to heavy metals such as lead, arsenic, mercury and cadmium. These highly toxic metals are naturally present in the metal ores, and contaminate the environment through the smoke and waste products (slag) produced by smelting. Even today, large smelting facilities in some countries cause widespread environmental pollution with heavy metals.

Badly chosen 'medicines' are also a common cause of health problems throughout history. In Chapter 6, I already discussed a plant called birthwort or *aristolochia*, which was in widespread use as a herbal medicine throughout the ages. Only quite recently it was found to cause liver damage and urinary tract cancer. In the same chapter, I also discussed the problem that many Ayurvedic and Chinese traditional medicines often contain dangerous amounts of heavy metals such as lead and mercury.

Then again, modern pharmaceutical products are not guaranteed safe either, as evidenced by well-known examples as Thalidomide and Vioxx, and by the opioid crisis in the US.

Occupational and industrial poisoning has been a growing problem from medieval times onward, as all sorts of crafts and home industries increasingly made use of toxic substances. Painters and paint makers were always looking for more durable paints with vibrant, non-fading colours. Unfortunately, the best pigments of those days were often based on mercury, lead, and arsenic, and poisoning was a very real danger. Another well-known example is the *mad hatter's disease*, or poisoning caused by a mercury compound used in the making of felt hats.

With the advent of the industrial revolution in the late eighteenth century, toxic products became more widespread and started affecting not just industry workers, but consumers as well—as the tragic story at the beginning of this chapter shows.

Air pollution as a result of human activities is another major problem of the past two hundred years, persisting up to this day. The widespread use of coal as the main industrial and domestic fuel claimed many lives. In homes, people were always wary of carbon monoxide ('coal gas'), while especially in cities and industrial areas, even the outdoor air was often anything but healthy. Only as recent as 1952, thousands of Londoners died from extreme smog caused by a combination of cold, windless weather and the use of coal for heating.

Up to this day, smog and air pollution still take a heavy toll on human health, with an estimated 8.7 million premature deaths worldwide in 2018 alone [47].

Toxins in Our Modern World

Over the past hundred years, scientific and industrial developments led to a huge surge in the production and use of all sorts of new, often toxic substances in numerous areas such as the manufacturing industry, agriculture (e.g. pesticides) and medicine. This of course also came with new risks.

Awareness about the hazards of chemical substances increased more or less in step with these developments. The beginning of the twentieth century saw the introduction of an increasing number of health and safety laws, intended to protect the general public and industrial workers from harm through poisoning, among other things. Over the course of the decades, these laws were extended to cover most things in our daily life, ensuring the safety of our food, our drinking water, our household products, our medicines, and the air we breathe.

Lead

Lead deserves its own mentioning, being both one of the most useful as well as harmful heavy metals. Lead has been used in numerous ways, dating back thousands of years. In the days of ancient Rome, it was extensively used for plumbing (hence the chemical symbol Pb for lead, from the Latin *plumbum*), domestic utensils and lots of other things. Lead has several handy properties: it is soft and corrosion-resistant, and has a low melting point, and thus is very easy to work with. Lead compounds were useful for pottery glazing, paints and cosmetics.

In later centuries, lead lay at the core of printing with movable type, and was still used for typesetting in the twentieth century. Lead was also highly valued by builders, who used it to waterproof roofs and seal off gaps in masonry.

One of the most controversial applications of lead however was in a so-called anti-knocking agent in petrol (gasoline), to make car engines run much smoother. This fuel additive was hugely successful right from its introduction in the 1920s, and almost overnight, all cars ran on leaded fuel. This lead of course had to go somewhere, and so it did—it went basically *everywhere*.

Even then, concerns were raised that all that lead belched out in the atmosphere could have detrimental health effects, as the toxicity of lead was well known by that time. However, critics were simply ignored, mostly because this lead additive was Big Business, and leaded gasoline would be the norm for the next half-century. Lead emissions increased in step with rapidly growing number of cars, and so did blood lead levels in people, especially in urban areas.

Only from the 1970s onwards did environmental concerns get the upper hand, and steps were taken to ban lead from car fuel. Also, evidence began to emerge suggesting that children were exceptionally vulnerable, with lead exposure causing developmental and behavioural problems even in minute amounts. As the 1990s saw a remarkable drop of violent crime rates in many countries, the idea began to take hold that decreasing lead exposure could play a role here. This *lead-crime hypothesis* surmises that childhood exposure to lead causes brain damage, learning disabilities and problems with impulse control. This public health problem would manifest itself in the form of increased crime rates some two decades later, when those children reached adulthood. By the same token, crime rates dropped some twenty years after the use of lead in car fuel was banned—a pattern that was observed in several countries.

However, there is not yet a consensus on the lead-crime hypothesis; not all countries show the same neat pattern with a 20-year shift, and scientists have also come up with other explanations, based on socio-economic factors.

What *is* clear, is that blood lead levels have returned to normal levels almost everywhere, and that is certainly a good sign.

The banning of lead, mercury and other hazardous chemical substances from our daily life has made our planet a safer place to live than it has ever been in many respects. Or has it? Some people still claim that we are constantly being poisoned in many different ways, and that this is what causes lots of vague health complaints. And very conveniently, many of these people also offer a solution: 'detox' products, which supposedly restore our health and well-being.

Detox

So-called *detox* treatments and products are a huge market, estimated to have an annual value of almost over 50 billion dollars worldwide.

Why Is Detox so Popular?

The huge popularity of the concept of detox and all its associated products and treatments is not some recent fad, but goes back thousands of years. The most compelling evidence for this is found in the world's religions and spiritual traditions: almost all religions have cleansing rituals of some sort, and usually also rules that stipulate what is considered 'clean' and 'unclean'. Personal hygiene plays an important role in holy scriptures such as the Bible. And just think of the saying 'Cleanliness is next to godliness.'

This idea of cleansing can take on many forms, ranging from literal washing as prescribed in Islam (e.g. before prayer) and submersion baptism as practised in several Christian denominations, to more abstract forms of cleansing such as Roman Catholic baptism with just a few drops of water, which according to the Catechism serves to clean the child's soul from sin. Catholic confession is supposed to achieve a similar periodic cleaning of the soul for people when they grow older.

Hindus believe that they clean themselves spiritually by drinking water from their holy river while standing immersed in it—but unfortunately, this holy river is the Ganges. Used by literally hundreds of millions of people as a sewer and garbage dump, the Ganges river is one of the most polluted rivers worldwide. As a result, this spiritual 'cleaning' takes a huge toll in physical disease, killing as many as several hundred thousand people every year by some estimates. Only recently, efforts were undertaken to address these problems, but with little effect so far.

However, a desire for cleanliness has its roots in far earlier times, and is probably an instinctive trait that evolved over millions of years. Just look at the animal kingdom: countless species exhibit some sort of grooming or cleaning behaviour. The evolutionary advantage is clear: keeping oneself clean helps to prevent disease and gets rid of parasites. Some animal species even specialized in grooming other species; examples are oxpeckers and pilot fish (although there is some debate whether oxpeckers are actually beneficial to their host species or not).

We humans took this whole cleanliness thing one very important step further with the invention of public hygiene: a structural, organised effort to dispose of our waste products in a safe manner, preventing it from contaminating our food and drinking water. Public hygiene has been instrumental in overcoming many infectious diseases, especially in densely populated areas.

In other words: hygiene and cleanliness, both personal and public, is generally a Good Thing, even though we've only known for the past few hundred years *why* this is so.

In our modern western world, we have largely abandoned the spiritual blemishes of the soul, returning to the more mundane concept of toxic substances actually poisoning us—after all, there really *are* lots of nasty chemicals out there. This idea is reinforced in no small way by the notion that it is an invisible threat. You can't usually see, taste or smell those toxins, so you can't tell if they're there or not. The logical next step is then to attribute any vague and chronic ailments to those invisible toxins. This is why the idea of periodical 'detox' is quite attractive, of course heavily supported by the alternative industry with its countless detox products and treatments. So let's now take a look at an actual example of a detox offering.

Detox Supplements

Herbs, minerals and other supplements are very often advertised for 'detox', usually in combination with other vague health claims such as 'boosting the immune system'. Most of these products are both useless and harmless: they don't do anything to 'detox the body' or 'cleanse the blood' or 'help the liver'.

Then again, some may be unhealthy. Let's look at some of the more common products, how they are marketed, and how they supposedly work—and also why none of these products actually does anything for us.

The following is paraphrased from a random Web page, found by searching for 'environmental toxins':

It is said that we are all loaded with environmental chemicals. Is this really true?

Alas, this is true. The CDC (Centres for Disease Control and Prevention) says that hundreds of foreign chemical substances and their breakdown products have been found in our blood, our tissues and even in breast milk!

Do these substances actually pose a health threat?

Many of those chemicals identified by the CDC are known to be harmful to people, while many others are still subject to toxicological research.

How do these chemicals end up in our body?!

It is a well-known fact that our whole environment is contaminated with toxic chemicals, so there is no way to avoid them. Our body simply can't keep these substances out.

There are many more claims on this Web page, effectively telling us that we are poisoning ourselves with every bite of food we eat, with every breath we take, and even with every sip of water we drink, and that this will almost inevitably damage our health if we don't do something about it.

This does not sound good. Actually, this sounds outright scary, and it would seem that the claims made here are even supported by America's most authoritative public health organization, the CDC! And there are lots of references to real science as well!

And this is only one of thousands of similar Web sites telling us similar things, so apparently, we should be really worried.

Luckily, a solution is only one mouse click away:

Protect yourself and your family with full-body detox: [activated charcoal]

Well, that *is* good news! Apparently, we only need to use a 'detox' product to get rid of all those nasty toxins that enter our body, simply by taking a daily dose of activated charcoal. And that for only $49.50 for 100 capsules! (Just a bit of a shame really, that you only get free shipping with orders from $50 upwards …).

Is this for real? Are we getting poisoned all the time, with all sorts of detrimental effects? And is the solution really this easy?

Are We Being Poisoned?

Let's start out by simply forgetting about all this alarming information, and look around us in the real world. Does it look like most people are suffering from poisoning? Are doctors finding toxic substances in their patients all the time? Are lots of people dying from mysterious, non-infectious conditions at a relatively young age? Are our children growing up weak, with all sorts of vague health problems?

Well, not really. In fact, not at all. Not only do we live longer on average than at any previous time in history, our health has never been better, and we even stay healthier longer when growing old. Also, child mortality has never been lower, and our children's health is better than even a mere 50 years ago, apart maybe from lifestyle-related issues such as obesity and lack of exercise. So what is going on here?

First of all, there is actually some truth in those claims: yes, all sorts of chemicals enter our bodies all the time, and yes, those chemicals can be detected in our blood, urine and even in breast milk. And yes, many of those chemicals are known to be toxic.

However …

- The *amount* (or dose, or concentration) of these chemicals is usually far too low to do any harm. Remember: the dose makes the poison (although this again is a bit too simplistic—small doses can be harmful too if they accumulate).
- Modern scientific analytic tools can find incredibly small amounts of substances, amounts that were not detectable even a few decades ago—so e.g. a water sample that would be considered '100% clean' 30 years ago can now be found to be contaminated with dozens of chemical substances.
- The toxic nature of the chemicals mentioned is often exaggerated or misrepresented.

As it turns out, the answer is no, we are not being poisoned all the time, as in: the chemical substances in our food, air and environment do not affect our health in a negative way. All this scaremongering has only one goal: separating you from your money. Web sites such as the one just mentioned follow a well-known strategy: scare people into believing that they have a serious problem, and then offer a simple solution to this problem—here in the form of 'detox' products, which promise to rid your body of all those nasty toxins. As it turns out, these products don't work as advertised, and may even be harmful. More about this in the Science section, later on in this chapter. But first, let's look at some other examples, just for the fun of it.

'But Toxins Accumulate in Your Intestines!'

This is a claim that is often heard wherever people try to sell detox products: that after years of eating processed food and red meat and of course exposure to 'toxic chemicals', our intestines are somehow caked with harmful toxic residues, causing all sorts of health problems.

This is completely untrue, as any doctor can confirm. Every day, doctors around the world examine the bowels of thousands upon thousands of people, and they never even once found accumulated waste products that have been stuck there for any length of time. In fact, it is physically impossible for this to happen, as the inside of the intestine is constantly renewed, with the complete lining being replaced every five to seven days. Anything that might be sticking to this lining is automatically expelled in the process.

What *is* true, however, is that some toxic substances such as lead can accumulate in the body through chronic exposure to these substances. But this doesn't happen under normal living conditions in western countries, as most sources of lead and similar hazardous chemicals have been removed from our environment.

Colon Cleansing

Regardless of what doctors and scientists say, colon cleansing in one form or another is one of the more popular treatments among alternative practitioners and their followers—not just for detox, but for lots of other purposes and conditions as well, up to and including cancer. But once again, these treatments don't do anything for your health. Treatments such as coffee enemas or the likes can even be harmful, as they can upset your mineral balance and cause intestinal damage. Yes, these treatments can remove chemicals from your body—but mainly the chemicals you actually need, such as minerals. They don't do anything about any 'toxins'.

Bentonite Clay

Another substance that is sometimes sold as a detox product is so-called *bentonite clay*, a very fine type of mineral clay, originating from volcanic ash. You may already know this type of clay as cat litter. Just like charcoal, bentonite clay can bind to all sorts of chemical substances. But unlike activated charcoal, bentonite clay also binds to heavy metals such as lead. So that is a good thing, right?

Alas, no. It is exactly this last property of bentonite clay that makes it unsuitable as a 'detox' remedy: in its natural state, it may already have adsorbed a fair amount of lead and other naturally occurring but unhealthy substances [48]. When bentonite clay enters the stomach, the exact opposite of detox may occur: the acid in the stomach may partly dissolve the clay, making lead compounds and other substances available for absorption into the body instead of removing them. So it is probably not a good idea to start munching kitty litter.

Detox Foot Baths and Footpads

Charcoal and bentonite clay are two 'detox' products that at least have a grain of truth to them, as both substances can indeed adsorb and bind toxic substances.

Rather sillier are footpads or foot baths that claim to 'draw out' toxins through the soles of your feet. Yes, when you finally take your shoes off after a long day, your feet may seem to emanate a vapour cloud of noxious fumes—but this is just the combination of moisture from sweat and bacteria on the surface of the skin. The only thing that can leave your body through your feet is water—read: sweat.

However, the manufacturers of these products use a smart gimmick: after a night under the soles of your feet, those footpads begin to show a distinct brown colour—that's them toxins being drawn out, that is! But no. The manufacturers put certain chemical substances such as iron compounds in their footpads, which turn brown when they come into contact with moisture. Just hold one of those footpads over a steaming kettle, and you will see them turning brown before your eyes. The water in those foot baths also turns brown, this time because a small electric current is passed through the water, dissolving iron compounds again.

And should you still be in doubt about these products, then just think for a moment: what do doctors and hospitals do when a poisoning victim is brought in? Do they cover them up in pads to 'draw out' the toxins? Do they come running with foot baths? Nope, nothing like that at all. They may administer activated charcoal (yes, the same stuff in the first detox product we mentioned), or they may make a patient throw up, or administer an antidote, or start chelation therapy—it all depends on the type of poison, the dose, and the timing of the poisoning. But at no point are pads or baths of any kind involved.

Poisoning Conspiracies

Most proponents of 'detox' believe that we are simply surrounded by toxins for no other reason than careless pollution by big corporations. There are however people who not only believe that we are constantly being poisoned, but also that this happens deliberately—usually through some sort of conspiracy by shady powers.

Still, those fears of surreptitious mass-poisoning have some legitimate origins: in historical times, the poisoning of drinking water was often considered one of the most heinous crimes thinkable. Especially in the Middle Ages, disease outbreaks were often attributed to deliberate poisoning of water and food supplies, with, alas, Jews often being blamed as the perpetrators of such 'poisonings'.

Water Fluoridation Conspiracies

Widespread water fluoridation was introduced from 1945 onwards as a way to improve dental health of children in particular, and as such it was very successful. But as could be expected, lots of people opposed the idea of 'forced medication with chemicals', coming up with an endless stream of reasons why fluoridation was a Really Bad Idea—most of which were not based on reality. And sure enough, water fluoridation conspiracy theories soon popped up, with the most common ones claiming that it was all a secret Russian/communist plot to poison the bodies and minds of western countries, all in proper Cold War style. The plot of Stanley Kubrick's film *Dr Strangelove* is also based on this very same conspiracy theory.

Water fluoridation was abandoned again in many western countries, mostly because of public resistance. Luckily, most toothpastes these days contain fluoride, and the importance of good dental hygiene is also common knowledge.

Chemtrails

Perhaps the most bizarre claim about 'toxins' says that the condensation trails we can see behind air planes passing overhead are not just condensed water vapour, but contain special 'chemicals' that are supposed to subdue the world's population. This way, a dark elite can enslave the entire human race for their own nefarious purposes. Or something like that, as this conspiracy 'theory' has many variants.

This conspiracy idea is of course quite crazy, and falls apart on even the slightest scrutiny. For one, dumping chemicals into the atmosphere from a height of ten kilometres is the single most ineffective and at the same time most conspicuous way to try and 'poison' our world. And, of course, there's the problem that tens of thousands of airline workers worldwide must be part of such a conspiracy—yet not a single one of them has ever blown the whistle on this in all those decades that this must have been going on. So chemtrails can be safely dismissed as complete nonsense.

What the Science Says

As should be clear by now, the alternative world's notion of toxins is pretty simple: we're all being poisoned by 'toxins', so we all need 'detox' once in a while. Never mind that they hardly even specify exactly *what* toxins they're talking about, let alone that they come up with doses or concentrations or such things. All those numbers and other fiddly bits of information are just things to keep the science folks busy and entertained. The only *really* important numbers are of course the numbers in the bank accounts of people selling all those detox products. Just buy our detox, and you'll feel a lot better!

However, when talking about real toxins, it absolutely matters *what* substance we're talking about, and also *how much* of that substance. There are lots of substances that are completely harmless (or even essential for our health) in lower doses, but become seriously toxic in higher doses. In a high enough dose, they can even kill you. What constitutes a harmless dose or a dangerous dose depends largely on the type of substance; one important measure of acute toxicity is the so-called LD50, which stands for 'Lethal Dose for 50% of organisms'. It is usually expressed in milligrams per kilogram body weight. For instance caffeine has an estimated LD50 of 150–200 mg (0.2 g) per kilogram of body weight in humans. This means that if someone weighing 80 kg takes in $80 \times 0.2 = 16$ g of caffeine in one go, then they have a 50/50 chance to survive.

Other things that matter with real toxins are the possibility of accumulation (especially with heavy metals and fat-soluble substances), the way that they end up in the body and much more. As said before: toxicology is a pretty big and complex field of science.

Luckily, we don't have to study all those thousands of substances ourselves to check if we can run into them (and in what doses). Every country has official organizations for protecting the general public from exposure to toxic substances from all thinkable sources. These organizations figure out what potentially harmful substances are used in agriculture, industry and households, and then set exposure limits that everyone has to observe. They take samples from the soil, drinking water supplies and food in supermarkets to see if they can find any traces of harmful chemicals, and if so, if these exceed the set limits. They specify maximum concentrations for certain household chemicals, and much, much more.[4]

The important thing to note is that there are *always* tiny amounts of 'toxins' in our food and water, both from natural and man-made sources. For instance rice is known to contain traces of arsenic, and fish contains mercury compounds—both substances known as deadly poisons, but basically harmless in the quantities that we normally consume. Still, rice cakes are not advised for very young children, and also certain types of fish should not be eaten more than once a week.

But unless you're actually working with concentrated toxic substances, there's no need to worry about any toxins in your food, your drinking water or your body. Still, let's take another look at those activated charcoal 'detox' capsules. What do they actually do in our body?

Detox Charcoal Revisited

Earlier on, we looked at a rather scary Web ad telling us that we're inevitably being poisoned all the time, but that we could get rid of all those toxins in our body by taking a couple of capsules with activated charcoal a few times a day.

Activated charcoal is actually used in cases of real poisoning because it can adsorb all kinds of chemical substances, including lots of toxic substances. The charcoal is then excreted from the body, together with the toxins. But this only works as long as the toxins are still in the stomach, so immediately

---

[4] A science blogger by the name of Credible Hulk has made an interesting comparison of the toxicity of the much maligned weedkiller glyphosate and a number of household products [49].

after an actual poisoning. And even then, it does not work for each and every toxic substance.

However, the directions for use of these charcoal capsules advise that they should be taken before bedtime, on a mostly empty stomach.

Just think about it for a moment: if there is nothing in the stomach, then there are also no 'toxins' in the stomach, so there is nothing for the activated charcoal to adsorb. The claim is made that toxins are 'drawn' from your body, but that is not how our body works. Anything we eat and drink is absorbed from our intestines into our bloodstream, after being broken down by our digestive system. This is mostly a one-way process, and toxins or other substances don't make their way from inside our body back into the intestines again. And, as already explained, most people don't have harmful amounts of toxins in their body in the first place, so there really isn't anything much to 'draw out'.

But perhaps it would be a good idea to take that detox charcoal right after meals, so it can protect us from toxins in our food before they are taken up by the body? Well, no. If anything, that would be even worse than taking it on an empty stomach. The problem is that activated charcoal does not distinguish between healthy substances and toxins. It will readily adsorb any vitamins and other healthy components in your food, if only because our food contains far more of those nutrients than toxins. Even worse, this charcoal may also adsorb prescription medicines such as contraceptives or heart medication, so it is important never to take charcoal together with any other medicine.

And then there's this: taking charcoal will turn your poo black, making it more difficult to spot potentially dangerous health problems such as intestinal bleeding (which can be a sign of intestinal cancer and other serious conditions).

Lastly, these things cost money. In the case of those charcoal capsules, you are advised to take three to four capsules every day, setting you back some $1.50 per day, for the rest of your life. That is well over $500 per year for something that does absolutely nothing for your health.

So in all, using activated charcoal is only advised in cases of real or suspected poisoning, and should then be taken as quickly as possible, preferably within an hour. Taking charcoal on a daily basis is useless and may even be harmful. In the end the only thing it'll give you is black (and expensive) poo.

Real Detox

Even though most people don't have to worry about 'toxins', real poisonings do happen, either accidental or deliberate.

Substance Detox

The most common types of poisoning are alcohol and drug abuse, and in the case of drugs, literal 'detox' is sometimes possible. When a person has overdosed on opioids (a class of drugs containing morphine, heroin, oxycodone and several other drugs), a special antidote by the name of naloxone can be administered to counter the most dangerous effects of those drugs, especially respiratory arrest. Naloxone works by occupying the same receptors in the body that opioids bind to, effectively blocking those opioids from having any effect.

The other, more common meaning of 'detox' from alcohol or drugs is not so much aimed at getting the actual substances out of the body, but at dealing with the addiction and handling the urge to take those substances in the first place. Some alternative treatments (mainly acupuncture) are said to be helpful in combating addictions, but the evidence is sparse and weak. Studies into acupuncture to help stop smoking found no clear effect [50].

Chelation Therapy

Another legitimate type of detox is *chelation therapy*. This is a treatment that comes closest to the popular concept of 'detox': the patient receives an IV with a special chemical substance that binds to heavy metals such as mercury and lead. This chemical is then excreted through the kidneys, together with the poisonous metal. In a way, this is similar to activated charcoal, with the difference that it adsorbs heavy metals in the bloodstream rather than the stomach and intestine.

Chelation therapy only works for certain metals, and must be carried out under close medical supervision, because it can have serious and sometimes even fatal side-effects. The main problem with chelating agents is that they also bind calcium, a metal that is vitally important for the functioning of our nerves, muscles and brain. Low blood calcium levels (a condition called *hypocalcemia*) can lead to heart problems, neurological problems and even death. Chelation therapy can also cause kidney and liver damage.

Unfortunately, alternative practitioners sometimes offer chelation therapy as a treatment for other conditions than heavy metal poisoning, such as heart disease and even autism. There is no evidence at all that these treatments are effective, and there *is* evidence that this treatment is dangerous [51].

Chelating agents will also cause a temporary rise in heavy metal levels in the urine, simply because everyone has very low, basically harmless amounts of these metals in their body. These so-called *provoked urine tests* are often carried out by alternative practitioners. The resulting false diagnosis of heavy metal poisoning then leads to (unnecessary) treatments, with the already mentioned risks of serious side effects.

If you are consulting an alternative practitioner who recommends chelation treatment, then walk out the door and find another practitioner who will not expose you to unnecessary, expensive and potentially very harmful procedures. If you suspect that you may be suffering from any kind of poisoning, consult a regular doctor and have some proper blood work done. This is the only reliable way to check if you are indeed laden with 'toxins'.

Antidotes

The third and last type of actual detox are *antidotes*. These are substances that are typically administered after acute poisoning, e.g. in case of snakebites. Many antidotes are *antibodies* that specifically bind to one type of poison or venom. These antidotes are made by injecting animals with harmless doses of the poison in question; the animal's immune system then responds by creating antibodies that neutralize the poison, at which point those antibodies are harvested from the animal's blood serum.

Other antidotes counteract the effects of a poison by binding to the same receptors in the body that the poison binds to. The already mentioned anti-opioid drug nalaxone is one such substance.

In all cases, time is of the essence: an antidote should be administered as fast as possible after poisoning, in order to minimize the damage done by the poison.

Let Toxins Be Thy Medicine

In Chapter 4, I already discussed the somewhat mangled quote from Hippocrates '*Let Food be thy Medicine*'. There I explained that yes, food is generally important to support good health and promote healing, but also that food is not medicine. However, toxic substances can be medicines, hence the caption of this section.

The most common example is chemotherapy, where toxic substances are used to kill off cancer cells. The general idea is that many cancer cells have a higher metabolic rate than most normal cells, and also a much higher, uncontrolled division rate (which is pretty much the definition of cancer). Many chemotherapy medicines try to take advantage of these characteristics, targeting rapidly dividing cells. Unfortunately, this means that certain body cells with high dividing rates (e.g. in the lining of the intestine and the hair follicles) also get hit hard. And cells with slower dividing rates don't get away scot-free either. This explains why chemotherapy often has very serious side effects and can take a heavy toll on a patient.

Still, chemotherapy has made much progress over the past decades in the form of individually tailored treatment regimens, more effective managing of side effects, and, more recently, immunotherapy. With immunotherapy, the immune system is 'trained' to recognize cancer cells and destroy them. This modern, highly targeted treatment form causes far less damage and side effects than the rather more crude approach of older types of chemotherapy, that affect far more types of healthy cells in the body.

A completely different example where a highly toxic substance can be used to the benefit of patients is digitoxin, already discussed in Chapter 6. Digitoxin can help control heart arrhythmia and other heart disorders. Unfortunately, the effective dose lies close to a toxic dose, so other, less dangerous medicines are preferred.

Perhaps one of the most perplexing examples may well be the use of the most potent toxic substance known to man: botulin toxin, better known under the brand name Botox. Botulin toxin is an extremely powerful neuro-toxin made by a bacterium named *Clostridium botulinum*. This bacterium is a cousin of the pathogen that causes tetanus, *Clostridium tetani*—which produces another toxin that is almost as powerful as botulin toxin.

Botulin toxin can cause fatal paralysis of the breathing muscles in doses as small as 100 nanograms, the smallest lethal dose of any known toxic substance. Or to put more comprehensible numbers to it: one teaspoon (5 grams) of the stuff is enough to kill about 50 million people.

This extremely potent substance is used daily in cosmetic treatments, paralysing the muscles in the skin that cause wrinkles. Apart from this what some might consider frivolous application, botulinum toxin also has thera-peutic uses. Examples are treatment of involuntary muscle spasms, excessive sweating and even migraine.

Conclusion

Our world is full of chemical substances, both natural and man-made, and many of these can be toxic under particular circumstances. And yes, those chemical substances are also found in our body—*everyone's* body—and include things such as mercury, arsenic, pesticides, solvents, and countless other substances that are often considered toxic. Many have a man-made origin, but many others are completely natural. All these potentially toxic substances are almost never a problem, and can be handled by our liver and our kidneys. As the old adage goes: *The dose makes the poison.* Also, strict environmental regulations prevent exposure of the general public to harmful substances in any significant amounts.

Yet lots of peddlers of alternative treatments try to convince us that we are in serious trouble, with (usually unspecified) 'toxins' destroying our health and well-being, and that we urgently need to 'detox'. An endless gamut of detox products and treatments is offered, from diets and herbal products to outright silly things such as footpads, but also potentially harmful treatments such as coffee enemas and chelation therapy. All these things have in common that they don't do anything for your health. At best, the placebo effect may make you feel better for a short while, but the only real effect they have is on your wallet.

Ironically, some real toxins have actual therapeutic value, with the most potent toxin of all being used no a daily basis in therapeutic and cosmetic treatments worldwide.

In the next chapter, we shall investigate a completely different phenomenon: energy—both the scientific kind and the alternative kind.

10

The Energy Problem

Party Tricks

Here's nice party trick: go to the kitchen sink, and slowly turn on the tap until you get a thin trickle. Make sure that the water still forms a continuous stream where it leaves the tap, so increase the flow if you only get droplets at first.

Then take an empty cup, and place it in the sink just next to the trickle, maybe 10 millimetres away.

*Now ask your friends or family if they can fill the cup from the tap, **without touching the tap, the water or the cup in any way**. And no, blowing at the water is also not allowed (although you might of course try and see if someone comes up with that solution). If they say that this is impossible, you could even bet that you can do it – if you're a betting person.*

Now what you do is take a balloon (hey, its a party trick, after all), rub it over your hair or over a woollen garment, and slowly bring it close to the trickle of water without actually touching it. Lo and behold, the stream of water magically bends towards the balloon, and now ends up in the cup! That calls for a drink!

(If you have no balloon, try a comb, a scrunched-up freezer bag – the semi-opaque crackly kind – or some bubble-wrap. Whatever you use, always check in advance if it actually works. You want to end up with water in the cup, not egg on your face.)

[Fast forward to the next morning]

The party was a great success, and your tricks went down well – as did a copious amount of drinks. Some of your overnight guests are now sitting around, bleary-eyed, nursing a cup of coffee and clearly not feeling very well.

© The Author(s), under exclusive license to Springer Nature
Switzerland AG 2023
R. Rasker, *Mind, Make-Believe and Medicine*,
https://doi.org/10.1007/978-3-031-29444-0_10

At which point a guest by the name of Alice suggests that she might be able to help. It turns out that she works in a integrative health clinic, and often uses Therapeutic Touch to take away pain and discomfort, make patients feel better and generally stimulate their healing. Her offer is met with some sniggers and low-key muttering about 'magical hangover cures', but one of the guys decides to give it a try anyway. After all, what does he have to lose? Alice explains that he should lie down on the couch (no problem there), after which she will try to sense his body energy with her hands, find blockades and stress points, and drain the negative energy that is making him feel miserable. This should help the body to get rid of those toxic after-effects of all that booze and hopefully lift the brain fog a bit. So our patient lies down amidst some jeering of his friends, and Alice starts hovering her hands over his body, closely following its contours. The rest of the company looks on in silence, with Alice occasionally commenting on what she is doing. After maybe 15 minutes, she concludes the treatment. She says that she can clearly feel that the body energy now has a much more free flow to it. When asked, our brave patient mumbles that he indeed feels a little better, although he is still a bit unsteady when getting up, and visibly winces when one of his friends slaps him on the shoulder ...

… and this is where we leave our merry friends to recover in peace, with their coffee, maybe an aspirin, and maybe some more Therapeutic Touch.

So what happened just now? The first half of our opening story shows a neat 'energy trick' that many people probably already know, but is still fun to watch: water being magically attracted to an object. At the end of the seventeenth century, people started to experiment with *electrical fluid* (static electricity) in much the same way as we did in our little anecdote. Little did they know that their tinkering almost literally sparked a development that profoundly changed our world. Ever more extensive scientific research into the nature and applications of electricity has made it the dominant factor in our society that it is today, with smartphones and all sorts of internet-based media and services being ubiquitous.

This chapter focuses on what is known as energy medicine and the 'energy' that it is based on. But first we will take a look at 'energy science', and in particular how electric energy has changed our world. This serves as a benchmark for comparison with the development of energy medicine.

Until about 1850, the greater public knew electricity mainly as a parlour trick, being able to 'magically' attract bits of fluff and paper, and of course to zap people—in the same way that we still get zapped when shuffling over the carpet, or getting out of a car in very dry weather. But all the while, scientists were working away at more serious applications, trying to figure out what this mysterious energy was and how it worked. Electrostatic attraction showed that it could have effects over a distance, and other experiments showed that it could also flow through metals and even wet objects.

One fascinating property was that electricity itself was completely invisible—until it made a spark, or produced other effects that gave away its presence. Again other experiments suggested that electricity (or at least electric charge) was literally everywhere, even inside living beings, and it was also discovered that electricity had some kind of connection with magnetism, and even with light.

By the late 1800s, both scientists and engineers began to get a grip on electricity. The electrical telegraph was the long-distance communication device of choice, and Thomas Edison invented and successfully marketed the electric light bulb, hugely increasing demand for electricity in homes. Electrically powered streetcars also became a common sight in towns and cities. By the 1920s, electrical household appliances were in high demand, and the roaring twenties would have been a whole lot less roaring without electricity to light music halls and other places of entertainment. From then on, developments succeeded each other at an increasing pace: telephone, radio, radar, TV, the first computers, and of course ever more electrically powered devices in our home to make our life more comfortable. The Internet really took off in the 1990s, and by the year 2000, cell phones enabled us to basically communicate with anyone we wanted, from any location we wanted, by means of handy[1] little devices that could fit in the palm of our hand.

And still, scientists keep on working at it. Electricity not only made it possible to build spacecraft that could navigate to the edge of our solar system and beyond, but even to *communicate* with those spacecraft, and receive pictures from a staggering 8 billion kilometres away—with a radio transmitter just slightly more powerful than your average cell phone. Scientists and engineers managed to build receivers to reliably pick up even those incredibly tiny signals, giving us high-resolution pictures of Pluto and its moon.

Modern medicine would also be unthinkable without electricity, especially for diagnostic purposes. One of the first medical breakthroughs in this respect was the discovery of X-rays more than a hundred years ago, which are still in use today. Nowadays, we also have MRI and CT scanning machines for creating even more detailed pictures of what's going on inside the body, all made possible by manipulating electricity in intricate ways.

Electricity is indeed an almost magical form of energy that almost invisibly powers an ever larger part of our life and society.

---

[1] Cell phones are even *called* 'Handy' in German.

Energy Medicine

The second half of our opening story also deals with energy, *life energy* to be precise, also known as *chi* or *qi* or *prana* in oriental traditions, and *anima* respectively *pneuma* ('life breath') in ancient Roman and Greek culture. There are some differences in the exact definition across cultures, but they all have two things in common: this energy is universal, and it is what makes living things alive. This also means that living creatures are fundamentally different from non-living things that are lacking this life energy. Another way to describe this life energy is as 'spirit'.

Energy medicine nowadays has varying definitions and descriptions for this life energy or qi. Most of these definitions follow the ancient wisdom that life energy is universally present, and that it can be tapped into for purposes of healing and gaining personal knowledge and insight. However, humans (and other living beings) also have their own personal energy field or energy flow, and this energy can get out of balance, become blocked or attain a negative nature, causing all sorts of health problems. Traditional Chinese Medicine (TCM) has a slightly different view, stipulating that in living creatures, a large part of this energy field flows along so-called *meridians* just below the body's surface.

Energy medicine practitioners claim that they can sense this field, usually with their hands, and then manipulate it in order to restore health, or at least, as they say 'stimulate the body's healing mechanism'. In most forms of energy medicine, this manipulation happens with the hands as well, handily combining diagnosis and treatment in one go (hey, who said alternative medicine can't be efficient?). Acupuncture uses needles to influence the flow of energy along the meridians, and *bioresonance* uses electrical equipment to measure and influence the body's energy.

Anja Chakra Energy

No doubt, you wondered what this 'energy' that lies at the basis of Reiki, therapeutic touch etcetera feels like, and how these practitioners experience it themselves. One problem here of course is that personal sensations are hard to describe adequately. This is especially the case with sensations that don't feel like anything you experienced before.

There is, however, a simple experiment that you can do to get an idea what it is all about. What you need is a metal object with some mass to it, but also a very sharp point. A needle is too small and flimsy, but a pair of compasses should work just fine. The only other thing that you need is a volunteer.

Now what you do is instruct the volunteer to sit still, looking straight ahead. Then you slowly move the sharp metal point towards the middle of the volunteer's forehead without actually touching it, while asking what sensations occur. Quite likely, the volunteer will describe a sort of tingling and even jarring sensation, getting stronger when the point gets closer. The point on the forehead is known as the *Anja chackra*, or the third eye, and it supposedly can see things that our normal eyes can't see. So in this case, it 'sees' the energy that you are channelling into the metal and focusing on the chakra by means of just a simple sharp pointed object!

Of course you should also switch places, so that you are the one experiencing this energy—or maybe you should be the guinea pig yourself the first time round. The effect can be quite amazing, and many people find it an eye-opener (third eye or otherwise).

So this proves that there certainly is some sort of energy there, right? After all, you can *feel* it, for crying out loud!

Well ... let's not spoil the fun right away, but just give a little hint: repeat the experiment, but now with the test subject blindfolded or having their eyes closed.

So this life energy, which is a pretty important phenomenon in the alternative world, has a history going back several thousand years—much further even than electricity. From ancient times onward, almost all cultures have discovered it and integrated it into their systems of philosophy and medicine. Even today it is still the foundation of several forms of alternative medicine, some of which are quite popular, such as acupuncture and Reiki.

All this gives rise to a rather puzzling question: if this life energy has been recognized and used for thousands of years already, then why isn't it being used everywhere in society, just like electricity? Or at least in regular medicine? Why is it only used in alternative medicine and in some esoteric and religious cultures, and nowhere else?

It turns out that there is a bit of a problem with this 'life energy': it does not exist.

Or maybe I should be a bit more precise: it seems to exist in some people's minds, but not in the real world. Even though thousands upon thousands of people claim that they can feel this energy, manipulate it, and clearly show its effects (such as improved health) to anyone, each and every attempt to objectively detect or observe it has failed so far.

Electric energy, in comparison, could be detected right from the moment it was discovered. Static electricity was detected by the way it attracted or repelled small objects, or even simpler by getting zapped; it could also be easily measured with so-called electroscopes. And, most importantly, literally anyone can repeat those experiments for detecting electricity, not just specially trained people or people who believed in the existence of electricity. Anyone can do the balloon-and-water trick, and anyone can experience the zap from static electricity when charged up. So-called *multimeters* are available for a couple of dollars in almost all hardware stores, enabling very accurate measurements of basic electrical phenomena such as voltage, current and electrical resistance. People unlucky or careless enough to touch live electrical wires *will* get shocked, no matter if they believe in electricity (or even in science) or not.

In comparison, qi or life energy can't be detected in any objective way. Only people who received special training or are otherwise made to believe in its existence can detect it—at least that is what they claim. But as soon as their claims are actually tested in experiments, their ability to feel this energy completely disappears.

What They Feel Is Real

Don't get me wrong: the people who claim that they can feel some sort of energy field are not lying. To them, the sensations they experience are perfectly real, just like the sensation our guinea pig experienced in the little home experiment I just described in the sidebar. The problem is that those sensations are not caused by any 'energy field', but by their own brain, much like people who lost a limb can experience sensations such as itching and even pain (so-called *phantom pain*) in a limb that is no longer there.

Conversely, people can also lose the sensation that a limb belongs to them. The late neurologist and best-selling author Oliver Sacks experienced this first-hand when he suffered a badly broken leg in an accident. He described his experience in his 1984 book *A Leg to Stand On*. One of his biggest surprises was how absolutely *real* this feeling of alienation from part of his own body was. His rational mind had a very hard time dealing with this completely altered bodily sensation that his own brain produced. It is therefore not strange at all that energy medicine practitioners are also convinced that what they feel is quite real.

The science part will get into this in more detail, describing several scientific experiments showing how people can feel things that are not real.

But Patients Feel It Too!

Well, yes, if practitioners can evoke special sensations, so can patients. Of course there is the placebo effect, where the mere expectation to feel something special causes the mind to, indeed, feel something special. If actual touching takes place, then this can have strong soothing and warming effects, especially since most people are not used to being touched in a very intentional and intense manner, certainly not by a stranger.

Even when no touching is involved, any sensations that do occur can be enhanced by heat radiated from a practitioner's hands, causing an ever so slightly warmer feeling there where those hands are. Subtle air movements can have a similar effect that 'something' is happening.

The Origins of Life Energy

Virtually all ancient cultures have come up with some sort of special 'life energy', usually associated with breath. This idea is not strange at all: living things are quite special when compared to inanimate objects. Living things can move about and seem to have a will of their own. This is completely different from, say, rocks or even trees.[2] Those inanimate things were just there, doing nothing much remarkable. And if these things did happen to do something dramatic, like fall on someone, then this was usually attributed to living(!) gods rather than the rock or tree itself.

Living things can also die, and then they become dead things, at which point they start behaving more or less like the aforementioned rocks and trees: they just lie there, slowly decomposing.

So clearly, there must be something inside living things that is not present in dead and inanimate things. Together with the observation that breathing is essential for life—the first thing any newborn must do is start breathing—the conclusion is almost inescapable that this special something is a kind of 'breath of life'. And sure enough, in creation myths around the world, gods make people come alive by literally breathing life into them.

Likewise, when a person or an animal dies, then its life breath leaves the body—but that means that it must go somewhere, right? So some cultures invented an omnipresent life energy, which is tapped into to make something alive, and to which the life breath returns when someone dies—which basically describes qi. In many cultures, this life energy also engenders the soul (at least in humans), which is considered to be the *personal* immaterial part that defines who we are, and what we think and believe (as opposed to the ubiquitous non-personal presence of life energy). To make thinking about life and especially death a bit less frightening, this soul is often thought to be immortal.

---

[2] It is not clear if those ancient cultures considered plants to be infused with qi in the same way as animals.

All this is once again a nice example of our human tendency to recognize patterns, link things together, and use our imagination while doing so, in order to explain important phenomena such as life and death—even if in reality, we had no clue what was going on.

All this neatly explains where qi comes from. But humans, never being content with just knowing things, also want to use it. If this life energy is essential for life itself, then it should also be possible to *do* something with it in cases where life is endangered, right? At which point this idea of life energy turns from a philosophy into a leading principle in medicine.

Once again it should be emphasized that this way of thinking about the world and human life is in no way stupid; the whole explanation is very logical—which is why most cultures have come up with it at one time or another. The main reason why it is outdated now is because through painstaking scientific work, we have found better explanations for how the world and the people in it function.

We now know that there is no fundamental difference between living creatures and dead matter. The only real difference is that living creatures have some insanely complex chemistry going on inside them, something that simple rocks can only dream of (if they could dream, which they can't—which is the whole point, really). We also identified lots of things that exist on the boundary of living and dead matter, such as viruses—and the scientific debate still goes on about whether viruses are alive or not. (The answer settled upon for now seems to be 'Somewhat'.) And yes, as expected, those 'somewhat living' things have less complicated chemistry than most living creatures, but still considerably more complex than inanimate things.

And even though our human mental processes and especially our consciousness and self-awareness have not been scientifically explained to the last detail, neurology has firmly established that these things are generated by and very tightly bound to our physical brain. No special, esoteric energy or even soul seems to be involved here.

Forms of Energy Medicine

Energy medicine is basically a modernized incarnation of the ancient concept of *vitalism*, the belief that all living creatures are somehow infused with a universal life energy, and that disease and suffering are caused by imbalances or other disturbances in this energy.

In spite of the fact that modern science can't find a trace of any special life energy, energy medicine in different guises is still very popular in alternative circles. So let's take a look at some of the most prominent forms. One of the more surprising findings is that although the concept of life energy or qi is thousands of years old, and many forms of energy medicine also emphasize their ancient roots, none of them is practised in its original form. All forms of energy medicine that are offered today are less than a century old—which is actually a good thing, given how some forms of energy medicine were *really* practised in the past.

Acupuncture

Even though acupuncture is usually seen as a separate type of alternative medicine or as an important part of Traditional Chinese Medicine (TCM), it is in essence a type of energy medicine.

Acupuncture is based on the concept that life energy or qi flows through the body through special conduits under the skin called *meridians*. The idea is that a lot of health problems stem from blockage of this energy flow. This can then be cured or at least improved by locating the meridians involved in the ailment, and inserting needles at certain special points (acupoints) along those meridians.

When we talk about acupuncture, most people nowadays envision these very thin needles (so-called *filiform* needles) that are gently inserted in the outermost layer of skin. However, these modern needles don't look like traditional needles at all—and the same goes for the actual acupuncture treatment.

Over a century ago, a Scottish physician by the name of Dugald Christie worked in China in a place called Moukden (now Shenyang). Not only did he introduce western medicine there, he wrote a book about his experiences aptly entitled *Thirty years in Moukden, 1883–1913, being the experiences and recollections of Dugald Christie* [52]. In his book, he describes how acupuncture was practised in those days:

The only mode of treatment in vogue which might be called surgical is acupuncture, practised for all kinds of ailments. The needles are of nine forms, and are frequently used red-hot, and occasionally left in the body for days. Having no practical knowledge of anatomy, the practitioners often pass needles into large blood-vessels and important organs, and immediate death has some- times resulted. A little child was carried to the dispensary presenting a pitiable spectacle. The doctor had told the parents that there was an excess of fire in its body, to let out which he must use cold needles, so he had pierced the abdomen deeply in several places. The poor little sufferer died shortly afterwards. For cholera the needling is in the arms. For some children's diseases, especially convulsions, the needles are inserted under the nails. For eye diseases they are often driven into the back between the shoulders to a depth of several inches. Patients have come to us with large surfaces on their backs sloughing by reason of excessive treatment of this kind with instruments none too clean.

This is how *real* traditional Chinese acupuncture was done. If anything, this looks nothing like the wishy-washy I-can-hardly-feel-a-thing acupuncture that is practised these days. And yes, many if not most people receiving acupuncture treatment were badly hurt, and some even died—if not from the stabbing itself, then from infections that must have regularly occurred. Unsurprisingly, acupuncture was not exactly a popular treatment, and at several points in Chinese history, it was almost completely abolished—not only because of its brutal nature, but also because there were often doubts about its efficacy already then [53].

Acupuncture as we now know it was conceived in the 1950s, as part of the politically motivated promotion of Traditional Chinese Medicine under Mao Zedong (also see Chapter 4). We will return to acupuncture in the Science section, further on in this chapter.

Bioresonance

In most forms of energy medicine 'life energy' is detected and manipulated by practitioners using their hands, or (in the case of acupuncture) needles.

A more technologically oriented variety of energy medicine is called *bioresonance*. Its basic premise is that every organ and even every cell in the body 'resonates' at a particular frequency. What's more: pathogenic microbes and even chemical substances also have their own resonance frequencies. The claim is that countless ailments and problems can be diagnosed by measuring these resonances and frequencies, pinpointing exactly what is wrong with a particular organ. These resonances are detected by a special bioresonance device, and processed by software on a connected computer.

The whole procedure is fast and simple: after entering the patient's name, age and gender into the computer, this patient just holds one or two metallic rods (the electrodes) in their hands, at which point a bioresonance scan is started. The scan takes a couple of minutes at most, after which the computer analyses the data and produces a diagnostic report. This report is highly detailed, showing health scores for all organs and dozens or even hundreds of physiological parameters.

The practitioner operating the bioresonance machine then discusses the results with the patient, and comes up with a treatment plan. This treatment plan often involves taking particular supplements for an extended period of time in order to treat any deficiencies found. Often, some sort of detox program is advised, or a treatment for parasites or chronic Lyme's disease. Some bioresonance machines are able to not only diagnose conditions, but even treat them. In this case, the patient once again holds the electrodes, after which the machine detects the troublesome resonance frequency and sends back an identical but opposite signal, so that it cancels out the disease-causing resonance.

After a couple of days or weeks, the patient returns, and the bioresonance scan is repeated. In most cases, the problems identified in the first scan have significantly improved, clearly showing that the diagnosis was correct and the treatment worked. OK, some new problems may be developing, but luckily, those are caught early, so they can be treated even before they cause symptoms.

This certainly sounds impressive!

Once again, please think about this for a moment. According to the claims made, these relatively small and cheap devices can perform an accurate diagnosis measuring dozens or even hundreds of health parameters, including levels of vitamins and minerals, the presence of microbial and parasitic infections, and the general state of health—all by holding an electrode for a couple of minutes. Then why doesn't every doctor have one of these in their office? They only cost a couple of thousand dollars, so they're far cheaper than all that hugely expensive, cumbersome scanning equipment in hospitals. In addition, they're much faster, safer and easier to use, with pictures showing each organ and what is wrong with it.

Unfortunately, they're also a total scam—but a pretty sophisticated, convincing scam. We'll explain in detail how the scam works in the science part of this chapter. There you can also read how you can test these devices if you're unlucky enough to have bought one yourself.

One important thing to note here is that bioresonance practitioners are just as much a victim of this scam as the patients they are 'diagnosing'— bioresonance practitioners have no knowledge of the actual technology; they simply trust the manufacturer on their word that these machines work as claimed. However, those manufacturers *absolutely know* that their products don't work, and literally get away with fraud. They go out of their way to design those machines in such a way that it creates the illusion of a functioning device without actually measuring or processing any real physiological data. Best case, their devices measure skin resistance, which might diagnose sweaty hands.

Hulda Clark's Zapper

Another noteworthy device in this category is the 'zapper', sold by the late Hulda Clark, a naturopath from Canada. Clark claimed that each and every disease was caused by a kind of parasitic flatworm, and that her 'zapper' could get rid of those parasites, effectively curing all thinkable diseases.

When you hear claims like this, all alarm bells should go off. All diseases have just one simple cause and one even simpler solution? Then why do doctors spend at least eight years in medical school?

Clark's claims are of course nonsense, and her zapper is useless. The most interesting thing about this zapper device is that the electronic schematic diagram can be found on the internet. This means that anyone can see how it is made and even build their own device. It turns out to be an extremely simple circuit[3] with just a few dollars worth of components. It produces an electrical signal (a so-called block wave) with a frequency of roughly 30 kilohertz (30,000 cycles per second, also see the next chapter) on a set of electrodes that should be held in both hands.

Completely contrary to its sweeping claims about eradicating parasites and diseases, it doesn't do anything at all in the body. Only by holding the electrodes against the tongue is it possible to feel an electric tingle, more or less like when touching the contacts of a 9-V battery against the tongue. The main difference is that a battery produces a steady direct current (DC), while the zapper produces 'chopped-up' direct current, with the voltage going to zero and then back to 9 V again some 30,000 times per second.

Still, lots of people build and buy these zappers, in the hope that they may help with particular health problems. And as always, placebo effects and other well-known mechanisms will give lots of users the illusion that it really works (at least for them), encouraging them to spread their positive testimonials on the Internet.

It must be noted that this zapper device is strictly speaking not 'energy medicine', as it is not associated with qi or another form of life energy. It produces an electrical signal that can actually be detected and measured. What it has in common with energy medicine is that it doesn't do anything for people's health, apart maybe from placebo effects.

---

[3] It is in fact the same circuit that most beginners in electronics start out with, based on a so-called 555 timer chip.

What the Science Says

In science, there is exactly one definition of energy: it is the capability to perform work, period. We distinguish several types of energy, which are in fact just systems in which energy is stored in one way or another. The standard unit of energy is the *joule*. For non-scientists: a 6 W LED lamp uses 6 J of energy per second, so one joule is not that much energy at all.

What Is energy?

In physics, energy is simply the capability to do work. One important property of energy is that it can't be created or destroyed, it can only be converted from one form of energy into another. This is why 'free energy machines' are fundamentally impossible, because that would mean that energy is created out of nowhere.

One of the simplest, most tangible forms of energy is kinetic energy. This is energy that is stored in moving objects. This is also the energy that can cause a lot of damage when two moving objects collide—because their kinetic energy can't just disappear, but has to go somewhere. Breaking and bending things absorbs a lot of energy, and ultimately turns it into heat energy.

There are also less tangible forms of energy. For instance chemical energy is energy that is involved when a chemical reaction takes place, and electrical energy is the energy that moves charged particles (usually electrons), which can then do useful things in all sorts of ways. A battery is a device that directly converts chemical energy into electrical energy. Then there is electromagnetic energy, which is capable of moving through empty space on its own—which is a Very Good Thing, because otherwise, we would not receive any light and heat (which are both electromagnetic energy) from the sun.

We will further discuss energy as defined in physics in the next chapter, when we talk about radiation energy in all its forms and guises.

It should be obvious by now that 'life energy', even if it would exist, is something completely different from energy as it is defined in physics.

Qi Questioned

If scientists would start investigating this qi or 'life energy', they would start out with a lot of questions that need to be answered before they would even begin to entertain the notion that it actually exists. How exactly is this life energy characterized? How can we objectively detect it? How can it be measured? If it can't be detected or measured, how do you know it is real? How does it interact with living creatures? And if it interacts with living creatures, then how can this interaction be reliably detected? How can a practitioner manipulate it, and use it to the benefit of patients? Can a practitioner make mistakes handling this energy? If so, what happens to patients? Is there research or even just some case reports to support any given answers?

There is an even more basic question: if this qi or prana or life energy is universally available as well as essential for the well-being of living creatures, then why haven't those living creatures evolved ways to deal with any 'energy problems' themselves? After all, living creatures have evolved ways to deal with virtually all conceivable health problems, as already explained in Chapter 4. Why is the intervention of a practitioner required for using qi?

One would also expect lots of people to be working with qi in a scientific way, exploring its character and its applications, just like all those scientists working in the fields of for instance genetics, biochemistry, quantum physics and electronics.

Strangely enough, energy medicine practitioners hardly ever ask these questions, nor do they do novel research into what they vehemently claim is a real phenomenon.

So one day, one Emily Rosa decided to do just that: research this mysterious life energy in a scientific experiment.

Rosa et al.

In 1996, Emily Rosa watched a television show where a Therapeutic Touch (TT) practitioner demonstrated her healing art, and said that anyone could be trained to feel the human energy field that she worked with. Emily wondered about this, especially since these people were so certain about what they felt. As a science fair was coming up at her school, she decided that she wanted to test these practitioners' abilities in a science project. The test was simple but elegant: first, she asked the practitioners who had agreed to partake in the experiment if they could feel the human energy field from her own hand if she held it 10 cm above the practitioner's hand, while facing each other. They all confirmed that, yes, they could clearly feel her hand's energy field.

Then the test was repeated, but this time, the practitioner was blinded, sitting behind a screen with two openings at the bottom. Emily would ask practitioners to extend their hands through those holes, palms up, and then she would hold her own hand over one of the practitioner's hands again, with a coin flip determining whether it would be the left or the right hand. The practitioner was then asked over which hand they detected Emily's energy field. This was repeated 10 or 20 times per practitioner. It turned out that the practitioners' guesses were no better than chance—they named the correct hand only half the time on average. In other words: they completely failed to detect a human energy field as soon as they could no longer see the other person's body. This is a strong indication that there is no human energy field, and that Therapeutic Touch is not based on any real phenomenon.

Rosa's research paper was written with the help of her mother and several other scientists, and published in 1998, in the prestigious *Journal of the American Medical Association* [54]. One interesting detail: to this day, Emily Rosa holds the record for the youngest person ever to have a scientific paper published in a peer-reviewed journal—she was nine years old when she carried out her research.

Another interesting detail: Rosa et al. also represents the most extensive research that has been done into Therapeutic Touch to date. There is virtually no other literature about TT, and there also is no scientific evidence that TT is beneficial for any medical condition.

Yet in spite of this rather strong (and widely publicized) evidence that Therapeutic Touch is no good, it continued to become more popular, and it is even used in hospitals in many countries. All without even the tiniest bit of evidence that it actually benefits patients.

Fake Limb Energy?

So what is going on with those people who claim that they can feel this energy field? It appears that their brain is somehow changing the processing of the sensory information from their hands. In other words: they trained their brain to 'extend' the range of feeling beyond their actual hands, and this extended sensation is triggered by what they see. When they visualise an energy field as a sort of aura around people, their brain also makes them *feel* something when their hands touch this invisible field.

This mechanism is also clearly demonstrated in the so-called *rubber hand experiment* [55]. In this experiment, healthy people have their left hand covered by a screen, with a realistic rubber hand visible and positioned in front of them. When the experimenters stroke the real left hand and the fake hand at the same time, test subjects begin to *feel* the rubber hand as if it were their own left hand; at the same time, the feeling of propriety of their real hand diminished. When asked to use their free right hand to point at their own left hand, they more often than not pointed to the fake hand.

This extended or transferred sensation also explains what happens in the little home experiment in the first sidebar, at the beginning of this chapter: when people see the sharp pointy end of the compasses held very close to their forehead, their brain tries to avert a dangerous situation by producing a sensation even without actual touching taking place, urging people to move their head away. When test subjects keep their eyes closed, they can no longer see the danger, so they won't 'feel' the proximity of the sharp point any more.

In effect, what those energy medicine practitioners feel are sensations that are produced by their own brain, not any elusive 'energy'. Extensive training can make these sensations feel quite real, and this makes it rather difficult for these people to accept the notion that no, they are not feeling any energy, and they certainly are not influencing anything that is happening inside their patients.

Acupuncture Research

More than any other type of alternative medicine, acupuncture has been the subject of a lot of scientific research in the past few decades. There are three main reasons for this:

- Acupuncture is one of the more plausible alternative treatments—after all, the intervention is real and physical: needles are actually being poked into the skin. Even without the underlying qi and meridian mechanisms (which are not plausible), there could well be some sort of interaction with nerves or the immune system, causing real effects such as the release of endorphins (natural painkillers).
- Acupuncture studies also seem to come up with positive results more often than other types of alternative medicine.
- Especially China produces a lot of acupuncture studies, to the greater glory of TCM and thus China. Unfortunately, the extremely high percentage of positive outcomes (as in: 100%) in these studies is suspect to say the least, so these studies are better dismissed [56].

Proper research into acupuncture really took off after the year 2000. While at first, outcomes suggested that it might be effective for pain relief in several conditions, the effects were mostly small and temporary, and placebo effects could not be ruled out. One of the problems with acupuncture was that double-blinded clinical studies were initially impossible because there was no good 'placebo acupuncture'; both the acupuncturist and the patient knew what was happening.

In more recent years, several methods for doing so-called *sham acupuncture* have been developed. The simplest way to perform sham acupuncture is to insert needles at random locations, away from meridians and acupoints. This helps to determine if there is actually some reason and reality to this idea of meridians. Another form of sham acupuncture is also pretty simple, and involves poking the patient's skin with pointed wooden sticks, without penetrating the skin. This would give the patient the sensation of needles being inserted. This type of sham acupuncture of course only works if the patient can't see the needles or sticks. Yet another form of sham acupuncture used needles with retractable points, which do not penetrate the skin at all [57].

Even though not a perfect acupuncture placebo, these studies with sham acupuncture showed that acupuncture was not effective for the overwhelming majority of conditions it was used for. Most studies found no difference between sham acupuncture and real acupuncture.

Around 2010, the totality of evidence at that point led scientists to believe that acupuncture was at best an elaborate placebo treatment—a pretty good placebo, but a placebo nonetheless. This means that acupuncture treatment can make people feel better—which may be helpful in managing pain—but it can't bring about any clinical improvement in any conditions [58].

This placebo effect can even be dangerous, as exemplified by studies into the use of acupuncture for asthma: asthma patients who were treated with acupuncture generally reported feeling better than patients who received no treatment. However, actual measurement showed no improvement in lung function at all, which means that these patients still ran an increased risk of a potentially deadly asthma attack. Only the group using real asthma medicine (albuterol) showed significant improvement in lung function [59].

So in all, acupuncture's relatively strong placebo effect may help (somewhat) with pain complaints, but it is not effective for any other conditions. Also, there is no scientific evidence whatsoever that meridians[4] or qi exist.

Bioresonance Revisited

Just to jog your mind about bioresonance, this is what a sales pitch for these machines looks like:

All cells in our body produce electromagnetic fields. These electromagnetic vibrations maintain their correct resonance while cells and organs are in good health. When disease occurs, these biological structures sustain damage and no longer function like they should. This structural damage causes the emitted energy pattern to change.

---

[4] One of the most important meridians in acupuncture is the so-called gallbladder meridian, in humans as well as animals. And sure enough, acupuncture for horses often focuses on this gallbladder meridian. There is just one tiny problem: horses don't have a gallbladder.

> *Bioresonance machines detect the electromagnetic fields produced by the cells inside the body, and register any deviations from the optimal frequency values. These resonances are then restored to their proper values. This is called* **bioresonance**.

No matter how scientific all this may sound, virtually every claim here is untrue. Let's look at the claims one by one to see what is wrong with them.

All cells in our body produce electromagnetic fields

Yes, this is fundamentally correct, but not in the way that these bioresonance peddlers mean. For most cells, those 'electromagnetic fields' are simply infrared radiation, a.k.a. heat. *Everything* with a temperature above absolute zero (-273.15 °C or 0 K) emits electromagnetic fields in the form of heat radiation (also see the next chapter). These electromagnetic fields are nothing special, and are fully identical for substances with the same temperature.

The only other type of electromagnetic fields that can be emitted by body cells comes from electrical activity in nerve and muscle cells. This electrical activity is measured by legitimate medical devices such as ECG and EEG machines, to monitor heart and brain activity, respectively. Ironically, bioresonance devices do NOT pick up or process these real electrical signals.

These electromagnetic vibrations maintain their correct resonance while cells and organs are in good health

Here it is suggested that the health of cells and organs can be directly measured by measuring their 'electromagnetic vibrations'. Which is simply nonsense, because most cells in our body produce no such vibrations.

When disease occurs, these biological structures sustain damage and no longer function like they should

Most of the conditions 'diagnosed' by bioresonance practitioners do not involve damaged or non-functional organs at all.

Bioresonance machines detect the electromagnetic fields produced by the cells inside the body ...

In reality, most bioresonance devices are a complete scam and don't measure anything. The ones that do measure something only pick up random noise, which can be filtered to produce any desired frequency or wavelength.[5] The only health indicator that these devices can measure is if someone has sweaty hands or not.

... and register any deviations from the optimal frequency values

How exactly is this done? And where can we find these optimal values? If cells in our body have very specific frequencies or wavelengths, then shouldn't there be lists or tables showing exactly *what frequency* a particular type of cell is associated with? A simple Internet search does turn up a few of those lists, but alas, hardly any two of them agree on actual values. Some mention a couple of hundred hertz, others talk about sixty million hertz (60 megahertz). That's quite a difference ...

For comparison: there are countless Web pages telling us which blood pressure values are healthy and unhealthy—and they all agree on the same values. The same goes for other health metrics such as heart rates and body temperature.

Also, there is no peer-reviewed scientific research at all describing that these frequencies were indeed observed, or how they were measured, how strong their signals were, where they originate in a cell, and what biological function they have—cells do not evolve to produce electromagnetic signals just for fun. Yet here it is simply posited that 'cells produce frequencies', period.

These resonances are then restored to their proper values

So let's get this straight. The device not only *measures* very special frequencies coming from all the cells and organs in our body, it also works the other way, *influencing* these frequencies? These things can actually cure conditions? This is as if you have a very special thermometer that not only tells you a patient's temperature, but at the same time can also *correct* fever or hypothermia. Which of course is nonsense.

Summarized: the devices peddled here, often costing well upwards of a thousand dollars, claim to be able to diagnose and even treat hundreds of health conditions. In reality, they are cheap pieces of digital junk electronics, mass-produced for just a couple of dozen dollars each, and the only effect they will ever have is to make a serious dent in your bank account.

---

[5] Frequency and wavelength of electromagnetic waves are basically each other's inverse. Frequency tells you how many waves per second pass by, and wavelength is a measure for the distances between each two wave crests. A long distance (wavelength) automatically means that it takes longer for each wave to pass by, resulting in a lower frequency. Also see the next chapter.

But even though these machines are a complete scam, they seem to produce pretty convincing and even repeatable results. They even show progress as a result from treatment! So how exactly does this scam work?

The Tricks Behind Bioresonance Machines

The first step in a bioresonance scan (or scam, if you will) consists of entering patient information into the computer: name, age, sex, and perhaps height and weight. This personal information is in fact an essential element of the scam, as it is used to help create the illusion of a functioning diagnostic device.

Then the patient is instructed to hold the electrode. The electrode has two electrical contacts, and the machine measures the so-called electrical *resistance* between the contacts. Human skin has a lower electrical resistance than air; this skin resistance tells the machine that someone is holding the electrode, and that a 'scan' can start.

The scan itself can take between one minute and a couple of minutes. Some bioresonance machines show a timer counting down the seconds; other machines just show one or more blinking lights. At the same time, the computer screen may show graphics of a human body, often highlighting the parts that are scanned at each moment, together with impressive-looking numbers and other data being recorded.

In reality, nothing is scanned, measured or recorded. The bioscan device only checks the electrode to determine if a person is actually holding it; everything else is just for show, creating the illusion that a complex scanning process is taking place.

When the 'scan' ends, the computer produces a highly detailed report about the state of health of the patient's organs, nutrient levels, any diseases etcetera.

This report is completely made up. The computer simply chooses more or less random values for each of the parameters it pretends to have 'measured', taking into account some of the previously supplied personal information. This way, it will not make the mistake of signalling e.g. prostate problems in women.

This report is then saved with the patient's name and other information, so that if you immediately repeat the scan with the same patient, you will get virtually identical results (suggesting that results can be replicated and are thus legitimate).

Now comes the clever bit: when, after a couple of weeks, a patient returns for a new scan, the computer looks up what parameters were less than optimal the previous time (for instance certain mineral levels or blood cholesterol). It then *makes up better values* for those parameters. Why does it do this? Simple: because the patient was almost certainly treated for those things, and everyone will be happy if that seems to have helped—even if in reality, the treatment was both unnecessary and without effect.

Another clever trick is that in the new scan, some *other* health parameters appear to be slipping somewhat—again requiring treatment. This way, patients can be turned into the best thinkable type of customer: a happy, returning customer who keeps paying good money in the illusion that these frequent bioresonance sessions benefit their health.

How to Test a Bioresonance Machine

If you own or have access to a bioresonance device, you can test it as follows:

* Enter your personal data and make a scan of yourself. Then wait 10 min, and scan yourself again—but now under a different name and with a slightly different age. The results of the second scan should be almost identical to those of the first scan, but most likely are completely different—because the computer sees a different name, and thus makes up a new and probably different random 'report'.
* Select your personal profile again (the one you entered first in the previous step), wrap a wet cloth around the electrode, and do another scan. The machine should come up with an error that no human body is detected. Instead it will not complain at all, and come up with a report that is almost identical to your first report. Congratulations! Your tea cloth appears to be in pretty good health, but it could do with some extra vitamin D and magnesium ...
* Enter your personal data again, but select the opposite gender to your own. Again a legitimate machine should immediately spot that certain organs are missing and others are present—but no: it will not complain at all and simply report a health status for organs you do not have.

A scientific study in Germany tested two of these machines, with the following results [60]:

* known serious illnesses in patients were not recognized at all,
* a corpse got a clean bill of health,
* completely healthy volunteers were diagnosed with numerous health problems,

- a wet towel and liver pâté were diagnosed with results similar to those of the healthy human volunteers.

If your bioresonance machine produces similar results, it is safe to say that you are the victim of fraud. You could try and ask for a refund from the manufacturer, or even file a legal complaint. After all, you probably spent thousands of dollars on a machine that claims to make trustworthy diagnoses, but in reality does nothing of the kind.

The *Real* Universal Life Energy

Qi as a universal life energy may be purely fictional, but there is something else that could be called 'universal life energy': ATP, short for *AdenosineT-riPhosphate*. ATP is a molecule that is present in all animals (including us humans), and is considered a kind of universal energy 'currency' in these living organisms. The vast majority of biochemical processes that involve chemical energy make use of ATP to carry and deliver that energy. The importance of ATP cannot be overstated: every day, our own body weight in ATP is synthesized and subsequently used to supply energy to countless chemical processes in our body. Apart from carrying energy, ATP is also base material for synthesizing DNA and RNA.[6]

Other Types of Body Energy

As already mentioned, bioresonance is in fact correct in one aspect: the human body indeed produces its own energy fields, and these fields can even be measured to tell us something about the functioning and the state of health of certain organs.

These fields are electric and magnetic fields, and they are produced by the activity of nerves and muscles. We can register the electrical activity of the brain in a so-called electro-encefalogram (EEG), which for instance shows brainwaves. With an electrocardiogram (ECG) we can see the electrical activity of the heart, for instance to detect any irregularities that may need treatment. Electromyography (EMG) is used to register the activity of muscles.

None of these electrical or magnetic fields is in any way related to bioresonance or 'life energy'.

---

[6] Part of the ATP molecule is a base called adenine, which is also one of the four 'letters' (C, G, A and T) of the genetic code.

Conclusion

There is no scientific evidence at all for the existence of *qi* or a similar kind of 'life energy', there is no way to objectively detect or measure it, and even the most experienced Reiki master or Therapeutic Touch practitioner can't explain what it is in any well-defined terms. Descriptions and explanations of qi are often contradictory, and there is no literature providing any consistent definitions either. Ostensibly, the only way to be able to 'feel' this qi is to accept its existence without any evidence.

Acupuncture, a very popular component of Traditional Chinese Medicine, is also based on the flow of qi through so-called meridians along which the needles are supposed to be inserted. But again, qi or meridians have never been found. Studies with sham acupuncture show that it doesn't matter where needles are inserted, or even if they're inserted at all. Acupuncture seems to be a placebo treatment, and as such may sometimes be helpful in managing pain.

About therapeutic touch and similar forms of energy medicine such as Reiki: there is no scientific evidence that these treatments do anything at all. An simple, elegant test carried out by a nine-year-old in 1998 showed that practitioners could not feel the body's 'energy field' when blinded, even though they were certain that they could before the test.

Bioresonance, which posits that cells and organs in the body naturally all have their own healthy (or diseased) frequency and uses various impressive-looking electronic devices, is even worse: not only does it not work, it is usually a scam.

The next chapter continues on the subject of energy, and this time *real* energy: radiation, in all its various forms, both the harmless and the harmful kind.

11

Radiation

The Neighbourhood Epidemic

Note: the events described are real, but people's names have been altered to provide a modicum of privacy.

September 2009, Fourways, Craigavon

Miranda was living with her husband in Craigavon, a nice residential area to the north of Johannesburg in the mild climate of South Africa, enjoying an active life running her business as a caterer.

One day in August 2009, she noticed to her surprise that a cell phone tower was erected on the plot right next to her residence. At first, she was just annoyed about this eyesore turning up without a warning. But within a few days of its installation, she also started noticing troubling symptoms: sleeplessness, brain fog and vague headaches, fatigue … And when she left town for business, she quickly felt better. Could that cell phone tower have anything to do with it?

She started asking around her neighbourhood to see if more people experienced any recent problems with their health, and sure enough, several other people reported symptoms as well, varying from generally feeling a bit under the weather to unpleasant tingling sensations, nausea, rashes, insomnia, tinnitus and lots of other vague complaints.

Miranda was not the person to just take things lying down, so she decided that something had to be done right away. After some searching, she found that the cell tower's owner was a provider by the name of iBurst – so she sent letters to this provider as well as her city council, protesting that the tower seemed to cause lots of health problems in its immediate vicinity, and that it had been erected without informing residents and without following the proper procedures. As both iBurst and the council could not be reached for comments, residents decided to organize themselves, and established the Craigavon Task Force. Soon thereafter protests were staged.

Weeks went by without an answer, and residents became increasingly frustrated as well as worried. By now, they were certain that their health complaints were linked to the tower's electromagnetic radiation, with some people noticing that symptoms subsided when they spent time with friends and relatives away from Craigavon. As still no official answer seemed to be forthcoming from iBurst, the residents decided to consult a legal firm, to see what more could be done. The main goal was to get the cell phone tower removed in order to restore people's peace of mind and (hopefully) health.

Several people living next to a newly erected cell phone tower in South Africa seem to have developed health problems, apparently because they were exposed to the radiation coming from that tower. Well, that sounds plausible, doesn't it? We all know that radiation can be pretty unhealthy, and if several people all get health problems around the same time that this cell phone tower is erected, then yes, that tower is a very good candidate for being the cause of those problems. But there's more to this story—to be continued ….

What Exactly Is Radiation?

In the previous chapter we explored the 'energy' that lots of alternative practitioners claim to use for healing people—energy that science has never been able to detect in any way, and almost certainly does not exist.

This chapter deals with real energy: radiation energy, to be precise. I will look at both the harmless types and not-so-harmless types of radiation. Also, I will discuss various beliefs, health scares and conspiracy theories involving radiation.

The definition of radiation is very simple: it is 'something' being emitted by a source. Usually, this something consists of electromagnetic fields such as radio waves or light. Another type of radiation is nuclear radiation, which is what most people think of as radiation. Both types come in harmless and dangerous varieties; some radiation is even healthy.

We're Bathing in Radiation!

Together with toxins, radiation is one of the alternative world's main buga-boos, often used to instil fear, uncertainty and doubt (FUD)—and of course to sell countless products and treatments that supposedly block or neutralize radiation, or heal people from its harmful effects.

In case you wondered: yes, the paragraph title is correct: we are literally bathing in radiation all the time. Luckily for us, most of this radiation is completely harmless, and consists of electromagnetic fields that are better known as heat (infrared radiation), light and radio waves.

We are also constantly exposed to nuclear radiation, mostly originating from natural sources such as the ground beneath our feet. This is because the earth's crust contains naturally occurring radioactive elements. Another natural source of nuclear radiation are so-called cosmic rays, which, as the name already suggests, come from space. All this radiation together is called *natural background radiation*. This nuclear background radiation level is theoretically harmful because it can cause damage (read: mutations) in our DNA; however, the actual risk is very small, mostly because we have evolved mechanisms to repair this kind of minor DNA damage.

What Makes Radiation Harmful?

Radiation is considered harmful if it is capable of damaging or destroying molecules in our body. When this so-called *ionizing radiation* causes signif-icant damage to the DNA in our cells, this can lead to cancer. The science section will discuss the difference between ionizing and non-ionizing radia-tion in more detail.

From a public health perspective, by far the most harmful type of natural radiation is ultraviolet (UV) radiation coming from the sun, causing well over a million cases of skin cancer worldwide each year, especially in people with a lighter skin colour [61]. Yes, there are much more dangerous kinds of radiation than UV light, but we are not normally exposed to those types.

Healthy Radiation?

From the same public health perspective, ultraviolet radiation is also quite *healthy*, as our body needs it to convert cholesterol into vitamin D. The trick is to get the optimal dose of UV exposure: enough meet our daily vitamin D requirement, but not more. The problem of course is that the amount of UV light can vary enormously depending on the time of the year, the geographic latitude, the weather, clothing, and other factors [62, 63]. As a rule of thumb, just spending 15 min a day in the summer sun in light clothing is enough for people with lighter skin. In the colder season at higher latitudes, vitamin D supplements or food fortified with extra vitamin D are advisable. The reason for this is that winter sunlight contains insufficient UV, and that dressing up warm also means that less skin is exposed.

Non-ionizing radiation can only be harmful by the heat it generates. We use this heating effect of certain types of non-ionizing radiation for cooking. One example is a microwave oven, which uses radio waves for heating up anything containing water; another example is the good old grill, which uses infrared radiation to cook food. In both cases, heating things up involves significant amounts of power (several hundred to several thousand watts). But generally speaking, all radiation that we are exposed to on a daily basis is low-power non-ionizing radiation, and thus completely harmless.

Then there's this: recent scientific research suggests that even the nuclear background radiation (the type that damages DNA) can actually be beneficial for our health, at least up to a certain (low) level [64]. The hypothesis is that occasional radiation damage activates the repair mechanisms mentioned earlier, which help prevent other damage to DNA and cell structures as well. This partially inverted dose-related response is called *radiation hormesis*.

Fun fact: we not only bathe in all sorts of radiation all the time, but we all are also a *source* of radiation—infrared radiation, or heat. You know those handy lights that automatically switch on when you come within detection range? Those lights are equipped with a sensor that detects the infrared radiation produced by you or any other warm-blooded animal. You can even make this radiation visible with a so-called *thermography camera*,[1] which translates different temperatures to different colours. So the next time someone says they don't want to be exposed to radiation, ask them if they want you to go away. After all, you are exposing them (as well as everyone else in your direct vicinity) to the infrared radiation coming from your body.

---

[1] Some unscrupulous practitioners offer thermography as an alternative for 'harmful' X-ray breast cancer screening, claiming that their thermal cameras can spot tumours by their slightly higher temperature. This does not work, and the small dose of X-rays in these screening procedures is completely negligible.

Why People Fear Radiation

One important reason why so many people are wary (or sometimes even outright scared) of radiation is that you can't see it or feel it, especially the dangerous kinds. Just like with toxins, you could be exposed to harmful radiation without knowing—and just like with toxins, there are lots of people out there trying to convince us that our health is indeed at risk because of radiation. And being humans, with a brain that creates associations all the time, we will associate *any* type of invisible radiation with danger, even the completely harmless types.

By the same token, the word *nuclear* is also automatically associated with nuclear radiation, i.e. invisible danger. For this reason (among others), the term Nuclear Magnetic Resonance (NMR) was changed to Magnetic Resonance Imaging (MRI) when this imaging technique was developed for use with patients—even though no nuclear radiation is involved here.

Electromagnetic Hypersensitivity

This fear of radiation seems justified by what is called *electromagnetic hypersensitivity* (EHS): the phenomenon that some people appear to be sensitive to electromagnetic fields. They experience all sorts of unpleasant symptoms when exposed to electromagnetic fields from wireless devices, smartphones, and of course cell phone towers. So maybe those Craigavon residents were unlucky enough to suffer from EHS? This question is explored in more detail in the science section.

First, let's take a look at one of the ways that people try to make money off these purported negative health effects of radiation (a.k.a. *radiophobia*): anti-radiation products.

Anti-radiation Products

It is of course a thoroughly human trait: wherever some people see danger and things to fear, others see opportunities. This is no different for the dangers of 'radiation', real and perceived. There is a veritable deluge of anti-radiation products out there, ranging from effective to useless to completely bonkers.

Real Anti-radiation Measures

The only effective way to block electromagnetic fields ('radiation') from cell phones, laptops, cell phone towers and other wireless sources is a so called *Faraday cage*, which is basically a fully enclosed metal shielding. As the name already implies, this metal shielding does not have to be solid, but can be a metal mesh, just as long as the holes in the mesh are significantly smaller than the wavelength of the electromagnetic field used. This is also how the metal mesh in a microwave oven door can block the electromagnetic radiation that is heating your food inside, while still allowing light to pass through.

You can test the principle of a Faraday cage for yourself using your cell phone. Simply wrap the phone completely in aluminium foil (or aluminum foil, or tinfoil,[2] as they say in the US), and try calling it. If the phone is fully covered without any gaps or slits, it can no longer receive any calls or communicate via a wireless connection.

Some people believe that they are suffering from severe electromagnetic hypersensitivity, and try to solve the problem by turning a room in their house (or sometimes even their complete house) into a Faraday cage. To this end, they cover the walls, the ceiling and the floor with aluminium foil or special electrically conductive paint. Now this should work in theory, but in reality, it turns out to be pretty difficult to get the shielding perfect, especially around doors (which of course still must open and close).

Shielding of nuclear radiation is a completely different kettle of fish, and depends on the type of radiation. More about this in the science section; suffice to say here that we normally are never exposed to nuclear radiation to any substantial degree, so we don't need shielding from it.

Fake Radiation Shielding

Converting even one room into an effective Faraday cage is not only a lot of work, but also doesn't make the living space any cosier. Everything, including any windows, must be covered up by (cheap) foil or (expensive) mesh, without any seams that could allow electromagnetic fields to leak through. And of course there should be no mains wiring which could still allow electromagnetic fields to enter the room—which means no lamps or other electrical and electronic equipment.

So to make life easier for those who still want to do something about 'radiation' without turning their house into a literal cage, there are lots of products

---

[2] This is also where the concept of 'tinfoil hat' comes from.

claiming to protect their users from radiation in one way or another. There is only one problem: none of those products work—and some even *produce* potentially harmful radiation.

One very popular (because relatively cheap) product category is **anti-radiation stickers**, which are meant to shield us from 'harmful electromagnetic pollution' from smartphones, laptops, tablets and other wireless devices, with 5G of course explicitly mentioned [65]. The idea is that you simply attach these stickers to the devices mentioned, after which they absorb or shield any 'radiation' coming from these devices.

This is one of those moments to pause and think, and ask a simple question: what does a smartphone (or any other wireless device) absolutely need in order to function? The answer is simple: radio signals, a.k.a. 'radiation'. So what happens to your smartphone if you block those radio signals? The earlier experiment with the cell phone wrapped in aluminium foil provides the answer: it stops working.

This alone tells us that these stickers and related products are probably bogus products. Yes, the companies selling these products claim that they block radiation but let through cell phone signals—but this claim is nonsensical: a cell phone signal *is* radiation. You can't block it and let it through at the same time. Products that decrease 'radiation' as claimed also have a negative impact on cell service, and the products that leave cell service intact simply don't work.

Ironically, radiation shielding products that actually do something by blocking part of a cell phone's signal, will likely expose the user to *more* radiation. The reason is simple: when a cell phone's signal gets weaker, the phone will automatically *increase* its transmission power to still reach the nearest cell phone tower.

What's even worse: those stickers are of course meant to be attached to the back of the phone, for the very simple reason that sticking them over the front side (i.e. the display) would render the phone useless. This means that the sticker is not normally between the phone and the user. In other words: it cannot shield the user from anything originating from the phone. Even worse still: any metal foil in such a sticker can act as a mirror, reflecting electromagnetic fields coming from the back of the phone to the front side, further increasing the exposure of the user instead of decreasing it.

Now these stickers are a relatively cheap scam, costing maybe a couple of dozen dollars at most. There are, however, far more expensive devices offered with claims that they block out or neutralize harmful radiation in a radius up to dozens of metres, creating a 'radiation-free bubble' or an invisible Faraday cage, as it were. These devices can set people back hundreds or even thousands of dollars—while in reality doing nothing at all. There are countless Web sites peddling such devices with sales pitches along the following lines:

Do you know that you and your loved ones are continuously irradiated by Electromagnetic Radiation (EMR)?

Every day, we are continuously exposed to a complex mix of electromagnetic fields from 5G, wireless and electrical appliances, digital TV and other sources in our environment.

EMR is a diffuse field with a positive polarization, affecting the body's biofield, ultimately leading to organ damage. This happens to everyone of us, with the amount of damage only depending on the measure of exposure and our initial health.

How our N-Field works

N-Field is short for 'Negative Frequency Field'. The N-Field device is made from a special material called Radinite, a hand-crafted energy-modulating crystal that has been tuned to counteract positive polarizations with a negative signal.

This negative frequency is introduced into the mains wiring system, which automatically carries it to sources of positive EMR (the harmful component of radiation fields). The N-Field's negatively polarized signal then neutralizes the positive EMR, eliminating the danger that EMR poses to your biofield, meridians, and organs. The effects of the N-Field are not restricted to the mains wiring system; the ground connection of the electrical wiring system enables its negative frequencies to enter the earth beneath the premises and build a protective shield that may stretch as far as twenty metres from the point of deployment.

For more extensive protection, we advise the use of separate N-Field devices at every twenty metres.

This may sound impressively scientific, but it is in fact a meaningless pseudoscientific word salad. Almost nothing of what is mentioned here is actually real, and the product itself is usually a lump of ordinary plastic, stuck to a mains plug that is not connected to anything. This useless hunk of plastic costs perhaps $5 to produce—but it is sold for almost $200. And this is just one of hundreds of similar products out there.

The way that all these bogus products are peddled usually follows this pattern:

1. Ask people if they sometimes experience headaches or insomnia or perhaps some other vague but quite common symptoms. (Almost everyone will answer 'yes'.)
2. Blame 'radiation' for causing those symptoms.

3. Offer a solution in for form of anti-radiation products.
4. Use lots of pseudoscientific gobbledygook to 'explain' how those products work, claiming that everything is 'scientifically proven'.
5. Ask a relatively high price for those products—because as consumers, we automatically associate a high price with advanced technology and high quality. The best price range for these products is several dozen to a couple of hundred dollars.

Harmful Anti-radiation Products?

The products just described may be a scam, but at least they are intrinsically harmless, as they simply don't do anything except drain your wallet. The same can't be said for another group of anti-radiation products.

These products (mostly bracelets, pendants and other trinkets, but also eye masks, sheets, stirring sticks and even children's products) are often advertised as 'negative ion' products, based on the pseudoscientific belief that so-called negative ions in the air are good for people's health and mood. In reality, these products do not benefit your health at all—quite the contrary: they contain radioactive thorium powder, which emits so-called alpha radiation (which, incidentally, is made up of *positive* ions, not negative). Several governments have warned consumers to stop using these products [66, 67].

Summarized, all of these 'anti-radiation' products are useless, regardless whether it is a $10 'Energy Dot' sticker or a $7000 '5G Fighter Plus'. Even the most expensive products consist of just some plastic resin, copper tubing or some bits of wire, and perhaps a handful of coloured metal shavings—worth maybe a buck or two in any scrapyard. There is nothing special or healthy about them, and some are even harmful.

Back to Craigavon

So far we've seen that there are people who seem to experience harmful effects from electromagnetic radiation. We also saw that there are lots of products offered that pretend to block or neutralize or 'harmonize' this radiation. However, most of those products don't do anything much, and the only effect that they may have on people is the placebo effect.

But perhaps it is still a good idea to avoid radiation? After all, a Faraday cage absolutely works, and many radiation-sensitive people claim that they feel much better inside one of those. And of course the fact that all those other products don't work doesn't mean that health effects from radiation are not real—many alternative treatments don't really work either, but that doesn't mean that people have no real health issues.

The second and final episode of the Craigavon saga will give us some more answers. Short recap: several residents in the vicinity of a newly erected cell phone tower developed health complaints, for which they blamed the tower. The also accused the cell phone provider of not following proper procedures. For several months, the provider did not respond to their complaints and questions, until one day ...

> *Finally, they got word that an iBurst representative would join the residents' meeting in mid-November, after three months of complaints and protests.*
>
> *And it was a bombshell: iBurst revealed that the tower had been switched off for almost two months prior to the meeting – which meant that it could not possibly have been the cause of the residents' health problems. Furthermore, iBurst offered to keep the tower switched off for several more weeks, to make certain that there was no link between the tower's electromagnetic fields and any symptoms.*
>
> *iBurst also showed that all necessary procedures had been followed to the letter, including informing neighbouring residencies in advance, and obtaining all the necessary permits.*

This certainly is a surprise! The tower had been switched off shortly after the first complaints were received, yet residents kept experiencing health problems for at least eight more weeks. This seems pretty definitive proof that those problems could not have been caused by the tower. It also could not have been that those health problems were somehow permanent, as these people themselves had reported that the symptoms abated when they were away from the area. Furthermore, all required procedures were followed.

So Craigavon residents were wrong, the cell phone provider was right, case closed, right?

Wrong. This time it was the provider who got an unpleasant surprise: instead of conceding that they were wrong and let matters rest there, Miranda and her neighbours became absolutely furious. They argued that they had been unwitting guinea pigs in an experiment with their health at stake, when iBurst secretly switched off the tower to see what would happen. Instead of accepting the situation, the Craigavon Task Force actually doubled down on their efforts to get the tower removed, threatening lawsuits if necessary.

In the end, iBurst decided that it wasn't worth the trouble, and settled with Craigavon residents to remove the tower—relocating it to a couple of hundred metres further on.

The remaining big question of course is what *was* causing those symptoms, if it wasn't the tower. What was going on here? All those people didn't fake their symptoms, now did they? No, they most likely didn't. The most probable answer is that they experienced a combination of three things: real but innocuous symptoms, the nocebo effect, and mass psychogenic illness.

First off, the symptoms that these Craigavon people reported are extremely common: headaches, insomnia, occasional dizzy spells, fatigue, slight nausea, tingling and lots of other unpleasant but not really alarming symptoms … almost everyone has experienced one or more of these at one time or other. Sometimes there are clear causes such as stress or too much coffee, but just as often, no cause can be found. People normally tend to ignore these very common, vague symptoms, but that changes when someone draws attention to them, after which they seem to occur far more often. This is the so-called *frequency illusion.*

Then there is the *nocebo effect*, which can be regarded as the evil twin brother of the placebo effect: the nocebo effect can make people feel sick or uncomfortable because they *expect* to feel something bad. This effect is also very common in pharmaceutical trials: many test subjects for a new type of medicine report side effects, not only those in the group that received the real medicine, but also the ones in the placebo group.

The last effect, *mass psychogenic illness*, is a social phenomenon. When someone in a group starts feeling sick, then quite often, others will soon start feeling unwell too. This may be an old evolutionary mechanism to protect tribes from food poisoning, as described way back in Chapter 1: if one individual gets sick all of a sudden, then it is safest if all others also stop eating, and perhaps even throw up what's already inside. Mass psychogenic illness (sometimes called mass hysteria) is quite common. News media regularly report about a classroom or other group of people all feeling unwell all of a sudden, sometimes complaining about a 'strange smell'. But when emergency services arrive on the scene, they almost invariably can't find any cause (or smell) at all, and the people involved almost magically recover within an hour or so.

All this of course still does not answer the question if the electromagnetic fields from cell phones etcetera can cause other health issues or not, but evidence is mounting that this is not the case. To get a more definitive answer, it is once again necessary to take a more scientific look at things.

What the Science Says

Up to this point, harmful (ionizing) and harmless (non-ionizing) radiation were mentioned, as well as several variants of both kinds. It also appears that people are not sensitive to electromagnetic radiation from cell phones and wireless devices—but we *are* of course sensitive to light and heat, which are also electromagnetic radiation. Then there is UV light, which is both harmful and healthy, depending on the dose. And oh, there was also some mention of nuclear radiation? In other words: the information so far is a bit of a confusing mishmash. In order to clear things up a bit, we'll have to look at some basic scientific properties of electromagnetic fields. This will get slightly technical, but it is not really difficult.

The Electromagnetic Spectrum

As already hinted at, radio signals, heat radiation, visible light and ultraviolet light are basically all the same; they are all vibrating electromagnetic fields (EMF), and they are all part of the so-called *electromagnetic spectrum*.

The only real difference between these forms of electromagnetic radiation is their *frequency*, which simply is the speed of the vibration, measured in cycles per second. One cycle per second is one hertz, abbreviated to 1 Hz. As the frequency goes up, prefixes are used; for instance 1000 Hz is 1 kilohertz (kHz), and 1,000,000 is 1 megahertz (MHz). When we run out of common prefixes long before we get to visible light, we will use powers of ten. This means that 1 kilohertz = 10^3 Hz, 1 megahertz = 10^6 Hz, 1 gigahertz = 10^9 and so on.

Electromagnetic fields are also described by their *wavelength*, in metres. This is simple to understand when you realize that those vibrating electromagnetic fields do not stand still, but travel through space at the speed of light. One frequency cycle of the field is associated with a certain distance travelled. This means that the wavelength of an electromagnetic field is the speed of light divided by the frequency (or $\lambda = c/f$, in symbols). The speed of light has a fixed value of almost 300,000,000 m per second.

This means that for instance an electromagnetic field with a frequency of 100 MHz (FM radio broadcast band) has a wavelength of 300,000,000/100,000,000 = 3 m. The general rule is that a higher frequency corresponds to a lower wavelength and vice versa.

The following table shows the frequency and wavelength ranges, with each higher range being ten times the previous one.[3] This puts the various types of radiation into perspective: only the highest frequencies (shortest wavelengths) of electromagnetic fields are ionizing radiation, and therefore harmful by definition. These are indicated by an asterisk (*). What's more, these types of

---

[3] The prefixes used in the frequency and wavelength ranges are defined and explained here: https://en.wikipedia.org/wiki/Metric_prefix.

ionizing radiation become more dangerous and penetrating with increasing frequency: ultraviolet radiation has little penetrating power, and only damages the upper layers of the skin. X-rays, on the other hand, can penetrate through the body—which is why they are used in medical imaging. X-rays can be blocked by a thin sheet of heavy metal such as lead. Gamma rays have more penetrating power still, and the 'hardest' gamma rays (i.e. those with the highest frequency) even make it through several centimetres of lead.

Frequency	Wavelength	Description/Examples
*30–300 EHz	10–1 pm	Gamma rays
*3–30 EHz	100–10 pm	Hard X-rays, gamma rays
*300 PHz–3 EHz	1 nm–100 pm	Hard X-rays
*30–300 PHz	10–1 nm	Soft X-rays
*3–30 PHz	100–10 nm	UV-C, extreme ultraviolet
300 THz–3 PHz	1 μm–100 nm	Consumer infrared (remote control), visible light, UV-A, UV-B
30–300 THz	10–1 μm	Near infrared
300 GHz–3 THz	1 mm–100 μm	Mid infrared
3–30 THz	100–10 μm	Mid to near infrared, thermal cameras
30–300 GHz	1 cm–1 mm	Microwaves, far infrared
3–30 GHz	10–1 cm	Microwaves, wireless routers, radar systems
300 MHz–3 GHz	1 m–10 cm	UHF TV, cell phones, wireless routers, microwave ovens
30–300 MHz	10–1 m	FM radio, VHF TV
3–30 MHz	100–10 m	Shortwave radio waves (SW)
300 kHz–3 MHz	1 km–100 m	Mediumwave radio waves (MW)
30–300 kHz	10–1 km	Longwave radio waves (LW), time code signals for clocks
3–30 kHz	100–10 km	Ultra low frequency radio waves
300 Hz–3 kHz	1000–100 km	Super low frequency radio waves
30–300 Hz	10,000–1000 km	50 Hz: Mains frequency for most of the world 60 Hz: Mains frequency for US and parts of Asia

The electromagnetic spectrum; the asterisk (*) marks ionizing radiation

What Makes Ionizing Radiation Harmful

It was already mentioned that ionizing radiation damages molecules. If those molecules happen to be DNA, then a cell can die or, even worse, become a cancer cell. The question now is how ionizing radiation causes this damage. Understanding this will take us a little further in the world of molecules and energy, so things will just get a bit more technical, although I'll try to keep it as simple as possible (and I won't mention the word 'quantum', promise!).

Alternatively, you can just takes this bit for granted and move on to the next paragraph.

Electromagnetic fields can behave like waves (which is how we looked at it up to this point), but also as a stream of particles moving with the speed of light. These particles are called *photons*, and every photon has an amount of energy that only depends on the frequency of the field. The higher the frequency, the more energy[4] the individual photons in that field have.

Why is this important? Because all molecules (including DNA) are made up of atoms held together by atomic bonds. These bonds can be broken (at which point the molecule is damaged or changed), but this requires a certain minimal amount of energy. And you guessed it: only photons with at least that amount of *binding energy* are capable of breaking that kind of bond.

As it turns out, the lowest binding energy in molecular bonds in our body, including the ones in DNA, is something in the order of 2.5 electronvolt. And this energy of 2.5 electronvolt turns out to be the photon energy of ultraviolet light.

This means that molecular bonds can only be broken by electromagnetic radiation from ultraviolet light and higher frequencies, such as X-rays and gamma rays. Visible light and fields with lower frequencies simply don't have photons with enough energy.

Nuclear Radiation

All man-made radio-frequency electromagnetic radiation such as cell phone signals is made by electronic circuits. Nuclear radiation is something different altogether, and originates from the nucleus of certain chemical elements. Those radioactive nuclei are inherently unstable, and when they *decay*, they emit certain particles and/or gamma radiation. In the process, they also change into the nucleus of another element—which in turn may be unstable as well. This so-called decay chain stops when a stable nucleus is reached; for many heavy radioactive elements such as uranium and thorium, this stable end station is lead.

Apart from the already mentioned background radiation and those somewhat radioactive 'anti-radiation health products',[5] nuclear radiation is not something that we encounter in daily life. This means that it is not really

---

[4] As we're dealing with very tiny quantities of energy, we're not using joules here (as in the previous chapter), but a much smaller unit called electronvolts. The formula is simple: $E = h f$, or in words: the photon energy (E) is a fixed number by the name of the Planck constant (h, about 4.14 electronvolt per hertz) times the frequency (f).

[5] Maybe someone should come up with special anti-radiation products to protect us from those radioactive products ….

an interesting (read: lucrative) phenomenon for makers of all those bogus 'radiation protection' products—and this also means that this topic is not explored any further in this book.

Cell Phones and Cancer

With all the latest information, we can simply look up the frequency used by cell phones in the electromagnetic spectrum, and see that these devices operate at frequencies that are roughly a million times lower than the lowest frequency of ultraviolet light. This also means that the photons in the electromagnetic fields of cell phones have an energy that is one million times lower than the minimum energy necessary it takes to damage DNA.

Based on this alone, it is *very* unlikely that electromagnetic fields from cell phones and other wireless devices can cause cancer or any other kind of harm. Still, there is a possibility that some kind of other, so far unknown mechanism is at play; some studies found a weak link between cell phone use and certain types of cancer, but other, similar studies found no link at all.

In 2002, one of the largest studies ever was done into health effects of electromagnetic fields. Around this time, cell phone adoption was growing fast—as was public concern about possible health effects, both short-term and long-term.

One problem of course was that cell phones had only been widely used for a couple of years, so how could they possibly investigate any long-term effects? The researchers came up with a solution: they looked at a group of 40,000 veterans who served as technicians in the US navy during the Korean war, some 40 years earlier [68]. Why navy technicians? Because about half of these people were exposed to high-intensity electromagnetic fields from radar installations, often for several years on end, while the other half received far less exposure. The frequencies used in radar and aviation electronics in those days are comparable to frequencies used in cell phones and wireless networking in 2002.

The study looked into the death rates of these groups of veterans, as well as the causes of death, and especially cancer. These figures were also compared to the same metrics in civilians in the same age group, so people who had *not* been exposed to high-powered radar fields.

The results from this study are quite interesting: those navy veterans were doing significantly *better* health-wise than civilians who did not serve in the navy. After 40 years, less veterans had died, and less has been diagnosed with cancer. Also, there was no significant difference between the two groups of navy technicians.

Now does this mean that being exposed to electromagnetic fields from high-powered radar is actually good for your health? No, of course not. The most likely explanation is that these navy people had an overall healthier lifestyle, with more exercise and less chances to develop obesity or bad lifestyle habits. This study *does* tell us that exposure to electromagnetic fields from radar and the likes does not appear to have any significant negative effects. These findings have been confirmed in the past decades: exposure to electromagnetic radiation from cell phones and (wireless) Internet does not appear to cause any health problems.

Cancer Statistics

Another way to investigate a possible link between cell phone use and cancer is to simply look up cancer statistics between about 1990 (when almost no-one had a cell phone) and 2020 (when virtually everyone in the western world was using a smartphone and/or other wireless devices). If cell phones pose a significant cancer risk, we would expect to see a distinct increase in the number of cancer diagnoses in the period mentioned. Now there has indeed been a slight but steady rise in the absolute number of cancer diagnoses—but that rise is almost certainly caused by the concurrent increase in life expectancy. After all, old age is by far the biggest risk factor for cancer. When corrected for age, there has not been a significant rise in the amount of cancer diagnoses overall [69].

Still, a link between cell phone use and cancer can't be completely ruled out. Some researchers claim to have found a link between some relatively rare types of brain cancer and long-term intensive cell phone use [70].

For this reason, the International Agency for Research on Cancer (IARC) has decided to include electromagnetic fields from cell phones and similar devices in their group 2B, which lists agents that are possibly carcinogenic to humans, but with no conclusive evidence yet [71]. Noteworthy: this list also contains foodstuffs such as pickles and certain occupations such as being a carpenter.

Electromagnetic Hypersensitivity Revisited

Earlier on, the term *electromagnetic hypersensitivity* (EHS) was briefly mentioned, together with the conclusion that those Craigavon residents probably did not suffer from this condition.

Now it is time to address the question if electromagnetic hypersensitivity actually exists. There are lots of people who claim to be sensitive to radio-frequency electromagnetic fields from e.g. cell phones and other wireless devices. But can they really feel those fields? Let's look at one case study ....

The case study of Mrs W.

Through the Internet, I came into contact with one Mrs W., who told me that she suffered from electromagnetic hypersensitivity. She said that she could instantly feel when she was near sources of electromagnetic fields (EMF), with unpleasant tingling sensations in her arms and upper body as symptoms. In particular, she could feel it when her neighbour returned home from work and switched on his laptop computer on his desk, located at the other side of the wall separating the two residences. She also experienced symptoms in other locations, such as a local hardware store with wireless networking pods mounted on the ceiling, and near cell phone towers.

As an electronics designer with expertise in biomedical engineering, I was intrigued, and asked her if she was willing to partake in a simple experiment to establish how accurate her sensitivity for EMF actually was. She agreed, and together, we drew up a protocol for the experiment. The idea was simple: I would come over and visit her at home, bringing a so-called field strength meter. This device measures the strength of any electromagnetic field we would be exposed to. In preparation, I also took a medical history of Mrs W.

After I arrived, we first had a cup of tea and a chat, and then it was time to get started. First, Mrs W. verified the functioning of the field strength meter by holding it near an active wireless router, and got a fairly high reading—and she confirmed that she could also feel this source of radiation. Both the meter's reading and her symptoms diminished when she walked to the opposite side of the room, so under unblinded conditions, her symptoms agreed with the meter's reading.

We then started the blinded part of the experiment. She would more or less go about her daily routine. Every ten minutes, she would jot down a score from 1 to 10, indicating the severity of symptoms she was experiencing. At the same time, I would measure and record the actual electromagnetic field strength, together with her husband. We would take care not to see each other's notes, or even look at or talk to each other as we wrote things down. For all the rest, we would enjoy a pleasant afternoon chatting, taking a walk outside, and visiting any 'hot spots' pointed out by Mrs W., all the while dutifully recording our data every ten minutes.

Then, after a very nice meal, it was time to lift the blinding, and see if her scores matched up with the meter readings from me and her husband.

Much to her surprise (but not mine), there was no correlation at all. Almost none of her high symptom scores matched my high meter readings and vice versa; only when we were visibly close to an active EMF source (e.g. someone close by using their cell phone) did both our observations agree. Mrs W. even felt somewhat embarrassed about it, and I reassured her that I was quite convinced that she was really experiencing symptoms, and that she really was sensitive in a way. Those symptoms were just not caused by any electromagnetic fields, but by a psychosomatic reaction (a nocebo effect, if you will) to the *idea* that she was exposed to EMF.

In the end, I told her that she could use the field strength meter for another couple of weeks, to keep on her person as she went about her business. Whenever she felt symptoms, she could take an actual reading of the real EMF level, and (hopefully) see that most of the time, there was no correlation. Even though this gave her some reassurance and made her less wary about sources of 'radiation', she is still not completely convinced that those electromagnetic fields are harmless.

Now the experiment described above is of course just an 'N = 1 study', but like the Craigavon story, it supports the notion that people can't actually feel electromagnetic fields in any way. Also, the medical history of Mrs W. revealed a clue why EMF was not the cause of her symptoms: she had undergone MRI scans without any trouble whatsoever.

Why this is a clue? An MRI machine uses very powerful radio-frequency electromagnetic fields, as in: many kilowatts, at just a few centimetres distance from the body. It is extremely unlikely that someone would suffer all kinds of symptoms when exposed to just a few milliwatts from a wireless device, yet notice nothing at all from thousands of watts produced by an MRI machine.

Looking at Nerve Signals

There is still another way to see how plausible the phenomenon of electromagnetic hypersensitivity is: by looking at how nerves work. It was already clear that radio-frequency fields are not energetic enough to cause damage to our cells and our DNA, but maybe those fields are capable of triggering nerves? After all, our nerve cells work with electrical signals, and disruption of those signals would in fact be an excellent explanation for all those strange and vague symptoms: tingling, itching, sleep disorders, restlessness and many more.

It is quite simple: a nerve cell in e.g. one of your fingertips has a long fibre (called *axon*), which is a kind of very thin hollow tube with that leads from to the fingertip to the brain. The circumference of this tube is the *membrane* of the axon. When in rest (so when the nerve cell is not triggered), the nerve cell maintains a voltage of −70 millivolts (−70 mV) across the membrane. This means that the inside voltage is 70 millivolts lower than the outside voltage, which is defined as zero volts; this −70 mV is the so-called *resting potential*.

When your fingertip touches something, so-called receptors trigger one or more nerve cells. This happens by raising the voltage to at least −55 mV, so by applying a voltage increase of 15 mV (−70 + 15 = −55). This −55 millivolts is the *threshold potential* of the nerve cell. As soon as this threshold potential is crossed, the nerve cell is triggered. From then on, the voltage will keep increasing all by itself, to top out at approximately +40 mV. This 40-millivolt peak is the *action potential*, and this is also the peak voltage that is transmitted along the nerve fibres. Within a few milliseconds, this peak rapidly drops off again, and after some 5 ms, the nerve cell returns to its rest potential of −70 mV, at which point it is ready for a new trigger to occur.

If the triggered nerve happens to be a pain nerve, this will produce a sensation of pain. If the nerve is linked to a pressure receptor, it will produce a sensation of pressure, and so on.

The key here is this 15 millivolts voltage increase: if you manage to change the resting potential by +15 millivolts, you can trigger the nerve cell, and thus cause the nerve to send a signal to your brain. So now the question is: can a cell phone signal cause this +15 mV across the membrane of nerve cells?

The answer is a resounding 'no', and the reason is simple: not only is the field strength of a cell phone far too low to induce the necessary voltage difference of 15 millivolts across the nerve cell's membrane, but nerve cells can't even respond to the high frequencies used by cell phones. The reason for this is that nerve signals are not propagated by moving electrons (small charged particles) as in electronics, but by moving ions, which are also charged particles, but far bigger and far more sluggish than electrons.[6] As a result, nerve cells only respond to frequencies up to a couple of kilohertz; they can't keep up at all with the many hundreds of megahertz used by cell phones, simply because their ions can't move that fast.

What all this means is that it is physically impossible that someone's nerves can respond to cell phone or Wi-Fi signals. The overall conclusion is therefore that electromagnetic hypersensitivity is not real; this is also supported by scientific research [72, 73]. Yes, the symptoms that these people experience are real, but they are not caused by electromagnetic fields, but by nocebo and other effects, as explained earlier on.

---

[6] And the reason why living creatures don't use electrons for propagating signals in their nerves is that those nerves then would have to be made of metal.

5G

Any discussion about radiation would of course not be complete without mentioning 5G. In certain circles, the term '5G' has somehow become synonymous with 'evil', with the wildest claims making the rounds. These range from the usual—but unfounded—claims that this radiation is somehow bad for your health, to the idea that 5G is used together with Covid-19 vaccinations to turn us all into mindless slave zombies. According to these conspiracy ideas, vaccines contain invisible microchips that can take full control over vaccinated people, and 5G is the channel by which those microchips (and thus the hapless sheeple[7]) are commanded and programmed. Unfortunately, these utterly crazy conspiracy ideas have led people all across the world to burning or otherwise vandalizing cell phone towers—many of which didn't even have any 5G equipment installed yet.

So What Actually *Is* 5G?

5G is short for '5th generation cellular network standard', as the successor to the 4G standard (and 3G and 2G and 1G before that). These standards define in detail how those wireless networks function in a technical sense, what frequencies are used and how digital data is structured and transmitted.

It lies beyond the scope of this book to go into all the details of the new 5G standard, but apart from a few clever tricks with how antennas are used and the possibility to use higher frequencies than 4G, there's nothing fundamentally different about 5G. It is still made up of non-ionizing electromagnetic fields with frequencies far below visible light and infrared. Scientific studies into the health effects of 5G so far have also found no evidence or even a plausible mechanism for any potential harm [74]. Admittedly, the quality of a lot of these studies leaves a lot to be desired, so more (and better) studies are planned and carried out; there is, however, no indication whatsoever that 5G technology is harmful in any way.

In all likelihood, things will just go as with previous generations cellular networking: there will be some initial upheaval and protests from people who believe that there's something wrong, followed by rapid adoption of the new standard, without any of the predicted problems or health effects materializing.

---

[7] For those unfamiliar with this term: it is a contraction of 'sheep' and 'people'.

How Smartphones *Are* Bad for People's Health

Even though electromagnetic fields do not appear to be harmful, intensive use of cell phones is still associated with real health issues. One of these is the increase in myopia (short-sightedness) in children, which occurs when a growing child spends a lot of its time looking at objects at a short distance—e.g. a smartphone screen or a book [75]. Another detrimental health effect is that intensive smartphone use usually means less physical exercise. Yet another problem has to do with the addictive nature of social media, where people (children and adults alike) are constantly eager for other people's messages and comments, and have a hard time turning off their cell phones because of 'Fear of Missing Out' (FOMO). This idea can cause several problems such as an overall lack of concentration, disturbed sleep, fatigue and other related symptoms. Also, the bright light from cell phone screens suppresses melatonin production, further contributing to sleeplessness. All this again looks a lot like some of the symptoms that some people attribute to 'radiation'. So in a way these people are right: radiation from cell phones can indeed cause significant health problems—not the radio-frequency radiation, but the light radiation from the screen.

Conclusion

Despite the fact that we are literally surrounded by natural and man-made sources of radio-frequency electromagnetic fields, there is no hard evidence that these fields cause cancer or are harmful in other ways. This notion is also supported by the fact that these fields are not energetic enough by far to break chemical bonds and cause damage to DNA.

Electromagnetic hypersensitivity, where people claim that electromagnetic fields cause all sorts of symptoms, also appears to be an imaginary condition. When properly tested, none of these people can actually sense the presence or absence of these fields.

The idea that electromagnetic fields are harmful is strongly propagated by people and companies who sell 'protection devices' against electromagnetic radiation—devices that are all bogus. Some are even the exact opposite of what is claimed: they don't block or neutralize radiation, but are *sources* of potentially harmful nuclear radiation.

All those scare stories about 5G can also be firmly relegated to the realm of fiction and conspiracy beliefs. There is nothing fundamentally different about 5G compared to its predecessors, and research so far has not found any harmful effects.

The next chapter goes full circle, returning to where we started out in this book: the very human ways of thinking (or, quite often, *not* thinking) that lead us astray, causing misunderstanding, distrust and even hatred for our fellow human beings. There, I will look for ways to keep talking to and hopefully understand each other—even if we don't agree on everything.

12

Our Very Human Brain

Packing Up

This chapter marks the end of my trip to the alternative world, and I want to thank anyone who joined me on this exploration, as well as those I met along the way. I have seen the sights, marvelled at some of the attractions, and was horrified by some of the others. In the course of this journey, I definitely got to know the inhabitants of this world a little bit better. It turned out that for the most part, they are very friendly people with all the best intentions.

Alternative Science?

However, no matter how friendly these people are, and no matter how good their intentions, and even despite their often considerable intelligence, there is one common denominator that I encountered time and again: lots of things that they firmly believe in are not supported by our current scientific knowledge, and often even contradict that knowledge. When confronted with this discrepancy, their reactions vary. Often, they simply ignore or dismiss the science. Some claim that science doesn't apply to what they believe. Others erroneously claim that their work is in line with science; others again come up with their own (pseudo)science.

© The Author(s), under exclusive license to Springer Nature
Switzerland AG 2023
R. Rasker, *Mind, Make-Believe and Medicine*,
https://doi.org/10.1007/978-3-031-29444-0_12

Why is this? Are all these people stupid? Or perhaps dishonest? No, I don't think so at all, especially after researching their work and ideas while writing this book. From what I can see, the overwhelming majority of those living in the alternative world are just as intelligent and honest as other people, driven by a desire to help their fellow human beings and do good things. This is not to say that they are saints—these people also make mistakes, they can be arrogant or blinded by their success, and some are driven by less sincere motives such as easy money, or getting respect and fame they don't really deserve. (Ghee, it almost sounds like they are real people …) But most of them are perfectly nice, trustworthy people, no different from the majority of people in other walks of life. It's just that in certain areas, they believe in things that are demonstrably wrong.

Honest People

One of the biggest problems with alternative medicine and other alternative systems of belief is the rejection of science associated with it—and often only the exact part of science that interferes with their beliefs. These people are perfectly happy to accept that science can work wonders when creating things such as computers and cell phones, or making air planes into a reliable, safe and cheap form of mass transport, or having doctors perform small miracles in treating for instance childhood leukaemia.

But when, for instance, the subject is vaccination or medicines, then all of a sudden science is Wrong, and not to be trusted. Then, contrary to all evidence and reason, they claim that vaccines injure and kill people in droves, that shaken water is a better medicine than Big Pharma's noxious products, and that you can heal people by simply waving your hands over their body. None of this is supported by proper science, and what is more: these people can *know* that what they're saying or doing has no scientific basis. Yet they ignore or dismiss the relevant scientific information. Sometimes they go one further and claim that there actually *is* scientific evidence for their beliefs, even if the vast majority of scientists themselves beg to differ. Why do they say this? Are all these people dishonest?

As it turns out, no. Alternative practitioners and believers are just as honest and trustworthy as other people—and people in general are in fact amazingly honest, as a very simple German experiment from 2014 shows [76]: over 650 people were asked by telephone to perform a coin toss in the privacy of their home, and tell the interviewer what side came up. Before the toss, they were told that they would receive a 15 euro prize if tails came up, but that they would get nothing when heads came up. One would expect a lot of people to lie about the outcome in order to get this €15 prize, and thus that many people would falsely report tails. After all, there was no way to verify the result of the toss.

The outcome was pretty amazing: *slightly more than half the people reported heads coming up*, and did not win the prize.[1] This is what you would expect if (almost) all people were telling the truth—after all, no-one would falsely report a losing toss. What this tells us is that yes, most people are inclined to be honest, even when this is less profitable than being dishonest.

We're All Fallible

If there is one thing that I learned when writing this book, it is that our brain plays tricks on us all the time—and that goes for my brain too. For me personally, one of the most annoying things was the continuous, often irresistible urge to be lazy and take short cuts, avoiding Kahneman's laborious System 2 thinking (see Chapter 1). All the time, I found myself writing stuff in an offhand manner, just relying on memory—and then, after realizing that I should actually *check* things, I often turned out to be wrong, mostly about details, but sometimes about quite important things. Even here, at the end of this book, I have this nagging feeling that there are still lots of things that are not quite right. It is even possible that I made some big whoppers along the way that I haven't noticed so far. No doubt, people will point these out to me, but it still means that I didn't exercise due diligence in getting the facts and the science straight. In any way, criticism is absolutely welcomed. I care rather more about getting my facts straight than about keeping up a personal delusion of being right.

Now there will of course also be lots of people who will think that I'm wrong about many things—maybe even about most of what I wrote. Alternative practitioners will no doubt say that I completely fail to understand their way of 'healing', and many people will accuse me of being a shill for Big Pharma, defending drugs in general and vaccines in particular. Some might even think I'm an agent of some conspiracy that they believe in, helping shadowy powers that rule the world to make their dominion of the world and the enslavement of ordinary citizens complete.

I'm perfectly fine with this kind of criticism too—in fact, people telling me that I'm completely wrong about homeopathy or energy medicine or the likes was an important motivation for writing this book. It stimulated me to investigate their beliefs and ideas, and why they hold them—and why they

---

[1] Interestingly, people were significantly less honest when almost identical coin-toss experiments were carried out in the lab instead of their own home.

will insist on holding them when science, logic, and even simple facts of life prove them wrong.

Still, I leave the door open to the possibility that I myself may be the one who is wrong—although someone would have to come up with lots of very good science-based evidence before I will change my mind on these subjects.

We're All Human

One might say that I paint a consistently bleak picture of our human brain, constantly focusing on the many ways that it can fool us and trick us in our modern, largely science-based world. I'd say that there is indeed some truth to this: I emphasize the positive role of science and reason, while pointing at emotions, beliefs and social traits as things that lead us astray from The Truth (pardon the exaggeration).

This of course does grave injustice to the fact that it is all those very human traits that give our life colour and meaning, and that we *all* largely rely on Kahneman's quick 'n easy System 1 thinking for our daily life. We are not like Mr Spock from *Star Trek*, being inhumanly logical all of the time. Even people who find Mr Spock's consistently logical world view appealing, do so for human reasons: knowing stuff and being right is *fun*, and gives us pleasant emotions of accomplishment and being in control.

The reason for me to give science the prominent place in this book is because this science has proven itself extremely helpful in dealing with universal problems such as disease and suffering; it can solve problems that we couldn't previously solve with our innate human traits. In the end, science provides all of us with much longer and healthier lives, with less suffering and loss, and much more opportunities to lead a rich and fulfilling life instead of just scraping by from day to day. Which in effect means that science, largely devoid of human traits as it is, can help us being human in no small way.

This is also why I think that rejecting science is undesirable, and why people should be discouraged to revert to and promote 'traditional' or otherwise unscientific forms of medicine—simply because they are not effective in combating disease and suffering, no matter if they give their adherents a warm fuzzy feeling of doing things 'natural' or 'taking control' of their own health, or belonging to a group of like-minded people.

The Believing Brain

One important driving force in our human world seems to be belief. In the alternative world, this usually boils down to belief in one or more forms of alternative medicine, often preceded by a special personal experience. This experience is often a seemingly spectacular healing through homeopathy or acupuncture or the likes. Others may have grown up in an environment where alternative medicine was the norm. In any case, the end result is a system of belief that prevails over critical thinking. From then on, this belief becomes the point of departure for any reasoning and decisions, at least where health and sickness are involved.

For an example of how belief can cause people to abandon reason, let's look at a religious group called Young Earth creationists. These are people who believe that everything written in one particular version of the Christian bible is the literal truth, period. This presents them with lots of problems, and big ones, at that: not only does the bible have quite a few internal contradictions (for starters, two different creation myths that can't both be the true at the same time), but it also contradicts almost everything that we know from prehistory and history. There is, for instance, Noah's flood, which, according to Young Earth creationists, happened around 4400 years ago, so 2400 BCE. One of the many huge problems with this is that during this alleged worldwide flood, there were several ancient civilisations around, such as Egypt's Old Kingdom and the Indus Valley Civilisation—both of which left uninterrupted written (or chiselled, if you will) accounts of their presence. None of these accounts even mentions a worldwide, devastating flood, let alone that those civilisations were wiped out by one.

There are many, many more insurmountable problems with reading bible texts as the literal truth. Yet these creationists will still assert that it is the literal, historical Truth, and that there is absolutely nothing that could ever make them believe otherwise. Maybe this mindset is best illustrated by the following quote from an American pastor:

> If somewhere within the bible I were to find a passage that said that two plus two equals five, I wouldn't question what I'm reading in the bible. I would believe it, accept it as true, and then do my best to work it out and to understand it.

This tells us two things: (1) these people do not believe in a god, but in a book, and (2) a strong enough belief can trump even the most fundamental human rationality and logic. Perhaps the scariest thing about this is that this can happen to almost anyone, even very intelligent people.

Just like everyone, I too will no doubt hold some beliefs that certain other people will look upon with puzzlement—beliefs that I find completely normal, and that are an integral part of my life. Now I have thought long and hard about coming up with a good example of such a belief, but it turned out that every example that I can come up with is not just a 'bare' belief, but is based on logical reasoning—or at least, so I believe(!). One example is that when it comes to establishing what is objectively true or not, I think that science is by far the best tool for the job. This, however, is not just a belief, but a logical conclusion based on how the scientific method works (see Chapter 2).

I used to wonder why not everyone would follow the same line of reasoning, but I think the answer is pretty simple: most people aren't as 'science-crazy' as I am. They are much more driven by automated human traits such as impulses, emotions and human social interactions—Kahneman's System 1 behaviour, in other words. Then again, I too have automated a lot of this scientific way of thinking, which of course increases the chance of errors creeping in.

So what is it in our mind that makes us susceptible to harbouring and even nurturing demonstrably false ideas and beliefs? I think that the single most important factor here is what I just mentioned: our heavy reliance on System 1 thinking, by which we tend to simply accept things without critical thinking. Once this acceptance has taken place, something interesting happens: it becomes logically impossible to think of those new ideas we believe in as bad or wrong. Also, the longer we live with particular emotions and beliefs, the more they become internalized—read: more difficult to abandon without upsetting the core of who we are as a person.

Smart People

One of the striking things about alternative medicine and pseudoscience is that, contrary to what one would expect, most people involved in it are in fact quite intelligent. The predominant education level among alternative practitioners and their clientele is higher education (BA or BS in the US). Then again, not many alternative believers have an academic education—but if they do, they are often among the fiercest proponents.

There are several good reasons why especially smart people can hold wrong beliefs and ideas. The basic reason is that nobody, not even the most highly educated scientist, is immune to fallacies, biases and emotion-driven beliefs. Many good scientists fall victim to the good old Post hoc fallacy, i.e. the human tendency to spot patterns and causal connections where there aren't any. And even when they realize that their remarkable observation or idea may be just a coincidence, the next trap already lies ahead: *confirmation bias*, where they subconsciously let additional observations confirming the first one prevail over contradicting evidence. This happens especially easily when the person having this particular idea is quite excited about it, and thinks that they're really on to something. This mechanism not only applies to alternative medicine and pseudoscience, but also in exactly the same way to conspiracy beliefs—more about this later.

I myself have seen many people get into projects doomed to failure because they were led by this exciting emotion of having a really good idea instead of by a thorough, rational assessment. And now that you ask: yes, I have been involved in such projects myself, often to my detriment. The sad thing is that even when harsh reality starts to kick in (hugely underestimated complexity and cost, realization that investors are not nearly as enthusiastic etcetera etcetera), people will often continue in fruitless but costly attempts to make things work, way beyond the point that rationally, they should have pulled the plug long ago already.

This irrational choice to continue with a failing endeavour involves several other fallacies and emotions. One of these is the *sunk cost fallacy*: 'We have invested so much now that we can't stop, and must continue to make it a success'—even when there are no realistic chances of success. Whole businesses have tanked because they kept believing in and thus pursuing projects that turned out to be duds fairly soon after the start. Another extremely human trait is involved here as well: most of us find it very difficult to admit when we are wrong, all the more when we have invested so much in something in terms of money and emotions. Suffering defeat or loss is seen as a humiliating weakness. This is often the point at which scientists or pharmaceutical companies start fudging data, and where alternative practitioners start denying reality, claiming and believing things that are clearly not true. Not good, but again quite human.

For alternative practitioners, their work is often an integral part of their life, especially if they work from home, as many do. They have committed fully to their chosen profession and the way that they work, investing lots of effort, time and money. Their reward, apart from a decent amount of money, is a steady stream of satisfied customers who seem to really benefit from what they do. All this together makes it extremely difficult to even contemplate that they might be wrong about what they do, no matter how smart they are.

Rationalization

Smart people are also good at rationalization, meaning that they can come up with rational explanations for the things they encounter and think about. This is of course a desirable trait for scientists and other problem-solvers—but the downside is that these smart people are also good at rationalizing *bad* ideas, once these ideas got a hold in their mind. Even worse, this ability to rationalize bad ideas can be pretty dangerous, as smart people are not only good at convincing themselves of bad ideas, but also others. This is further enhanced by things such a good academic credentials, previous successes and seniority.

Dunning-Kruger

Then there is the so-called *Dunning-Kruger effect*. This is a cognitive bias by which people with a limited amount of knowledge tend to overestimate the knowledge and abilities that they have. Now this may appear to apply only to not-so-smart people, or people with a limited education, but nothing could be further from the truth. Regardless of our intelligence level and education, each and every one of us is only really knowledgeable in certain limited areas. None of us is an expert in everything, and we all have areas that we have some knowledge about, but not very much—our very own 'Dunning-Kruger areas'.

This is why even Nobel laureates sometimes fall victim to the Dunning-Kruger effect: being absolutely brilliant in their field of expertise gives them great (and justified) confidence in their knowledge and skills—but only in that particular field of expertise. When these very smart people set out in a completely new direction, they mistakenly believe that they can easily tackle any questions and problems there as well. They base this confidence on their current knowledge—knowledge that in fact is woefully inadequate for that new field of expertise. This has happened to several Nobel prize winners, which is why it is sometimes called the *Nobel disease*.

However, as mentioned already, it is mostly people with a higher education who get caught up in all sorts of alternative things. The main reason why they are extra susceptible to the Dunning-Kruger effect is that they have gathered quite a bit of knowledge in the course of their education, but without the scientific mindset to judge the *validity* of that knowledge. In other words: they are mostly trained to take knowledge at face value, instead of critically evaluating it, e.g. by means of the scientific method.

Alternative Medicine on Trial

The first principle is that you must not fool yourself, and you are the easiest person to fool.

Richard Feynman (1918–1988)

Throughout this book, I explored several types of alternative medicine. The conclusion was that most are ineffective, but at the same time mostly harmless, at least in a direct sense. There is also the fact that the overwhelming majority of patients is satisfied with the treatment they received and the outcome. So why not live and let live, and stop harassing alternative practitioners with all that science-based criticism?

This is an understandable argument, but it is wrong in several respects. The fundamental problem is that alternative medicine is based on deception: patients are told that the treatment they receive can benefit their health, but this is not supported by science. The scientific consensus is that most forms of alternative medicine have no real effect beyond placebo (which, almost by definition, is deception). It should, however, be noted that this deception is not deliberate: almost all alternative practitioners first and foremost deceive themselves. They really believe that what they do has therapeutic effects.

This self-deception is also evident from some of the more common tropes encountered in discussions with alternative practitioners and their followers. '*Think for yourself!*' and '*Do your own research!*' are two often-heard exhortations in alternative circles. The suggestion is that people should not take for granted whatever doctors, scientists and other experts say, but find out things for themselves. This sounds reasonable, but is actually a quite silly: most people can't possibly reach well-informed conclusions about complex matters such as the risks and efficacy of for instance vaccines by just 'thinking for themselves'. What of course is *meant* is 'listen to us [anti-vaccine people], and not to scientists, experts, politicians, mainstream media etc.' In other words: people are invited to deceive themselves by rejecting solid scientific expertise and replace it with 'own research'.

Alternative medicine is also harmful in that many of its practitioners have no medical or scientific education. Many if not most of the diagnoses in alternative medicine are wrong, and by extension, so are any treatments based on those diagnoses. The fact that there is nothing seriously wrong with up to 80 or 90% of patients seeking help from alternative practitioners does not detract from this. People with harmless ailments are often diagnosed with conditions that in reality they do not have,[2] resulting in unnecessary and often costly treatments—and, depending on the diagnosed 'condition' itself, substantial stress and worry for the patient. It's even worse for those unlucky enough to really have a serious condition without knowing. They run a substantial risk of harm and even death as a result of delaying proper diagnosis and treatment by a regular doctor.

Then there are still several popular but inherently harmful types of alternative medicine: oriental herbal medicines containing toxic heavy metals, chiropractic neck manipulations that can cause strokes, and unnecessary chelation therapy that can send patients into cardiac arrest, to name just a few. And, of course, paying for something that is promised but not actually delivered (i.e. effective healthcare) is by definition harmful, if only in a financial sense.

But even though alternative medicine *does* harm people on a regular basis, one could argue that the far larger number of satisfied customers more than makes up for this.

What to do?

The Dilemma

The logical question is if alternative medicine should be tolerated or not, given that it is in fact not 'medicine' in the sense that it can really make sick people better. This question is however a false dichotomy: there are many more ways to look at and deal with alternative medicine than to either leave it alone or try to ban it.

To be clear about one thing: yes, there are some types of alternative medicine that should absolutely be banned, simply because they do a lot of harm to people. At the top of this ban list of mine are alternative cancer treatments. Not a single alternative cancer treatment has ever been proven to work. Yet the practitioners offering these bogus treatments are selling desperate, scared patients false hope, robbing them not only of sometimes large sums of money, but often also their last weeks or months of life. There are several other types of alternative medicine that deserve banning, mostly those involving children (who can't give informed consent), or inherently harmful alternative treatments.

Banning all of alternative medicine, however, is an impossible proposition for practical reasons, and would cause some serious societal repercussions and

---

[2] Very few alternative practitioners will tell their clientele that they can't find anything wrong with them and thus need no treatment.

upheaval. It is simply not a viable option to put thousands[3] of people out of work—especially with an even greater number of customers holding them in high regard.

So far, the main course of action of scientists and sceptics was trying to educate the public about the true nature of alternative medicine and pseudoscience. I suppose this book also falls into this category. This education is only partially effective, among other things because most people cannot make a truly informed choice on whom to believe. They lack the background knowledge to judge if they should listen to what a homeopath says, or to what scientists or sceptics say. After all, homeopaths have *also* written countless books with lots of explanation and details about how their system of medicine works—at least from their point of view.

Open Mind

I think that it is important to at least try to engage alternative practitioners themselves in a constructive dialogue, in order to see if they are willing to open their mind to the possibility that they might be wrong about what they believe. This is no doubt a tricky and delicate process, especially since both sides tend to accuse each other of dogmatic positions, but there are ways to at least come nearer to one another; these are discussed in the next section.

The goal is not so much to put alternative practitioners out of business, but just to make them rethink and hopefully abandon the whole medical context. I for one would be perfectly fine with homeopaths presenting their art as a 'feelgood treatment', without the pretence that they can cure medical conditions. There are lots of other respectable professions and institutes dedicated to making people feel good—think spas, beauty parlours, hairdressers, the whole wellness industry, and yes, even pubs, restaurants[4] and other places where people pay good money to simply have a good time. So why can't alternative medicine practitioners just drop the whole 'medicine' part, and stick to the truth? What they do makes people feel good, and that should already be worth the money.

There are of course problems with this approach. Many alternative practitioners are fervent believers in every aspect of what they do, and to them, even doubting their *modus operandi* is pure sacrilege. These people simply will never admit that their alternative 'medicine' is in reality not medicine at

---

[3] Here in the Netherlands, there are approximately 25,000 alternative practitioners on a total population of some 18 million.

[4] The word 'restaurant' literally means 'place to restore [strength and vigour]'.

all. Others will come up with all sorts of reasons and excuses why science is wrong—and, ironically, often present scientific studies to support this point of view.

Still, I think it often can't hurt to start at least communicating and see if there is some common ground to be found. That is, if we really want to try and find out what motivates 'the other side'—regardless of which side we're on ourselves. Not only is it all too easy to simply dismiss anything that is said and done by those you disagree with, but it doesn't contribute to any meaningful solution to the underlying question: how to make (and keep) people healthy and happy as much as possible. There is enough polarization in society and politics as it is already.

Communication Across the Divide

In the course of the years, I came across lots of proponents and advocates of alternative medicine, and also quite a few practitioners. As one would expect, most resulting discussions did not really go all that well, especially when taking place on Internet forums and the likes. Quite often, these discussions were best described as 'trench warfare'. Based on these sometimes rather frustrating experiences, I assembled a list of dos and don'ts. Yes, most of these things are no-brainers—but it is still surprising how easy it is to descend into mud flinging contests and other unwise behaviour. Just screaming and throwing stuff at the monkey opposite us still seems to be deeply ingrained in our human brain—and alas, I too speak from lots of personal experience of Doing it Wrong.

The best way to go about discussions of course also depends on who you're talking to, where the discussion takes place (social media, Internet forums, or in person), and what your goals are. An exchange of opinions and points of view will usually be much easier than any attempts to 'win' a discussion.

These are some points to keep in mind:

* Stay cool and composed at all times. Don't ever let emotions take the driver's seat, as this will cloud your judgement and make you say and do stupid things. Also don't follow suit if the other side becomes emotional (e.g. angry or rude or disdainful). Remember: these discussions should never be personal, but revolve around facts and generalized opinions.
* Be honest and open about your motives. Hidden agendas or sly tactics to steer a discussion in a certain way will only raise suspicions and antagonize participants as well as any audience.

* As a first point of order, try to establish facts that both sides agree upon, and work the discussion from there. Return to this 'safe base' if things threaten to derail or escalate in any way.
* Try to create some form of common ground based on these facts. Beware, however, of fallacies such as false balance or the truth 'lying in the middle'. If there is an overwhelming scientific consensus that something is untrue (e.g. claims that vaccines cause autism), then it is a mistake to concede this point to any degree. If there is no credible evidence for certain claims that are made, then stick with your point.
* Ask questions instead of making assertions—but beware of the tactic of *'Just asking questions'* (which in reality are controversial assertions or accusations disguised as questions).
* Check regularly if you understand the other person's point. Many discussions derail because of minor misunderstandings. Also make certain that the other side doesn't misrepresent your point (e.g. as part of a *straw man* tactic).
* Related to the previous point: regularly try to shift your point of view to the other person's position, to try and see how *you* may come across in their eyes. Remember that the person on the other side is often just as genuinely convinced of the truth of their position as you are of yours.
* Don't be afraid to call out mistakes or obvious untruths from the other side, but keep any comments polite, to-the-point and impersonal.
* Don't be afraid to concede good points made by the other side.
* Resist any urge to use strong language; especially name-calling will only serve to make you look silly. No-one was ever persuaded to change their position by being called stupid.
* Beware of certain debating tactics such as the *Gish gallop*[5] whereby someone is flooded with a rapid succession of unimportant arguments, with the goal to have the opponent floundering to address each and every one of them—something that is usually impossible.
* Ignore trolls and others who are clearly trying to sow chaos and confusion.
* Don't expect anyone to change their mind. The best you can hope for is a better mutual understanding, and maybe to make the other side think about your point of view instead of blindly rejecting it.

---

[5] Named after a young-earth creationist by the name of Duane Gish, who routinely used this tactic to 'disprove' evolution in debates.

Why Debates Are Not Recommended for Scientific Topics

Public debates are usually not a very good way to have a scientific exchange of opinions, as there are many tricks and strategies to 'win' debates regardless of the merits of the arguments and topics presented. Some of these were already mentioned, such as burying the opponent under a heap of often weak and spurious arguments (the Gish gallop), or drawing the debate into the realm of emotions. Other successful tactics are to simply ignore valid criticism, and instead go off on a tangent that is not related to the question at hand (a so-called *red herring*), or resort to *whataboutism* (turning criticism around, e.g. to defend the inefficacy of homeopathy by claiming that pharmaceutical medicines often don't work either—even though this is irrelevant for establishing the efficacy of homeopathy).

For instance anti-vaccine groups often hold public debates featuring several 'experts', with the aim to spread their views among a greater audience. The quotation marks are there for a reason: the debating panels are usually stacked with people who hold anti-vaccine views, but are rarely if ever actual experts on the subject of vaccines, immunology or epidemiology. Quite often, regular pro-vaccine doctors and scientists are invited for these events as well. These real experts are usually wise enough decline such invitations, for reasons already mentioned—which of course is then spun by the anti-vaccine crowd as a victory. Any counter-invitations to take part in a purely scientific discussion (i.e. by exchanging papers and commentaries with carefully researched arguments) are in turn rejected by the anti-vaccine people—who have no acceptable scientific arguments or evidence on their side.

'Don't Trust Anyone!'

Belief in alternative medicine and pseudoscience usually stays limited to the topic of medicine itself, even though this belief often involves some vague conspiracy, e.g. that vaccine makers can't be trusted, or that a simple, universal cancer cure is kept secret by pharmaceutical companies, in order to protect their profits from existing cancer medicines.

Things get taken to another level when mistrust in everyday societal institutions (and sometimes even fundamental, well-established knowledge) becomes a core belief for people. Examples are the rejection of news from mainstream media in favour of more obscure sources, or the belief that you can't trust (most) doctors to act in your best interest. Of course politicians on 'the other side' are also not to be trusted—in fact, they are increasingly portrayed as pure evil, especially in the United States with its highly polarized political landscape. All these beliefs, hate and mistrust can amalgamate into one 'super-conspiracy' that encompasses literally everything that is supposedly wrong with the world—with QAnon as the most prominent example.

Real Conspiracies

Just to get this out of the way: conspiracies are a real thing. Over the course of history, there have been lots of conspiracies, often linked to power struggles—just think of all those attempts to overthrow governments, or for instance the Watergate scandal. Maybe the closest thing to those many Covid-19 and anti-vaccine conspiracies was the Tuskegee Syphilis Study, a hugely unethical scandal involving medical science [77].

However, almost all of these conspiracies came to light sooner rather than later, in most cases because someone spilled the beans, or because the goal of the conspiracy had been attained (e.g. a coup). The Tuskegee Syphilis Study, lasting 40 years, was an exception, mainly because there were relatively few people involved, and because those involved believed that what they did was justified from a scientific point of view. But even this scandal became public through a leak from the inside. Only very rarely is a conspiracy revealed by outsiders—and not a single widespread conspiracy idea such as those spread by QAnon was ever found to be true.

How Do They Know?

For the sake of the argument, suppose there really could be something horrible going on, orchestrated by a relatively small group of people, and that these people are extremely successful in keeping their conspiracy secret. Nobody suspects a thing: not scientists, not politicians, not the general public … And not a single conspirator so far has broken their silence and spilled the beans.

This then raises a very simple question: *how do conspiracy believers know about it?*

In fact, they don't. What they do is what was already explained in Chapter 1: when trying to make sense of certain events, they look for patterns and clues—and even insignificant coincidences can be interpreted as such. They then 'connect the dots', make up a more or less logical story about the whole thing, and voilà, there is your conspiracy! The mental process behind this is explained in more detail further on.

The interesting thing is that these conspiracy ideas (I think that 'theory' is too much honour) often look highly implausible or sometimes even plain crazy to outsiders. Quite often, it is difficult to imagine that someone would actually believe those things. Then there is of course the hard evidence—or rather: the total lack of any hard evidence. Most of the time, these things hinge on some minor events or coincidences that happen on an almost daily basis. Sometimes they can even be tracked back to just one misinterpreted quote from some public figure.

Saint or Satan?

A famous example of a misinterpreted quote is a 2010 TED Talk with Bill Gates saying that carbon emissions could be curbed by slowing down the growth of the world population, most of which takes place in developing countries. Gates speculated that a reduction in population growth of 'perhaps 10 or 15%' could be brought about by improving healthcare, including vaccination. What Gates meant was that improving healthcare and reducing child mortality in poor countries eventually leads to lower birth rates and thus a smaller future population.

However, conspiracy believers immediately took the quote and ran with it, claiming that Gates accidentally spilled the beans on a sinister plot to kill off 15% of the world population through vaccines—which to them, also proved that vaccines are lethal poison. They were right all along!

To us outsiders, perhaps the most bizarre thing about this is that Gates has dedicated his life to philanthropy for the past decades, spending billions of dollars on (indeed) improving healthcare for people in the poorest countries on the planet. So it seems that the man behaves like a saint, yet is vilified as one the most evil people on the planet, all because of one mangled quote. Now of course Gates made all that money in a not-so-nice way, by abusing the dominance of his computer software, deliberately stifling any competition by unsavoury business practices instead of competing on product quality. There are in fact quite a few pretty good reasons not to like the man. But these past business practices are almost never mentioned, so they don't seem to play any role in the conspiracy narratives.

According to professor Joseph Uscinsky from the University of Miami, author of several books and articles on conspiracy theories, it is much simpler: a combination of money and power is already enough for someone to become a target of distrust, hatred and, eventually, conspiracy beliefs. The idea is that extremely rich and powerful people can do pretty much anything they want—also to other people—and get away with it. Which has a kernel of truth in it, given numerous, only recently uncovered cases of serious abuse perpetrated by rich and powerful people, crimes that went unpunished for many years.

What also might play role is the fact that many people find it hard to believe that rich people such as Gates indeed give away huge sums of money to the poor. This perceived contradiction suggests hypocrisy, making them more a target of hate than 'ordinary' greedy rich people.

Spilled Beans: Best Before Date

Three can keep a secret if two of them are dead.
                                    Benjamin Franklin (1705–1790)

One defining characteristic of a conspiracy is secrecy. Openly planning to take control of groups of people, a whole country or even the world is not a conspiracy, but politics.

The more people are involved in a conspiracy and the longer this conspiracy exists, the bigger the chance that the whole thing comes to light. Scientist David Grimes even devised a formula to predict the 'expiry date' on any particular conspiracy [78]. For instance, suppose that the 1969 moon landing was not real but a hoax, a conspiracy as some people believe. Grimes's formula predicts that this conspiracy would likely have been exposed in less than 4 years, mostly because of the large number of people involved (some 411,000).

Another inherent problem with many presumed conspiracies is the fact that they simply don't make sense. In the chapter on vaccines, I already mentioned the conspiracy belief that vaccine makers are conspiring to sell harmful vaccines. To this end, they bribe scientists and doctors into silence about this mass poisoning, and falsify studies to fool governments and the public. Such a conspiracy doesn't make sense in several respects. For one, it would be far more expensive and risky to pay off those millions (!) of doctors and scientists than to simply produce a safe and reliable vaccine. Another reason is that countless scientists and government agencies worldwide are coming up with more or less the same results when studying the safety and efficacy of vaccines—which would mean that the conspiracy would not only cost insane amounts of money, but also involve very elaborate co-ordination to make certain that the falsified data from all those different organizations in all those different countries matched up.

Where Conspiracy Beliefs Start

Belief in conspiracies starts out in much the same way that belief in alternative medicine and even discoveries in real science starts: people try to find a solution to a problem, or want to make sense of certain events or observations. When they think they stumbled upon something, they start building a story explaining what they found—and this is where our human brain gets in the way of things such as truth and reality:

- Just a few facts and cues from the world around us are enough to fire up our story-making machinery, which actively tries 'connecting the dots' (read: find a pattern). This means that almost by definition, every form of reasoning starts out as a product of our brain, with only a few links to the real world.
- To make matters worse, our innate tendency to prefer Kahneman's 'fast and sloppy' System 1 thinking almost inevitably introduces things such as confirmation bias, where we tend to accept things we already believe far more readily than contradicting information. The same goes for information from people we know and trust—even though they are not experts on the subject matter.
- To muddy the waters even more, our brain tends to let salience (e.g. things that trigger our emotions rather than our rationality) prevail over truthfulness.

What all this means is that even the most absurd conspiracy beliefs come into existence in much the same way as well-researched scientific hypotheses. The most important difference is that scientists are trained to critically examine and verify every single step in the story they come up with. They constantly check if what they're doing is compatible with objective reality.

Conspiracy believers, on the other hand, tend to take giant, mostly unwarranted steps from one fact or cue to the next. Their 'checks' mostly boil down to disseminating their ideas and beliefs among their peers, and see what they think about it. This may resemble the scientific process of peer review to some degree, but the problem is that at no point, those ideas and beliefs are verified against objective facts and reality. The result is a particular 'conspiracy bubble', made up of lots of individual facts, factoids and interconnecting stories, most of which are completely detached from reality.

Conspiracy belief also has a lot in common with cults and religions: both serve as a way to explain things that are hard to understand and/or outside of our control. Both involve social bonding with a group by professing and sharing those beliefs, and carrying out group 'rituals'—read: protest gatherings in the case of conspiracy believers. And just as with religion, people are more drawn to conspiracy beliefs in times of chaos or disaster, such as the recent Covid-19 pandemic.

Conspiracy belief is nothing new, and has been with us probably from the dawn of mankind. As already mentioned before in this book, people find it very difficult to accept that things 'just happen'; they always want to find *causes* and *reasons*. Science has been extremely successful in finding causes, especially for natural phenomena. Pointing out reasons, however, is quite a different matter, because 'reason' presupposes human actors or agents. Whenever something bad happens, people have a tendency to try and find other people who can somehow be blamed for this bad thing.

What is new, however, is the unprecedented speed and scale at which conspiracy belief managed to spread in the past few years. Popular social media and in particular the algorithms behind those media play an important role here. Through these algorithms, people are almost irresistibly drawn into one of many 'rabbit holes' with all sorts of extreme (mis)information.

In this light, it is not surprising that rumours about the Covid-19 virus being 'man-made' and 'released from a secret Wuhan lab' were spreading considerably faster than the actual disease itself. These two notions have since been instrumental in a much larger conspiracy narrative, where obscure but extremely powerful forces released the virus upon us unsuspecting sheeple in order to achieve their nefarious goals—one of which is supposedly a 'New World Order', where all people are enslaved to do the bidding of those mysterious forces.

Which is a bit strange when you come to think of it: yes, there exists a relatively small group of extremely rich and powerful people. However, these multi-billionaires don't need any shady schemes to 'enslave' people—because they *already have maximum control* over almost anyone and everything they want: they simply pay people or businesses or other organizations to do whatever it is they want them to do. Trying to exert even more control over people would only make things more difficult for themselves. Then of course there is the problem that releasing a deadly disease on mankind does not turn them into slaves. At the most, it turns them into sick and dead people, who are not only rather unprofitable, but also not known for their propensity to follow orders. So there is still no good reason why this virus would be deliberately released. At which point conspiracy believers of course came up with all sorts of new mini-conspiracies to shoehorn their 'Wuhan lab theory' into the greater scheme of things after all.

Some popular narratives say that the virus was released in order to have an excuse to vaccinate all of mankind, and that those vaccines[6] contained invisible microchips[7] that could control the human victim, receiving its commands through the new 5G network[8]—which, incidentally, was just about to be rolled out in Wuhan when the pandemic hit. No way that all this was a coincidence!

---

[6] Made by Bill Gates of course.

[7] Also made by Bill Gates.

[8] No doubt linked to Bill Gates as well.

Another quite popular but even more insane conspiracy belief said that many (democratic) American political leaders were members of a satanic cult that was routinely abusing and murdering children, drinking those children's blood to make them immortal. Oh, and that Donald Trump would expose these evildoers and use his presidential powers to arrest them all on a 'day of reckoning'. For various reasons, this particular conspiracy seems to be no longer in vogue.

Social Traits and Social Media

Social media and the algorithms they use form a very fertile breeding ground for conspiracy beliefs. As the name already implies, social media work by allowing users to create or join groups where they will meet like-minded people—appealing to one of the oldest human traits to survive in a hostile environment. Finding and joining such groups takes no effort at all. Quite often, all it takes is just *one* search for a particular subject (e.g. 'Wuhan lab leak') in order to get presented with an endless list of social media messages, groups and articles that all point users towards platforms, groups, videos and Web sites promoting the 'lab leak' narrative. What's worse: both the search history and the Web pages someone visited are remembered by the algorithm in order to present them with *more* of this content—and not just the same, but increasingly extreme content, because that is what grabs (and keeps) users' attention.

This almost fully automated mechanism sucking hapless Internet users down rabbit holes is only half of the problem. The other half are the users themselves. Once someone has joined a group dedicated to, say, anti-vaccine conspiracies, then cult-like social dynamics can make things even worse. Those social media groups extend a warm welcome to anyone showing interest in the group's subject and willingness to accept whatever the group's main topics are. This welcome is all the warmer when someone comes up with their own contributions to the group, in the form of 'news' items or other bits and pieces of a particular conspiracy idea. The only requirement is that it matches the group's ideology; it doesn't have to be true—these stories or comments are often liked even better the more extreme they are.

Conversely, this warm welcome immediately turns cold when someone starts asking sceptical questions, points out that a particular bit of news is not true, or fails to fully embrace the group's mores and ideas. These people are more likely than not banned from the group right away. So what you end up with is a self-sustaining echo chamber of extreme ideas—or rather: a network of echo chambers, as of course a huge amount of the (mis/dis)information in such groups consists of links to other, very similar groups. This is not called *viral information* for nothing: all those titbits of false information behave very much like viruses, infecting susceptible people, damaging their healthy world view, and using these infected people to spread to others again.

Most major social media platforms are nowadays trying to curb at least the worst of this endless spread of disinformation, but so far, they do not appear to be hugely successful. Also, new media channels have jumped into the gap, catering to conspiracy believers and other spreaders of disinformation and misinformation. These media channels present themselves as protecting the people's right to free speech, even if that free speech almost completely consists of false information, hate propaganda and death threats.

If the flood of conspiracy belief has abated somewhat in recent times, then this is most likely the result of most western countries abandoning Covid-19 countermeasures and life returning back to normal as a result. When people can once again go about their life as they used to, then there is no real need any more to question day-to-day events and speculate about sinister plots that supposedly try to take away their freedoms.

The Dangers of Disinformation and Misinformation

Conspiracy belief and its associated misinformation and disinformation are harmful in that they erode one essential element of our modern human society: the trust that we have in each other. This has a negative impact at every thinkable level in society, from families falling apart to groups of people planning violence against politicians. There was even one certain US ex-president who consistently spread conspiracy-based disinformation in an attempt to subvert democracy, for no other reason than to stay in power.

Our society runs on trust—not just trust in our own family and friends as in most of human history, but also trust in countless others, mostly experts, most of whom we'll never know personally (also see the sidebar *Who must you trust* in Chapter 2). This should not be taken lightly: virtually everything in our life requires *lots* of experts. Those experts are people like you and me, earning their living by doing things that other people want or need, but can't do for themselves.

Healthcare is one such field of expertise where we absolutely need to trust the experts—at least, if we want to maintain the current status quo, with low child mortality, high life expectancy and ever more conditions that can be treated effectively. Unfortunately, the stream of disinformation caused by the

Covid-19 pandemic has seriously damaged public trust in medical science and healthcare experts.

One major problem is that belief in all sorts of nefarious conspiracies also incites believers to threaten or even commit violence: on December 4, 2016, a heavily armed man entered a pizzeria named Comet Ping Pong in Washington D.C., fired several shots, and demanded to be shown the basement. According to the 'Pizzagate conspiracy theory', Hillary Clinton and other high-ranking politicians were torturing and abusing children in that basement. It took a while before the gunman was convinced that the pizzeria did in fact not have a basement …

The most horrible example of the dangers of misinformation and conspiracy thinking is of course what happened in Germany in the 1930's, with Nazi politicians spreading all sorts of lies and rumours about Jewish conspiracies to destabilize Europe and take control in the ensuing chaos. In reality, it was of course the Nazi leadership conspiring against Jews and other minorities, in what is considered the biggest, most evil crime against humanity ever. Unfortunately, even nowadays dictators all over the world use disinformation and incite conspiracy beliefs in order to keep in power and justify heinous acts of war and suppression.

What Can We Do?

The problem with conspiracy belief and is that it is not limited to just certain aspects of healthcare or lifestyle such as alternative medicine, but affects all aspects of society. It causes sweeping distrust in almost every institution, ranging from politics to 'mainstream media' to almost all of healthcare.

This distrust can even extend to family members and friends: someone who is entrenched in conspiracy beliefs will often no longer trust anyone who tries to tell them that they're wrong, even if it is their own child or parent or close friend. Any criticism is countered by arguments that 'You don't understand it', or 'You don't know what I know'. Critics are often even accused of being part of the alleged conspiracy.[9]

Unfortunately, there is no simple solution. As already said before, a strong enough belief can trump everything, even the most basic rationality. Contrary to reason, it also seems that the more outlandish a belief is, the more fervently it is defended by the believer—probably because there are fewer *real* reasons for propping up this belief.

---

[9] This is particularly common in anonymous online forum discussions, where for instance proponents of vaccination are accused by anti-vaccine activists of being 'Big Pharma' shills, who earn 'blood money' by promoting vaccinations.

The communication tactics discussed earlier in the paragraph *Communicating across the divide* still apply, but are in most cases even less effective with conspiracy believers than with proponents of alternative medicine. This is because conspiracy belief is largely based on not trusting or even listening to whatever 'unbelievers' say, and because it involves making up a different reality, where nothing is what it seems. This makes it extremely difficult to agree on even simple facts, find common ground, and to convince the other side at least of your own good intentions. The only person who can talk someone out of a strong belief is that person self.

In my opinion, the best way to deal with this problem is to try and immunize people by making them familiar with certain characteristics and patterns of conspiracy ideas, misinformation and disinformation. The most important characteristic to look out for is if something tries to appeal to people's emotions—in particular negative emotions such as indignation, anger and fear. If you encounter a headline saying 'BIGGEST vaccine scandal EVER', then the article is almost certainly trying to tell you things that aren't true.

About conspiracy believers themselves: I pity most of them. It must be pretty horrible to live in a world where you feel that you can't trust anyone or anything, and must be ever vigilant in order to avoid becoming a zombie slave or something similar. The sad thing is that these people *have* become zombie slaves—of their own extreme beliefs, making their life difficult at almost every step.

Yet I still think that we should not give up on trying to communicate with them. They are, after all, people—often seriously misguided people, but people nonetheless.

Then of course there are also the people who actively spread and encourage disinformation and conspiracy nonsense for their own personal and/or political gain. These are people who have made spreading distrust and hatred not only their personal life mission, but also their business, hurting countless others by what they do. One such example is Alex Jones, who caused immense grief by persistently claiming that the Sandy Hook elementary school shooting (where twenty children were killed) never happened, and that the grieving parents were liars and actors—causing his followers to harass those parents for many years. Jones claimed that this mass shooting was made up by the government in order to have an excuse to take away people's guns. Jones was recently convicted of paying Sandy Hook parents over a billion dollars in damages—a sum that also reflected the hundreds of millions of dollars he made peddling merchandise and products in his conspiracy-laden talk show, effectively turning conspiracy mongering into a successful business model.

It is to be hoped that this verdict is a turning point in a worrisome trend, where just a handful of loud voices spreading chaos, disinformation and distrust can cause lots of scared and insecure people to turn their back on normal society—and thus on most of their fellow human beings. Which is in fact not all that different from those baboons way back in Chapter 1, huddling together on a rock because their leader saw a threat that wasn't really there.

Conclusion

We have come full circle: in this final chapter, I discussed how our human brain favours quick 'n easy beliefs and jumping to conclusions over meticulous but arduous reasoning processes to determine what is true and what isn't.

One of the problems here is that belief tends to be self-affirming, and often sets off a positive feedback loop: supporting information is integrated in the belief ever more easily, while contradictory information is increasingly ignored and discarded. This can lead to a situation where the concept of being wrong about a certain belief is almost literally unthinkable to the person or persons involved. This is why it is so hard to convince for instance staunch anti-vaccine activists that there is nothing wrong with vaccines. Their rock-solid central belief is that vaccines are evil—and from there, they will try to interpret any information as a confirmation of that belief.

The same goes with conspiracy believers. The Internet is rife with stories about whole families falling apart because people start believing conspiracy ideas that are based on the premise that you can't trust anyone who contradicts those ideas—not even your own children or parents.

Still, there are some positive things to note: most conspiracy ideas eventually peter out when whatever started and kept them going (e.g. Covid-19 countermeasures such as lock-downs, social distancing and vaccination mandates) stops, and life returns back to normal without any doomsday predictions coming true. The most important thing to do in my opinion is to keep communicating with people, even if they are wrong about certain things.

The point is that we all make mistakes, and that we are all wrong about things some time or other—but most of us are also trying to live our lives the best we can, being kind, helpful and trustworthy to others. After all, the alternative world described in this book is in fact the same world we all live in, but just viewed with another mindset.

So let's be respectful when pointing out when other people are wrong, and always have an open mind to the possibility that we ourselves may be wrong as well.

Appendix

A.1 Common Biases, Fallacies and Bad Practices

Our human brain is by no means perfect when it comes to observation and reasoning, and there are many pitfalls and errors on the road to gathering knowledge and understanding.

Here, an overview is provided of the most important biases, bad practices and fallacies; many of these are discussed in this book. Note that this is by no means an attempt to provide an exhaustive list—there are hundreds more.

Literally *everyone* is susceptible to these biases and fallacies, simply because they are the result of how our brain has evolved. The scientific method tries to avoid these pitfalls by means of strict rules for the collection and processing of information, and by explicitly encouraging scientists to try and *disprove* a new hypothesis. This means that scientists are slightly less at risk (but by no means immune!) for these cognitive pitfalls.

Most adherents and practitioners of alternative medicine and pseudo-science are not scientists, and as such do not follow the scientific method. Therefore, it should come as no surprise that most ideas and practices in the alternative universe are based on biases, fallacies and false beliefs. This is also the main reason why most alternative treatments are found to be placebo treatments at best, and harmful at worst—even though the latter is of course not the intention of its practitioners.

A.2 List of Common Biases and Bad Practices

Biases and bad practices are typically flaws in observation or experimentation that can lead to a wrong study outcome. Biases can be subtle and hard to spot, while bad practices are more visible, but can still be overlooked. This is why it is important that scientific research is as transparent as possible, to enable other scientists to check every detail of a particular study.

A versus A + B study design. This is a study design whereby a combined treatment A + B is compared to just treatment A. As an additional treatment B will introduce an extra placebo effect, the A versus A + B study design will often turn out positive for the combined treatment, even if B has no real effect at all.

Confirmation Bias. This bias is based on our tendency to favour information that matches our preconceived beliefs, while at the same time disregarding or playing down information contradicting those beliefs.

Expectation Bias. The name says it all: we erroneously think we see something because we expect to see it. It is in other words false pattern recognition, often amplified by the mental excitement of anticipation/expectation itself.

Frequency illusion. This is a bias where drawing the attention to a particular occurrence or phenomenon makes you see it around you far more often than before.

P-hacking, also known as **Fishing Expedition**. This is a bad practice in studies whereby a significant result is achieved by either comparing many variables (resulting in one or more significant correlations by chance alone), or by increasing the sample size after the fact until the significance threshold (usually $p < 0.05$) is reached.

Selection bias. When taking a small sample to say something about a larger population, one should be very careful to ensure that this sample is representative for the larger population. Failing to do so introduces selection bias, potentially resulting in a wrong outcome.

Survivorship bias. This bias looks only at the group reaching a certain goal, ignoring the group that did not make it. If you want to know if for instance a particular cancer treatment works, you should not just look for patients who received the treatment and survived, but also for those who died *despite* receiving the treatment.

A.3 List of Common Fallacies

A *fallacy* is best described as a flawed line of reasoning. Like biases, fallacious reasoning leads to false conclusions, but often causes more widespread effects in the form of false beliefs. Fallacies are generally less subtle and thus easier to spot than biases.

Anecdotal fallacy. See: Personal experience fallacy.

Cherry picking. This fallacy boils down to just seeking out isolated pieces of evidence that support a case or argument, while ignoring the often much larger amount of evidence against that case or argument. This is related to confirmation bias and expectation bias.

Correlation implies causation. This fallacy, related to the Post hoc fallacy, says that if two things seem to happen together, then one must cause of the other. The flaw here is that there may be a *third* phenomenon causing both other phenomena. This fallacy is caused by our tendency to see patterns and connections.

False balance. False balance occurs mostly in news reporting, where a journalist or media channel presents 'both sides' of a story or subject as more or less equal, even if they're not equal at all. An example is when a scientist is quoted about the need to vaccinate our children against deadly disease, followed by allowing an anti-vaccine group to present their claims that vaccines cause grave harm to children. There is ample evidence for the scientist's claims, but no good evidence at all for the anti-vaccine claims.

False dichotomy or **false dilemma**. The false dichotomy consists of presenting two things as mutually exclusive, while in reality there are more options. The most well-known false dichotomy is the adage 'Whoever is not with us, is against us', designating anyone who does not join the speaker's group as the enemy. Creationists also use the false dichotomy a lot: they try to disprove evolution, because they believe that the biblical creation event is then the only remaining alternative.

Galileo gambit. This fallacy applies when pseudoscientists or alternative practitioners are criticized by mainstream science, and then compare themselves with Galileo Galilei, who was prosecuted because his observations contradicted religious dogma. One big mistake here is that Galileo was actually correct, whereas everyone who invoked the Galileo gambit so far turned out to be wrong. Another big mistake is that Galileo was prosecuted by the church, not by other scientists.

'Just asking questions'. This is a tactic by which someone frames accusations or controversial assertions as (leading and loaded) questions, in order to come across as inquisitive or sceptical rather than aggressive.

Mechanistic fallacy. The mechanistic fallacy occurs when a particular treatment solves a certain aspect of a problem, without in fact contributing to solving the problem as a whole. An example is using supplements to normalize someone's vitamin and mineral levels, without actually improving someone's quality of life or susceptibility to disease.

Moving the goalposts. This is a fallacy whereby certain agreed-upon criteria or definitions are later changed to support an untenable argument after all. An example is to 'save' a negative study by watering down the quality of the evidence used.

Natural fallacy (appeal to nature). This fallacy implies that anything 'natural' is automatically good, whereas 'unnatural' things are deemed bad. It appeals to our idea of an idyllic past, where everyone was healthy and happy in the warm embrace of Mother Nature. This mostly false image is often used to sell us all sorts of things that, ironically, are often quite unnatural. And, of course, there are many natural things that are distinctly bad for us, while many unnatural things are highly beneficial to our health, well-being and even survival.

Nirvana fallacy. This fallacy applies when something must be perfect in all respects, or else it is no good at all. It is often used by anti-vaccine people claiming that a vaccine should fully protect all vaccinated people for the rest of their life without any side effects whatsoever, or else it is a 'failed' vaccine.

Nobel disease. This is not so much an isolated fallacy as well as a tendency of highly respected scientists (and often even Nobel laureates, hence the name) to seriously overstep their areas of expertise and embrace pseudoscience. This generally happens later in their life and/or career.

Personal experience fallacy. This very common fallacy occurs when one or more personal experiences or anecdotes are taken as evidence for a particular phenomenon. Many types of alternative of medicine as well as individual practitioners have started out as a result of a single, often revelation-type personal experience. One notable example is Samuel Hahnemann, who based his whole idea of homeopathy on just one personal experience with cinchona bark (which later turned out to be a fluke, when other doctors were unable to replicate his findings).

Post hoc ergo propter hoc. This Latin phrase can be translated as 'After = Caused by': when event A is followed by event B, we assume by default that event A also caused event B. This extremely common fallacy is again the result of our human propensity to recognize patterns and connections, even if there aren't any.

Science was wrong before. This fallacy is used when claims from pseudo-scientists or alternative practitioners contradict established science. Instead of coming up with proper evidence supporting their own claims, they take the far easier route of claiming that science was wrong in the past, so it may well be wrong now. Which means that they may well be right. Which, as a line of reasoning, is wrong.

Straw man fallacy. In this fallacy, an unwelcome position or argument is misrepresented in such a way that it is easier to refute or criticize than the original position.

Sunk cost fallacy. This fallacy describes how it becomes increasingly difficult for people to abandon a certain failing endeavour the more they invested in it (in terms of money, effort and emotions). Also known as 'Throwing bad money after good money'.

Tradition, appeal to. Appeal to tradition says that if something has been used for a long time, it must be good. This is not necessarily true. For example blood-letting has been practised for thousands of years, yet we now know that it was not effective for any condition it was used for. In fact, it harmed and killed countless patients.

Literature and Web References

1 The Hindu. (2019, November 6). *Indian cow's milk has gold,* says BJP leader. https://www.thehindu.com/news/national/other-states/indian-cows-milk-has-gold-says-bjp-leader/article29892587.ece

2 Fanelli, D. (2009, May 29). *How Many Scientists Fabricate and Falsify Research? A Systematic Review and Meta-Analysis of Survey Data.* PLOS ONE. https://journals.plos.org/plosone/article?id=10.1371/journal.pone.0005738

3 Hawley, B. C. (2014, October 3). *The story of the fake bomb detectors.* BBC News. https://www.bbc.com/news/uk-29459896

4 *The ultimate homeopathic remedy* | ScienceBlogs. (2011, September 1). https://scienceblogs.com/insolence/2011/09/01/the-ultimate-homeopathic-remedy

5 Elsevier (2014, January). *Retraction notice to "Long term toxicity of a Roundup herbicide and a Roundup-tolerant genetically modified maize" [Food Chem. Toxicol. 50 (2012) 4221–4231].* https://doi.org/10.1016/j.fct.2013.11.047

6 Chuong, E. B. (2018). *The placenta goes viral: Retroviruses control gene expression in pregnancy.* PLOS Biology, *16*(10), e3000028. https://doi.org/10.1371/journal.pbio.3000028

7 E number. (2020, April 24). Wikipedia. https://en.wikipedia.org/wiki/E_number

8 Garrison, S. R., Korownyk, C. S., Kolber, M. R., Allan, G. M., Musini, V. M., Sekhon, R. K., & Dugré, N. (2020). *Magnesium for skeletal muscle cramps.* Cochrane Database of Systematic Reviews. https://doi.org/10.1002/14651858.cd009402.pub3

9 Levine, M. (2011, March 3). *Vitamin C: A Concentration-Function Approach Yields Pharmacology and Therapeutic Discoveries.* [*Advances in Nutrition*, Volume

2, Issue 2, 01 March 2011, Pages 78–88]. https://doi.org/10.3945/an.110. 000109

10 Adler, J. (2013, June). *Why Fire Makes Us Human*. Smithsonian; Smithsonian.com. https://www.smithsonianmag.com/science-nature/why-fire-makes-us-human-72989884/

11 *"living without eating for NINE YEARS" BUSTED*. (n.d.). www.youtube.com. Retrieved January 7, 2023, from https://www.youtube.com/watch?v=iwOX7vOf0_s

12 Singer, T. (2004). *Empathy for Pain Involves the Affective but not Sensory Components of Pain*. *Science*, 303(5661), 1157–1162. https://doi.org/10.1126/science. 1093535

13 *Early humans may have cared for disabled young*. New Scientist. Retrieved January 7, 2023, from https://www.newscientist.com/article/dn16873-early-humans-may-have-cared-for-disabled-young/

14 Moseley, J. B., O'Malley, K., Petersen, N. J., Menke, T. J., Brody, B. A., Kuykendall, D. H., Hollingsworth, J. C., Ashton, C. M., & Wray, N. P. (2002). *A Controlled Trial of Arthroscopic Surgery for Osteoarthritis of the Knee*. *New England Journal of Medicine, 347*(2), 81–88. https://doi.org/10.1056/nejmoa013259

15 *Alternative Medicine for Cancer Treatment Raises Mortality Risk - National Cancer Institute*. (2017, September 12). www.cancer.gov. https://www.cancer.gov/news-events/cancer-currents-blog/2017/alternative-medicine-cancer-survival

16 Singh, H., Meyer, A. N. D., & Thomas, E. J. (2014). *The frequency of diagnostic errors in outpatient care: estimations from three large observational studies involving US adult populations*. *BMJ Quality & Safety*, 23(9), 727–731. https://doi.org/ 10.1136/bmjqs-2013-002627

17 Poprom, N., Numthavaj, P., Wilasrusmee, C., Rattanasiri, S., Attia, J., McEvoy, M., & Thakkinstian, A. (2019). *The efficacy of antibiotic treatment versus surgical treatment of uncomplicated acute appendicitis: Systematic review and network meta-analysis of randomized controlled trial*. *American Journal of Surgery, 218*(1), 192–200. https://doi.org/10.1016/j.amjsurg.2018.10.009

18 US Preventive Services Task Force. (2022). *Aspirin Use to Prevent Cardiovascular Disease: US Preventive Services Task Force Recommendation Statement*. *JAMA, 327*(16), 1577–1584. https://doi.org/10.1001/jama.2022.4983

19 Onakpoya, I. J., Heneghan, C. J., & Aronson, J. K. (2016). *Post-marketing withdrawal of 462 medicinal products because of adverse drug reactions: a systematic review of the world literature*. *BMC Medicine, 14*(1). https://doi.org/10.1186/ s12916-016-0553-2

20 Earnest, M. (2020). *On Becoming a Plague Doctor*. *New England Journal of Medicine, 383*(10), e64. https://doi.org/10.1056/nejmp2011418

21 *Echinacea*. (2020, July). NCCIH. https://www.nccih.nih.gov/health/echinacea

22 *NCCIH*. (n.d.). NCCIH. https://www.nccih.nih.gov/

23 *List of medicinal plants*. (n.d.). *RationalWiki*. Retrieved January 7, 2023, from https://rationalwiki.org/wiki/List_of_medicinal_plants

24 Schippman, U., Leaman, D.J., Cunningham, A.B. (2002). *Impact of Cultivation and Gathering of Medicinal Plants on Biodiversity: Global Trends and Issues.* https://www.researchgate.net/publication/265157471

25 Mayo Clinic. (2017). *St. John's wort.* Mayo Clinic. https://www.mayoclinic.org/drugs-supplements-st-johns-wort/art-20362212

26 Chen, C.-H., Dickman, K. G., Moriya, M., Zavadil, J., Sidorenko, V. S., Edwards, K. L., Gnatenko, D. V., Wu, L., Turesky, R. J., Wu, X.-R., Pu, Y.-S., & Grollman, A. P. (2012). *Aristolochic acid-associated urothelial cancer in Taiwan. Proceedings of the National Academy of Sciences, 109*(21), 8241–8246. https://doi.org/10.1073/pnas.1119920109

27 Mikulski, M. A., Wichman, M. D., Simmons, D. L., Pham, A. N., Clottey, V., & Fuortes, L. J. (2017). *Toxic metals in ayurvedic preparations from a public health lead poisoning cluster investigation. International Journal of Occupational and Environmental Health, 23*(3), 187–192. https://doi.org/10.1080/10773525.2018.1447880

28 Ching, C. K., Chen, S. P. L., Lee, H. H. C., Lam, Y. H., Ng, S. W., Chen, M. L., Tang, M. H. Y., Chan, S. S. S., Ng, C. W. Y., Cheung, J. W. L., Chan, T. Y. C., Lau, N. K. C., Chong, Y. K., & Mak, T. W. L. (2017). *Adulteration of proprietary Chinese medicines and health products with undeclared drugs: experience of a tertiary toxicology laboratory in Hong Kong. British Journal of Clinical Pharmacology, 84*(1), 172–178. https://doi.org/10.1111/bcp.13420

29 FDA. (2019). *Step 1: Discovery and Development. U.S. Food and Drug Administration.* https://www.fda.gov/patients/drug-development-process/step-1-discovery-and-development

30 Wikipedia Contributors. (2019, December 15). *List of largest pharmaceutical settlements.* Wikipedia; Wikimedia Foundation. https://en.wikipedia.org/wiki/List_of_largest_pharmaceutical_settlements

31 *CAPSICUM ANNUUM - HOMOEOPATHIC MATERIA MEDICA - By William BOERICKE.* (n.d.). www.homeoint.org. Retrieved January 8, 2023, from http://www.homeoint.org/books/boericmm/c/caps.htm

32 Lewindon, P. J., Harkness, L., & Lewindon, N. (1998). *Randomised controlled trial of sucrose by mouth for the relief of infant crying after immunisation. Archives of Disease in Childhood, 78*(5), 453–456. https://doi.org/10.1136/adc.78.5.453

33 Stolberg, M. (2006). *Inventing the randomized double-blind trial: the Nuremberg salt test of 1835. Journal of the Royal Society of Medicine, 99*(12), 642–643. https://www.ncbi.nlm.nih.gov/pmc/articles/PMC1676327/

34 *NATRIUM MURIATICUM - HOMOEOPATHIC MATERIA MEDICA - By William BOERICKE.* (n.d.). www.homeoint.org. Retrieved January 8, 2023, from http://www.homeoint.org/books/boericmm/n/nat-m.htm

35 *The Proving of Cynomorium Coccineum "I was a hidden treasure and I wanted to be known, so I created this" - Mike Andrews.* (2015, November 21). https://hpathy.com/materia-medica/proving-cynomorium-coccineum-hidden-treasure-wanted-known-created/

36 *Interhomeopathy - Trituration Proving of the Light of Saturn.* (n.d.). www.interh omeopathy.org. Retrieved January 8, 2023, from http://www.interhomeopathy. org/trituration_proving_of_the_light_of_saturn

37 *Interhomeopathy - Berlin Wall.* (n.d.). www.interhomeopathy.org. Retrieved January 8, 2023, from http://www.interhomeopathy.org/berlin_wall

38 *File: The cow pock.jpg.* (2014, January 29). Wikipedia. https://en.wikipedia.org/ wiki/File:The_cow_pock.jpg

39 Giusti, R. M. (1995). *Diethylstilbestrol Revisited: A Review of the Long-Term Health Effects. Annals of Internal Medicine, 122*(10), 778. https://doi.org/10. 7326/0003-4819-122-10-199505150-00008

40 Wise, J. (2001). *Finnish study confirms safety of MMR vaccine. BMJ: British Medical Journal, 322*(7279), 130. https://www.ncbi.nlm.nih.gov/pmc/articles/ PMC1173183/

41 Kahneman, D., & Tversky, A. (1979). *Prospect Theory: An Analysis of Decision under Risk. Econometrica, 47*(2), 263–292.

42 Washington, D. (2019). *As filed with the Securities and Exchange Commis-sion on UNITED STATES SECURITIES AND EXCHANGE COMMIS-SION.* https://s21.q4cdn.com/488056881/files/doc_financials/2018/Q4/2018-Form-10-K-(without-Exhibits)_FINAL_022719.pdf

43 *The Vaccine Adverse Event Reporting System (VAERS) Request.* (n.d.). Wonder.cdc.gov. https://wonder.cdc.gov/vaers.html

44 Jain, A., Marshall, J., Buikema, A., Bancroft, T., Kelly, J. P., & Newschaffer, C. J. (2015). *Autism Occurrence by MMR Vaccine Status Among US Children With Older Siblings With and Without Autism. JAMA, 313*(15), 1534. https://doi.org/ 10.1001/jama.2015.3077

45 Madsen, K. M., Hviid, A., Vestergaard, M., Schendel, D., Wohlfahrt, J., Thorsen, P., Olsen, J., & Melbye, M. (2002). *A Population-Based Study of Measles, Mumps, and Rubella Vaccination and Autism. New England Journal of Medicine, 347*(19), 1477–1482. https://doi.org/10.1056/nejmoa021134

46 Uchiyama, T., Kurosawa, M., & Inaba, Y. (2006). *MMR-Vaccine and Regression in Autism Spectrum Disorders: Negative Results Presented from Japan. Journal of Autism and Developmental Disorders, 37*(2), 210–217. https://doi.org/10.1007/ s10803-006-0157-3

47 Vohra, K., Vodonos, A., Schwartz, J., Marais, E. A., Sulprizio, M. P., & Mickley, L. J. (2021). *Global mortality from outdoor fine particle pollution gener-ated by fossil fuel combustion: Results from GEOS-Chem. Environmental Research, 195*(110754), 110754. https://doi.org/10.1016/j.envres.2021.110754

48 U.S. Food & Drug Administration (2018). *FDA Warns Consumers Not to Use "Best Bentonite Clay." FDA.* https://www.fda.gov/drugs/drug-safety-and-availabil ity/fda-warns-consumers-not-use-best-bentonite-clay

49 *Glyphosate toxicity: Looking past the hyperbole, and sorting through the facts. By Credible Hulk.* (2018, June 30). The Credible Hulk. https://www.credibleh ulk.org/index.php/2015/06/02/glyphosate-toxicity-looking-past-the-hyperbole-and-sorting-through-the-facts-by-credible-hulk/

50 White, A. R., Rampes, H., Liu, J. P., Stead, L. F., & Campbell, J. (2014). *Acupuncture and related interventions for smoking cessation. Cochrane Database of Systematic Reviews.* https://doi.org/10.1002/14651858.cd000009.pub4

51 *Doctor charged in autistic boy's death.* (n.d.). NBC News. Retrieved January 8, 2023, from https://www.nbcnews.com/health/health-news/doctor-charged-autistic-boys-death-flna1c9468718

52 Christie, D., Christie, I. I., & University of California. (1914). *Thirty years in Moukden, 1883–1913, being the experiences and recollections of Dugald Christie. In Internet Archive.* London, Constable and company ltd. https://archive.org/details/thirtyyearsinmo00chrigoog

53 *A true history of acupuncture.From online Information.* (2011, November 3). Virginia Institute of Traditional Chinese Medicine. https://arthuryinfan.wordpress.com/2011/11/03/a-true-history-of-acupuncture-from-online-information/

54 Rosa, L. (1998). *A Close Look at Therapeutic Touch. JAMA, 279*(13), 1005. https://doi.org/10.1001/jama.279.13.1005

55 Botvinick, M., & Cohen, J. (1998). *Rubber hands "feel" touch that eyes see. Nature, 391*(6669), 756–756. https://doi.org/10.1038/35784

56 Vickers, A., Goyal, N., Harland, R., & Rees, R. (1998). *Do Certain Countries Produce Only Positive Results? A Systematic Review of Controlled Trials. Controlled Clinical Trials, 19*(2), 159–166. https://doi.org/10.1016/s0197-2456(97)00150-5

57 Park, J., White, A., Stevinson, C., Ernst, E., & James, M. (2002). *Validating a New Non-Penetrating Sham Acupuncture Device: Two Randomised Controlled Trials. Acupuncture in Medicine, 20*(4), 168–174. https://doi.org/10.1136/aim.20.4.168

58 Vickers, A. J., Cronin, A. M., Maschino, A. C., Lewith, G., MacPherson, H., Foster, N. E., Sherman, K. J., Witt, C. M., Linde, K., & Acupuncture Trialists' Collaboration. (2012). *Acupuncture for Chronic Pain. Archives of Internal Medicine, 172*(19), 1444. https://doi.org/10.1001/archinternmed.2012.3654

59 *Should Acupuncture Be Used For Asthma? | Asthma.net.* (2016). Asthma.net. https://asthma.net/natural-remedies/acupuncture

60 Dorsch, W., & Kolt, A. (2019). *Einfache Testverfahren zur Überprüfung der Aussagekraft von Bioresonanz-basierten medizinischen Befunden — der Leberkäse-Test. Allergo Journal, 28*(4), 22–30. https://doi.org/10.1007/s15007-019-1859-0

61 *Ultraviolet radiation.* (2022, June 21). www.who.int. https://www.who.int/news-room/fact-sheets/detail/ultraviolet-radiation

62 Hawk, J. L. M. (2020). *Safe, mild ultraviolet-B exposure: An essential human requirement for vitamin D and other vital bodily parameter adequacy: A review. Photodermatology, Photoimmunology & Photomedicine, 36*(6), 417–423. https://doi.org/10.1111/phpp.12584

63 Wacker, M., & Holick, M. F. (2013). *Sunlight and Vitamin D. Dermato-Endocrinology, 5*(1), 51–108. https://doi.org/10.4161/derm.24494

64 David, E., Wolfson, M., & Fraifeld, V. E. (2021). *Background radiation impacts human longevity and cancer mortality: reconsidering the linear no-threshold paradigm. Biogerontology.* https://doi.org/10.1007/s10522-020-09909-4

65 *SmartDot radiation-protection phone stickers "have no effect."* (2021, January 11). *BBC News.* https://www.bbc.com/news/technology-55613452

66 *Scalar energy products and health.* (2017, April 26). *ARPANSA.* https://www.arpansa.gov.au/understanding-radiation/radiation-sources/more-radiation-sources/pendants

67 *Anti-5G necklaces found to be radioactive.* (2021, December 17). *BBC News.* https://www.bbc.com/news/technology-59703523

68 Groves, F. D. (2002). *Cancer in Korean War Navy Technicians: Mortality Survey after 40 Years. American Journal of Epidemiology, 155*(9), 810–818. https://doi.org/10.1093/aje/155.9.810

69 Siegel, R. L., Miller, K. D., & Jemal, A. (2020). *Cancer statistics, 2020. CA: A Cancer Journal for Clinicians, 70*(1), 7–30. https://doi.org/10.3322/caac.21590

70 Khurana, V. G., Teo, C., Kundi, M., Hardell, L., & Carlberg, M. (2009). *Cell phones and brain tumors: a review including the long-term epidemiologic data. Surgical Neurology, 72*(3), 205–214. https://doi.org/10.1016/j.surneu.2009.01.019

71 *IARC group 2B.* (2022, August 26). Wikipedia. https://en.wikipedia.org/wiki/IARC_group_2B

72 Rubin, G. J., Munshi, J. D., & Wessely, S. (2005). *Electromagnetic Hypersensitivity: A Systematic Review of Provocation Studies. Psychosomatic Medicine, 67*(2), 224–232. https://doi.org/10.1097/01.psy.0000155664.13300.64

73 Dieudonné, M. (2020). *Electromagnetic hypersensitivity: a critical review of explanatory hypotheses. Environmental Health, 19*(1). https://doi.org/10.1186/s12940-020-00602-0

74 Karipidis, K., Mate, R., Urban, D., Tinker, R., & Wood, A. (2021). *5G mobile networks and health—a state-of-the-science review of the research into low-level RF fields above 6 GHz. Journal of Exposure Science & Environmental Epidemiology, 31*(4), 585–605. https://doi.org/10.1038/s41370-021-00297-6

75 Foreman, J., Salim, A. T., Praveen, A., Fonseka, D., Ting, D. S. W., Guang He, M., Bourne, R. R. A., Crowston, J., Wong, T. Y., & Dirani, M. (2021). *Association between digital smart device use and myopia: a systematic review and meta-analysis. The Lancet Digital Health, 3*(12). https://doi.org/10.1016/s2589-7500(21)00135-7

76 Abeler, J., Becker, A., & Falk, A. (2014). *Representative evidence on lying costs. Journal of Public Economics, 113*, 96–104. https://doi.org/10.1016/j.jpubeco.2014.01.005

77 Alsan, M., & Wanamaker, M. (2017). *Tuskegee and the Health of Black Men. The Quarterly Journal of Economics, 133*(1), 407–455. https://doi.org/10.1093/qje/qjx029

78 Grimes, D. R. (2016). *On the Viability of Conspiratorial Beliefs. PLOS ONE, 11*(1), e0147905. https://doi.org/10.1371/journal.pone.0147905

Index